AF574364

Cancer Treatment and Research

Volume 175

Series editor

Steven T. Rosen, Duarte, CA, USA

This book series provides detailed updates on the state of the art in the treatment of different forms of cancer and also covers a wide spectrum of topics of current research interest. Clinicians will benefit from expert analysis of both standard treatment options and the latest therapeutic innovations and from provision of clear guidance on the management of clinical challenges in daily practice. The research-oriented volumes focus on aspects ranging from advances in basic science through to new treatment tools and evaluation of treatment safety and efficacy. Each volume is edited and authored by leading authorities in the topic under consideration. In providing cutting-edge information on cancer treatment and research, the series will appeal to a wide and interdisciplinary readership. The series is listed in PubMed/Index Medicus.

More information about this series at http://www.springer.com/series/5808

Siamak Daneshmand
Kevin G. Chan
Editors

Genitourinary Cancers

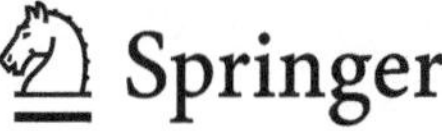

Springer

Editors
Siamak Daneshmand
Norris Comprehensive Cancer Center
University of Southern California
Los Angeles, CA, USA

Kevin G. Chan
City of Hope National Medical Center
Duarte, CA, USA

ISSN 0927-3042 ISSN 2509-8497 (electronic)
Cancer Treatment and Research
ISBN 978-3-319-93338-2 ISBN 978-3-319-93339-9 (eBook)
https://doi.org/10.1007/978-3-319-93339-9

Library of Congress Control Number: 2018944327

This Springer imprint is published by the registered company Springer Nature Switzerland AG
The registered company address is: Gewerbestrasse 11, 6330 Cham, Switzerland

Contents

New Imaging Techniques in Prostate Cancer

Karim Marzouk and Behfar Ehdaie

Contents

Abstract

Rapid advances in diagnostic imaging have been developed in parallel with the changes in the contemporary management of prostate cancer. Increasingly, clinical management and decision making in prostate cancer are influenced by

K. Marzouk · B. Ehdaie (✉)
Urology Service, Department of Surgery, Memorial Sloan
Kettering Cancer Center, 353 East 68th Street, New York, NY 10065, USA
e-mail: ehdaieb@mskcc.org

K. Marzouk
e-mail: marzoukk@mskcc.org

S. Daneshmand and K. G. Chan (eds.), *Genitourinary Cancers*, Cancer Treatment and Research 175, https://doi.org/10.1007/978-3-319-93339-9_1

technologies such as magnetic resonance imaging-targeted prostate biopsies for men with elevated PSA, imaging for active surveillance, and nuclear medicine studies for men with advanced or recurrent prostate cancer. Furthermore, novel imaging techniques have been developed such as hyperpolarized MRI, choline and prostate-specific membrane antigen positron emission tomography that exploit features like the unique metabolism in prostate cancer tissues, as well as altered glycoprotein conformation. These technologies have allowed for the identification of tiny foci of prostate cancer in men with early biochemical recurrence, greatly surpassing the limitations of traditional morphological imaging. With promising findings, studies are ongoing to uncover the clinical application of these imaging modalities. Ultimately, several factors such as cost-effectiveness and the overall reduction in disease mortality will dictate the implementation of these imaging technologies in the future. This chapter provides an overview on new and emerging prostate imaging techniques that can be used in the diagnosis of primary cancer as well as the staging and detection of metastatic disease.

Keywords
Prostate cancer · Imaging · Detection · Magnetic resonance imaging
Hyperpolarized MRI · PSMA · Choline-PET

1 Introduction

Prostate cancer is the most common malignancy in men in the USA, with an estimated 161,000 new cases and 27,000 deaths expected in 2017 [1]. Recent advances in translational research have allowed for the introduction of an array of new imaging technologies aimed at improving the diagnostic accuracy of prostate cancer detection. Several factors such as cost-effectiveness and the overall reduction in disease mortality will ultimately dictate the implementation of these imaging modalities in the future. This chapter provides a brief overview on new and emerging prostate imaging techniques that can be used in the diagnosis of primary cancer as well as the staging and detection of metastatic disease.

2 Multiparametric Magnetic Resonance Imaging

Magnetic resonance imaging (MRI) has become the cornerstone for imaging in prostate cancer. Initially employed for disease staging, the use of MRI has expanded to include primary tumor detection and treatment planning. Unlike traditional morphological imaging, multiparametric magnetic resonance imaging (mp-MRI) combines T2-weighted imaging with the functional sequences of diffusion-weighted imaging (DWI) and dynamic contrast enhancement (DCE). The incorporation of functional imaging has substantially improved the diagnostic capabilities of MRI, not only in detecting prostate cancer but also in characterizing disease aggressiveness. Currently, the most common form of evaluating mp-MRI is through the Prostate Imaging Reporting and Data System (PIRADS) which was updated with a second version in 2015 [2].

T2-Weighted Imaging

T2-weighted imaging (T2WI) is the staple of mp-MRI as it provides the best picture of prostate gland anatomy. In mp-MRI protocols, T2 images are obtained in 3 planes, providing excellent zonal imaging that clearly illustrate the peripheral and transition zones. In this phase, the peripheral zone demonstrates high signal intensity (bright), opposite to the transition and central zones that demonstrate lower signal intensity (dark). Prostate cancer is typically detected as an area of low signal on T2WI, or dark areas, in contrast to the normal peripheral zone. The high-quality resolution of T2WI makes it the most useful sequence in determining aggressive features such as extra-capsular extension or seminal vesicle invasion. However, the use of T2WI alone to diagnose prostate cancer is confounded by other conditions, including prostatitis, post-biopsy changes, or radiation which can result in anatomical changes that mimic cancer on T2WI.

Diffusion-Weighted Imaging

Diffusion-weighted imaging (DWI) uses the differential movement of water in the interstitial space as a method to reflect the architectural features of the prostate. The apparent diffusion coefficient (ADC) is the quantitative measurement of the movement of water in the interstitial space. Prostate cancer has high cell densities, therefore restricting the diffusion of water compared to normal tissues and resulting in areas of cancer demonstrating high signal (bright) with high b-value sequences, and low signal (dark) on ADC map. DWI is an essential part of mp-MRI because it increases the sensitivity of MRI and relates information about tumor aggressiveness [3]. Studies have demonstrated that ADC values can be used to differentiate aggressive cancers versus lower-grade cancer due to the highly restricted diffusion illustrated with higher Gleason grades [4].

Dynamic Contrast Enhancement

Dynamic contrast enhancement (DCE) consists of imaging sequences obtained before, during, and after the rapid infusion of gadolinium-based contrast material. DCE imaging improves the sensitivity of MRI by detecting abnormal areas of enhancement that are typical of prostate cancer. Conversely, specificity of DCE is limited since abnormal enhancement can also result from benign conditions such as

BPH and inflammation. The utility of DCE is heightened in diagnosing disease recurrence after primary treatment of prostate cancer with radiation therapy.

Localized Disease

Primary disease detection

The evaluation of mp-MRI as an adjunctive tool to PSA is an important step toward improving the detection of high-grade prostate cancer. With numerous studies on the topic, there are conflicting reports on the fundamental role of MRI in men with suspected prostate cancer prior to biopsy. In the most recent systematic review, mp-MRI followed by targeted biopsy (TB) aided in the detection of 2–13% of clinically significant cancers that were missed by conventional transrectal ultrasound (TRUS)-guided systematic biopsy [5]. However, the same publication also highlighted that MRI TB missed 0–7% of clinically significant cancers that were detected by systematic TRUS biopsy. Adding to the uncertainty, two systematic reviews concluded that MRI-ultrasound TB increased the detection of clinically significant cancer versus TRUS biopsy [6, 7], whereas another two systematic reviews failed to identify any significant benefit to utilizing MRI and targeted biopsy [8, 9]. Substantial heterogeneity in the definitions of clinically significant cancer, variability of radiographer experience in interpreting mp-MRI, as well as differing technical experience when performing targeted biopsies all hamper a clear interpretation of the existing literature. Large prospective studies such as the *PROstate MRI Imaging Study* (PROMIS) and the ongoing *Goteborg Randomized Screening Trial* have shed light on the potential role of mp-MRI in biopsy naïve men with suspected prostate cancer [10–12]. However, further evidence from high-quality prospective studies is needed prior to the routine and widespread use of mp-MRI in all men with elevated PSA prior to biopsy. With these limitations in mind, there is consensus that in patients with suspected cancer and a history of a negative prostate biopsy, mp-MRI is beneficial and should be considered prior to repeat biopsy. MRI and targeted biopsies in this setting have resulted in improved detection of clinically significant prostate cancer [5, 8, 9]. This position is supported by the latest consensus statement from the American Urological Association and Society of Abdominal Radiology [13].

Staging & Disease Characterization

The use of mp-MRI in the clinical staging and characterization of prostate cancer is reported to be clinically useful, especially given its predilection for detecting aggressive disease. In a prospective study of 183 men that underwent mp-MRI before surgery, it was shown that the detection of prostate cancer on MRI was significantly dependent upon tumor size and Gleason grade [14]. As tumor size increased ≥ 1 cm^3 as did the ability to detect them on T2WI. Also, the detection of cancer was significantly greater for lesions with Gleason grade ≥ 7 in smaller foci of disease [14]. The apparent diffusion coefficient (ADC) from diffusion-weighted imaging has also greatly improved the sensitivity of MRI. It has been shown that a significant inverse correlation exists between lower ADC values and higher Gleason scores and that combining DWI to T2WI improves the overall characterization of prostate cancer aggressiveness [15]. When combining all the features of multiparametric imaging together, MRI has excellent specificity in detecting adverse pathological features of prostate cancer. In a large systematic review assessing the diagnostic accuracy of MRI for local staging, it was found that MRI had a high specificity for extra-capsular extension (ECE), seminal vesicle invasion (SVI), or overall stage T3 disease: 0.91 (95% CI, 0.88–0.93), 0.96 (95% CI, 0.95–0.97), and 0.88 (95% CI, 0.85–0.91), respectively [16]. However, the imaging sensitivity to detect microscopic extension was low: ECE 0.57 (95% CI 0.95–0.97), SVI 0.58 (95% CI, 0.47–0.68), and overall stage T3 0.61 (95% CI, 0.54–0.67).

Overall, multiparametric MRI is a established modality that improves the detection of higher-grade prostate cancer and reduces misclassification in staging and characterization of prostate cancer. Implementing mp-MRI in management of men with prostate cancer must be approached cautiously being mindful of known limitations. First, although the PIRADS system is a means for standardizing the interpretation of mp-MRI, the assessment criteria is subjective and substantial inter-reader variability can exist. Second, limitations in the sensitivity for MRI detecting high-risk disease highlight the importance of not dismissing negative studies, especially in the presence of other indicators of clinically significant cancer such as elevated PSA or abnormal rectal examination. Additionally, the diagnostic accuracy of MRI is impaired in men with post-biopsy inflammatory changes and hemorrhage. Serious consideration should be given for delaying MRI for 3 months following prostate biopsy to limit the impairment of potential inflammatory changes.

Metastatic disease

The use of MRI in the assessment of metastatic prostate cancer is most studied in disease metastases to bone. Technetium 99 (Tc-99) bone scans have historically been regarded as the gold standard for evaluating the presence of metastatic disease to the bone. The use of whole body mp-MRI (WBMRI) is emerging as viable alternative to Tc-99 bone scans. With no radiation exposure and no need for intravenous contrast agents, functional DWI sequences in addition to whole body MRI are more sensitive to detecting metastatic lesions within bone and also improve the detection of lymph node and soft tissue metastases. In one prospective study of 100 patients with high-risk prostate cancer, WBMRI outperformed Tc-99 bone scans for detecting bony metastatic disease and performed as well as CT for enlarged lymph node detection [17]. A meta-analysis of 27 studies also revealed that WBMRI had a higher sensitivity for detecting bone metastasis than choline-PET/CT and Tc-99 bone scans [18]. Overall, on per-patient analysis, MRI had a pooled sensitivity and specificity of 97 and 95%, respectively.

3 Hyperpolarized Magnetic Resonance Imaging

Hyperpolarized ^{13}C MRI is a novel imaging technique that monitors the uptake and metabolism of endogenous molecules in prostate cancer tissues. The application of hyperpolarized ^{13}C in cancer imaging relies on the ***Warburg hypothesis***, where malignant tissues can reprogram metabolic pathways resulting in increased glycolysis and shunting of pyruvate to lactate [19]. Pre-clinical models using transgenic adenocarcinoma of the mouse prostate (TRAMP) have demonstrated that hyperpolarized ^{13}C MRI can track the real-time dynamic conversion of ^{13}C-pyruvate to ^{13}C-lactate in mouse cancer tissues [20]. TRAMP studies have also established that more aggressive and advanced cancers can be correlated with the magnitude of ^{13}C-lactate generation from ^{13}C-pyruvate [21].

Hyperpolarized ^{13}C MRI is performed through the use of commercially available MRI scanners that are coupled with specialized pulse sequences and radiofrequency coils [22]. Using magnetic fields, ^{13}C-labeled compounds are hyperpolarized and administered to patients as an intravenous injection, allowing for the real-time detection of signals generated from the flux of hyperpolarized ^{13}C-pyruvate to lactate in prostate cancer tissues. The first human study of hyperpolarized MRI in prostate cancer was conducted by Nelson et al., which verified the safety and feasibility of this technology in 31 men with localized prostate cancer [22]. Similar to pre-clinical evaluations, this study confirmed that signals from ^{13}C-lactate accurately distinguished the location and size of prostate cancer lesions from surrounding non-cancerous tissues. Moreover, hyperpolarized MRI highlighted signals from areas of tumor involvement that were not visible with mp-MRI.

By exploiting the altered metabolic properties of cancer cells, hyperpolarized ^{13}C MRI represents the future in imaging technology. With the ability to project high-quality images with signal intensities of greater than 50,000 fold at 3 T, hyperpolarized MRI can dramatically enhance our current ability to stage prostate cancer and detect early disease recurrence. Studies examining the clinical application of this technology in prostate cancer are ongoing.

4 Choline Positron Emission Tomography

Choline-PET is a nuclear medicine imaging modality that utilizes ^{11}C-choline or ^{18}F-choline in order to generate 3D images produced from gamma ray emissions. Choline is a substrate for the synthesis of phosphatidylcholine in the prostate cell membrane. Its uptake in is upregulated in prostate cancer, making it a suitable radiotracer for PET scans [23]. Radiolabeling using choline is favored over the traditional fluorodeoxyglucose (FDG) radiotracer since FDG lacks specificity for prostate cancer. Currently, ^{11}C-choline-PET is approved for use by the FDA for the detection of recurrent prostate cancer [24].

Localized disease

There appears to be a limited role for ^{11}C-choline-PET in the initial detection and characterization of primary tumors. Two studies have highlighted the relatively poor performance of choline-PET in this setting. Watanabe et al. compared the use of choline-PET, FDG-PET, and mp-MRI in 43 patients suspected of having prostate cancer prior to biopsy and surgery [25]. The sensitivity, specificity, and accuracy of choline-PET detecting prostate cancer were 73, 59, and 67%, respectively, which was significantly inferior to the performance of mp-MRI; 88% for all. In another review of 26 men with biopsy proven prostate cancer that underwent radical prostatectomy, the sensitivity, specificity, and accuracy of choline-PET were 55, 86, and 67% respectively [26]. Based on evidence from the available literature, the role of choline-PET in the initial detection and characterization of prostate cancer is unclear and requires further study.

Metastatic Disease

Primary Staging

Similar to findings from initial disease detection, the use of choline-PET in primary lymph node staging appears to be inadequate. A European study prospectively evaluated ^{11}C-choline-PET in 36 patients with prostate cancer prior to undergoing prostatectomy and bilateral extended pelvic lymph node dissection. All patients had negative preoperative CT scans and a nomogram-calculated risk of lymph node metastasis between 10 and 35%. The performance of choline-PET in this setting was poor, with a lymph node region-based sensitivity of only 9.4% and a patient-based sensitivity of 18.8% [27]. Therefore, more evidence is needed before choline-PET can be considered for routine primary lymph node staging.

Recurrent Disease

The detection of metastasis in patients with biochemical recurrence is well studied using choline-PET imaging. In a recent systematic review, 22 articles were indentified that evaluated recurrence of prostate cancer using choline-PET. Overall, the detection rate was found to be greater than 80% if the median PSA was 2 ng/ml or greater; however, choline-PET detection rates were less than 30% in men with median PSAs less than 1 ng/ml [28]. This highlights the major pitfalls of choline-PET imaging, its strong dependency on PSA levels. A meta-analysis of 14 articles examined the relationship between the detection rate of choline-PET and PSA kinetics [29]. When restaging patients with prostate cancer, ^{11}C-choline-PET was found to have an overall pooled detection rate of 58%. However, this increased to 65% when the PSA doubling time was less than 6 months; and to 71% and 77% when PSA velocity was greater than 1 and 2 ng/ml/year, respectively.

Overall, 11C-choline-PET can be a valuable tool in restaging patients with recurrent prostate cancer. With accuracy linked to PSA levels, recommendations have been made that ^{11}C-choline-PET should only be used when PSA levels are 2 ng/ml or greater [30]. Given the findings from the existing literature, implementation of choline-PET may be restricted to restaging patients with higher PSA values and short PSA doubling times.

5 Prostate-Specific Membrane Antigen

Prostate-specific membrane antigen (PSMA) is a type II transmembrane glycoprotein with domains in the extracellular, transmembrane, and intracellular environments [31]. The altered expression and transformation of PSMA in prostate cancer has made it the target for imaging research aimed at enhancing prostate cancer detection. In non-neoplastic tissues, PSMA is expressed in the apical region surrounding the prostatic ducts, an area which is not amenable to ligand binding [32–34]. In prostate cancer however, neoplastic transformation of prostate tissues results in the transfer of the glycoprotein to the luminal surface of cells, making PSMA a susceptible target for binding [35]. Expression of PSMA has been shown to increase according to grade and stage of malignancy and also has been found in androgen-independent disease as well as distant metastatic prostate cancer [36–38]. With these properties, PSMA provides an excellent target for isotope radiolabeling.

Developed in Heidelberg, Germany, the binding of PSMA with Gallium-68 (^{68}Ga-PSMA) is currently the most popular form radiolabeling PSMA for PET scans [39, 40]. The use of ^{68}Ga has many potential advantages over other ligands; it is rapidly cleared from the bloodstream and has a low background activity, generating high image quality [41]. Additionally, ^{68}Ga demonstrates a high affinity to inhibitors of PSMA, and on biding to prostate cells, internalization occurs and radiotracer can be exhibited even in small areas of metastasis [39, 40].

Localized Disease

The nature of PSMA's enhanced expression with aggressive disease precludes its utility in low-risk prostate cancer. Additionally, it has been identified that approximately 10% of primary cancers do not overexpress PSMA, theoretically limiting its application in low grade prostate cancer [42, 43]. However, one potential use for PSMA staging localized disease may be in the setting of patients with suboptimal mp-MRI due to artifact resulting from post-biopsy inflammation and hemorrhage or patients who have undergone partial gland ablation. There are preliminary indications that the interpretation of the PSMA-PET is not impaired by reactionary inflammation such as that demonstrated in MRI after prostate biopsy [44]. However, due to the lack of clinical evidence at the time of this writing, the routine use of PSMA-PET scans for the detection of localized disease cannot be recommended at this time.

Metastatic Disease

Primary staging of lymph node metastasis

A prospective study by Herlemann et al. evaluated the ability of ^{68}Ga-PSMA-PET/CT to detect metastatic lymph nodes in a group of 20 patients undergoing radical prostatectomy with intermediate and high-risk disease [45]. Additionally, 14 patients with biochemical recurrence were also included in the study prior to undergoing secondary lymph node dissection. Accuracy of the PSMA-PET and CT scans was analyzed separately relative to the lymph node pathology. Overall, the sensitivity and specificity of PSMA-PET for the detection of lymph node involvement were 84 and 82%, respectively, compared to 65 and 76% for CT [45]. Another study by Maurer et al. [43] evaluated 130 patients with intermediate- and high-risk disease that underwent staging with ^{68}Ga-PSMA-PET prior to radical prostatectomy. Nodal metastasis was present in 41 of 130 patients (31.5%). On patient-based analysis, sensitivity and specificity of 65.9 and 98.9%, respectively, were demonstrated for lymph node staging using PSMA-PET. This was in comparison with CT and MRI that demonstrated a combined sensitivity of 43.9% and specificity of 85.4% [43].

Overall, preliminary evidence indicates that ^{68}Ga-PSMA-PET outperforms traditional imaging (CT & MRI) in the staging of metastatic lymph nodes prior to surgery. Although still lacking high-level evidence from clinical trials, PSMA may improve preoperative staging, especially in patients with high-risk disease. Ultimately, how this will impact overall disease recurrence and survival is still unknown.

Recurrent Prostate Cancer

Advancements in treatments for patients with recurrent prostate cancer have stimulated research in metabolic imaging and improving classification of patients with biochemical recurrence. Preliminary data is emerging that shows promising results for PSMA-PET in secondary staging. A pivotal study by Afshar-Oromeih et al. first illustrated the statistically superior detection of metastatic lesions with ^{68}Ga-PSMA-PET compared to ^{18}F choline-based PET scans in 37 patients with biochemical recurrence [46]. Comparably, another retrospective study of 66 patients selected for salvage lymphadenectomy compared the findings of PSMA-PET against choline-PET using post-lymphadenectomy histology. PSMA illustrated significantly better accuracy (92%) and higher negative predictive value (97%) versus choline-PET, accuracy 83% and NPV 89% [47]. The use of sequential imaging in another report of 125 patients with biochemical recurrence established that PSMA scans after negative choline-PET increased the overall detection rate of recurrent cancer by 11% [48]. A large summary of the diagnostic performance of PSMA-PET was illustrated in a systematic review and meta-analysis of 16 studies with 1309 patients. PSMA demonstrated an 86% overall sensitivity and specificity on per-patient analysis [49]. The sensitivity and specificity for per lesion analysis were 80 and 97%, respectively. However, similar to choline-PET, PSMA demonstrated a trend for increased positivity with higher PSA levels in patients with biochemical recurrence. Pooled estimates for PSMA-PET positivity were highest (95%) when PSA was greater than 2 ng/ml, but this dropped to 58% when PSA was between 0.2 and 1 ng/ml [49]. Patients with PSA doubling times less than 6 months were found to have a pooled PSMA positivity of 92%.

Overall, ^{68}Ga-PSMA-PET has emerged as a promising imaging modality to detect metastatic prostate cancer. Several limitations preclude the widespread use of this technology at this point in time. First, well-designed prospective clinical studies are still lacking. The impact of enhanced metastasis detection on overall survival is not clear, especially in patients with very early stages of biochemical recurrence. Second, the high costs and the requirement of onsite generators to obtain ^{68}Ga will likely limit the use of this technology to larger medical centers.

6 Conclusions

During the past two decades, the diagnosis and management of prostate cancer has undergone significant advancements in which men are detected earlier with less aggressive tumors due to PSA screening. Additionally, outcomes after radiation and surgery have improved with the incorporation of robotic technology and targeted radiation therapy. Advances in imaging have been developed in parallel with the changes in management of prostate cancer, including MRI-targeted prostate biopsies for men with elevated PSA, imaging for active surveillance, and nuclear medicine studies for men with advanced or recurrent prostate cancer. Several studies are underway to establish the role of modalities described in this chapter for routine use in clinical practice. Imaging is emerging as an important complement to clinical and pathologic characteristics to classify which patients with prostate cancer to treat and others to monitor more effectively.

References

1. Siegel RL, Miller KD, Jemal A (2017) Cancer statistics, 2017. CA Cancer J Clin 67(1):7–30
2. Barrett T, Turkbey B, Choyke PL (2015) PI-RADS version 2: what you need to know. Clin Radiol 70(11):1165–1176
3. Barentsz JO, Richenberg J, Clements R et al (2012) ESUR prostate MR guidelines 2012. Eur Radiol 22(4):746–757
4. Nagarajan R, Margolis D, Raman S et al (2012) Correlation of Gleason scores with diffusion-weighted imaging findings of prostate cancer. Adv Urol 2012:374805
5. Haider MA, Yao X, Loblaw A, Finelli A (2016) Multiparametric magnetic resonance imaging in the diagnosis of prostate cancer: a systematic review. Clin Oncol [Royal College of Radiologists (Great Britain)] 28(9):550–567
6. Valerio M, Donaldson I, Emberton M et al (2015) Detection of clinically significant prostate cancer using magnetic resonance imaging-ultrasound fusion targeted biopsy: a systematic review. Eur Urol 68(1):8–19

7. Gayet M, van der Aa A, Beerlage HP, Schrier BP, Mulders PF, Wijkstra H (2016) The value of magnetic resonance imaging and ultrasonography (MRI/US)-fusion biopsy platforms in prostate cancer detection: a systematic review. BJU Int 117(3):392–400
8. van Hove A, Savoie PH, Maurin C et al (2014) Comparison of image-guided targeted biopsies versus systematic randomized biopsies in the detection of prostate cancer: a systematic literature review of well-designed studies. World J Urol 32(4):847–858
9. Schoots IG, Roobol MJ, Nieboer D, Bangma CH, Steyerberg EW, Hunink MG (2015) Magnetic resonance imaging-targeted biopsy may enhance the diagnostic accuracy of significant prostate cancer detection compared to standard transrectal ultrasound-guided biopsy: a systematic review and meta-analysis. Eur Urol 68(3):438–450
10. El-Shater Bosaily A, Parker C, Brown LC et al (2015) PROMIS–Prostate MR imaging study: A paired validating cohort study evaluating the role of multi-parametric MRI in men with clinical suspicion of prostate cancer. Contemp Clin Trials 42:26–40
11. Grenabo Bergdahl A, Wilderang U, Aus G et al (2015) Role of magnetic resonance imaging in prostate cancer screening: a pilot study within the goteborg randomised screening trial. Eur Urol
12. Ahmed HU, El-Shater Bosaily A, Brown LC et al (2017) Diagnostic accuracy of multi-parametric MRI and TRUS biopsy in prostate cancer (PROMIS): a paired validating confirmatory study. Lancet
13. Rosenkrantz AB, Verma S, Choyke P et al (2016) Prostate magnetic resonance imaging and magnetic resonance imaging targeted biopsy in patients with a prior negative biopsy: a consensus statement by AUA and SAR. J Urol 196(6):1613–1618
14. Vargas HA, Akin O, Shukla-Dave A et al (2012) Performance characteristics of MR imaging in the evaluation of clinically low-risk prostate cancer: a prospective study. Radiology 265(2):478–487
15. Vargas HA, Akin O, Franiel T et al (2011) Diffusion-weighted endorectal MR imaging at 3 T for prostate cancer: tumor detection and assessment of aggressiveness. Radiology 259(3):775–784
16. de Rooij M, Hamoen EH, Witjes JA, Barentsz JO, Rovers MM (2016) Accuracy of magnetic resonance imaging for local staging of prostate cancer: a diagnostic meta-analysis. Eur Urol 70(2):233–245
17. Lecouvet FE, El Mouedden J, Collette L et al (2012) Can whole-body magnetic resonance imaging with diffusion-weighted imaging replace Tc 99 m bone scanning and computed tomography for single-step detection of metastases in patients with high-risk prostate cancer? Eur Urol 62(1):68–75
18. Shen G, Deng H, Hu S, Jia Z (2014) Comparison of choline-PET/CT, MRI, SPECT, and bone scintigraphy in the diagnosis of bone metastases in patients with prostate cancer: a meta-analysis. Skeletal Radiol 43(11):1503–1513
19. Wilson DM, Kurhanewicz J (2014) Hyperpolarized 13C MR for molecular imaging of prostate cancer. J Nucl Medicine Official Publ Soc Nucl Med 55(10):1567–1572
20. Lupo JM, Chen AP, Zierhut ML et al (2010) Analysis of hyperpolarized dynamic 13C lactate imaging in a transgenic mouse model of prostate cancer. Magn Reson Imaging 28(2):153–162
21. Albers MJ, Bok R, Chen AP et al (2008) Hyperpolarized 13C lactate, pyruvate, and alanine: noninvasive biomarkers for prostate cancer detection and grading. Cancer Res 68(20):8607–8615
22. Nelson SJ, Kurhanewicz J, Vigneron DB et al (2013) Metabolic imaging of patients with prostate cancer using hyperpolarized [1-(1)(3)C]pyruvate. *Science translational medicine.* 5(198):198ra108
23. Schuster DM, Nanni C, Fanti S (2016) PET Tracers Beyond FDG in Prostate Cancer. Semin Nucl Med 46(6):507–521
24. US Food and Drug Administration (2012) FDA approves 11C-choline for PET in prostate cancer. J Nucl Med 53(12):11N

25. Watanabe H, Kanematsu M, Kondo H et al (2010) Preoperative detection of prostate cancer: a comparison with 11C-choline PET, 18F-fluorodeoxyglucose PET and MR imaging. J Magn Reson Imaging 31(5):1151–1156
26. Testa C, Schiavina R, Lodi R et al (2007) Prostate cancer: sextant localization with MR imaging, MR spectroscopy, and 11C-choline PET/CT. Radiology 244(3):797–806
27. Budiharto T, Joniau S, Lerut E et al (2011) Prospective evaluation of 11C-choline positron emission tomography/computed tomography and diffusion-weighted magnetic resonance imaging for the nodal staging of prostate cancer with a high risk of lymph node metastases. Eur Urol 60(1):125–130
28. Evangelista L, Briganti A, Fanti S et al (2016) New clinical indications for (18)F/(11) C-choline, new tracers for positron emission tomography and a promising hybrid device for prostate cancer staging: a systematic review of the literature. Eur Urol 70(1):161–175
29. Treglia G, Ceriani L, Sadeghi R, Giovacchini G, Giovanella L (2014) Relationship between prostate-specific antigen kinetics and detection rate of radiolabelled choline PET/CT in restaging prostate cancer patients: a meta-analysis. Clin Chem Lab Med 52(5):725–733
30. Heidenreich A, Bastian PJ, Bellmunt J et al (2014) EAU guidelines on prostate cancer. Part II: treatment of advanced, relapsing, and castration-resistant prostate cancer. Eur Urol 65(2): 467–479
31. Leek J, Lench N, Maraj B et al (1995) Prostate-specific membrane antigen: evidence for the existence of a second related human gene. Br J Cancer 72(3):583–588
32. DeMarzo AM, Nelson WG, Isaacs WB, Epstein JI (2003) Pathological and molecular aspects of prostate cancer. Lancet (London, England) 361(9361):955–964
33. Eder M, Eisenhut M, Babich J, Haberkorn U (2013) PSMA as a target for radiolabelled small molecules. Eur J Nucl Med Mol Imaging 40(6):819–823
34. Ghosh A, Heston WD (2004) Tumor target prostate specific membrane antigen (PSMA) and its regulation in prostate cancer. J Cell Biochem 91(3):528–539
35. Maurer T, Eiber M, Schwaiger M, Gschwend JE (2016) Current use of PSMA-PET in prostate cancer management. Nat Rev Urol 13(4):226–235
36. Silver DA, Pellicer I, Fair WR, Heston WD, Cordon-Cardo C (1997) Prostate-specific membrane antigen expression in normal and malignant human tissues. Clin Cancer Res Official J Am Assoc Cancer Res 3(1):81–85
37. Bostwick DG, Pacelli A, Blute M, Roche P, Murphy GP (1998) Prostate specific membrane antigen expression in prostatic intraepithelial neoplasia and adenocarcinoma: a study of 184 cases. Cancer 82(11):2256–2261
38. Chang SS (2004) Overview of prostate-specific membrane antigen. Rev Urol 6(Suppl 10): S13–18
39. Banerjee SR, Pullambhatla M, Byun Y et al (2010) 68 Ga-labeled inhibitors of prostate-specific membrane antigen (PSMA) for imaging prostate cancer. J Med Chem 53(14):5333–5341
40. Eder M, Schafer M, Bauder-Wust U et al (2012) 68 Ga-complex lipophilicity and the targeting property of a urea-based PSMA inhibitor for PET imaging. Bioconjug Chem 23(4):688–697
41. Bouchelouche K, Turkbey B, Choyke PL (2016) PSMA PET and radionuclide therapy in prostate cancer. Semin Nucl Med 46(6):522–535
42. Eiber M, Weirich G, Holzapfel K et al (2016) Simultaneous 68 Ga-PSMA HBED-CC PET/MRI improves the localization of primary prostate cancer. Eur Urol 70(5):829–836
43. Maurer T, Gschwend JE, Rauscher I et al (2016) Diagnostic efficacy of (68) Gallium-PSMA positron emission tomography compared to conventional imaging for lymph node staging of 130 consecutive patients with intermediate to high risk prostate cancer. J Urol 195(5): 1436–1443
44. Eiber M, Nekolla SG, Maurer T, Weirich G, Wester HJ, Schwaiger M (2015) (68)Ga-PSMA PET/MR with multimodality image analysis for primary prostate cancer. Abdom Imaging 40(6):1769–1771

45. Herlemann A, Wenter V, Kretschmer A et al (2016) 68 Ga-PSMA positron emission tomography/computed tomography provides accurate staging of lymph node regions prior to lymph node dissection in patients with prostate cancer. Eur Urol 70(4):553–557
46. Afshar-Oromieh A, Zechmann CM, Malcher A et al (2014) Comparison of PET imaging with a (68)Ga-labelled PSMA ligand and (18)F-choline-based PET/CT for the diagnosis of recurrent prostate cancer. Eur J Nucl Med Mol Imaging 41(1):11–20
47. Pfister D, Porres D, Heidenreich A et al (2016) Detection of recurrent prostate cancer lesions before salvage lymphadenectomy is more accurate with (68)Ga-PSMA-HBED-CC than with (18)F-Fluoroethylcholine PET/CT. Eur J Nucl Med Mol Imaging 43(8):1410–1417
48. Bluemel C, Krebs M, Polat B et al (2016) 68 Ga-PSMA-PET/CT in patients with biochemical prostate cancer recurrence and negative 18F-Choline-PET/CT. Clin Nucl Med 41(7):515–521
49. Perera M, Papa N, Christidis D et al (2016) Sensitivity, specificity, and predictors of positive 68 Ga-prostate-specific membrane antigen positron emission tomography in advanced prostate cancer: a systematic review and meta-analysis. Eur Urol 70(6):926–937

Targeted Ablative Therapies for Prostate Cancer

Jared S. Winoker, Harry Anastos and Ardeshir R. Rastinehad

Contents

J. S. Winoker · H. Anastos · A. R. Rastinehad
Department of Urology, Icahn School of Medicine at Mount Sinai, New York, USA

A. R. Rastinehad (✉)
Department of Radiology, Icahn School of Medicine at Mount Sinai, New York, USA
e-mail: Art.Rastinehad@mountsinai.org

S. Daneshmand and K. G. Chan (eds.), *Genitourinary Cancers*, Cancer Treatment and Research 175, https://doi.org/10.1007/978-3-319-93339-9_2

Abstract

Men diagnosed with low- to intermediate-risk, clinically localized prostate cancer (PCa) often face a daunting and difficult decision with respect to treatment: active surveillance (AS) or radical therapy. This decision is further confounded by the fact that many of these men diagnosed, by an elevated PSA, will have indolent disease and never require intervention. Radical treatments, including radical prostatectomy and whole-gland radiation, offer greater certainty for cancer control, but at the risk of significant urinary and/or sexual morbidity. Conversely, AS preserves genitourinary function and quality of life in exchange for burdensome surveillance and the psychological impact of living with cancer.

Keywords

Focal therapy · Prostate cancer treatment · Biochemical recurrence
High-intensity focused ultrasound · Radiofrequency ablation · Photodynamic therapy · Electroporation

1 Introduction

Men diagnosed with low- to intermediate-risk, clinically localized prostate cancer (PCa) often face a daunting and difficult decision with respect to treatment: active surveillance (AS) or radical therapy. This decision is further confounded by the fact that many of these men diagnosed, by an elevated PSA, will have indolent disease and never require intervention. Radical treatments, including radical prostatectomy and whole-gland radiation, offer greater certainty for cancer control, but at the risk of significant urinary and/or sexual morbidity [1, 2]. Conversely, AS preserves genitourinary function and quality of life in exchange for burdensome surveillance and the psychological impact of living with cancer [3, 4]. Current trends demonstrate that more than 40–50% of men with low-risk disease initially opt for AS [5, 6]. However, approximately one-third of them will ultimately come off surveillance because of disease upstaging, disease progression, or the psychological burden of cancer [7]. Further, it has been shown that a significant percentage of men who meet the criteria for AS at diagnosis, but elected to undergo radical prostatectomy, were found to have higher risk disease [8].

Focal therapy (FT) has emerged as a middle ground to AS and radical therapy, providing oncologic control for localized disease while mitigating the urinary and sexual morbidity of more aggressive treatments [9]. By definition, FT encompasses any targeted treatment modality that preserves part of the prostatic tissue, including focal ablation and hemiablation patterns. Technological advancements in prostate imaging are at the cornerstone of FT. The advent of multiparametric magnetic resonance imaging (mpMRI) and the subsequent incorporation of fusion biopsy platforms have significantly improved the pretreatment identification and characterization of suspicious lesions as well as the diagnostic accuracy of biopsies. With respect to detection of clinically significant (CS) PCa, mpMRI has a sensitivity of 44–87% with a negative predictive value of 63–98% for CS disease [10]. Siddiqui et al. presented level 1 evidence that MR fusion biopsy outperforms standard 12-core biopsies for cancer detection [11]. In a phase III trial, MR fusion-guided biopsy detected moderate or high-risk lesions at a rate of 72% and detected 87% of lesions missed by standard 12 core biopsy [12]. Growing collective proficiency in interpretation of mpMRI and targeted biopsies for PCa detection and staging have naturally given way to a renascent interest in FT by application of these technologies.

Widespread support for FT in PCa has been met with considerable resistance as up to 80% of cancers feature multifocality, of which nearly 80% feature bilateral foci of disease [13, 14]. However, radical prostatectomy morphometric studies have shown that despite the multifocality and clonal heterogeneity of PCa, all lesions do not harbor the potential for metastatic progression. Based on genomic analyses from 94 cancer sites in 30 men who had died from metastatic PCa, Liu and colleagues demonstrated that most metastases originate from a single precursor cancer cell [15]. Classically, clinically insignificant disease has been defined by lesions <0.5 cc in volume without any grade 4 or 5 [13, 16]. Villers et al. found that 80% of

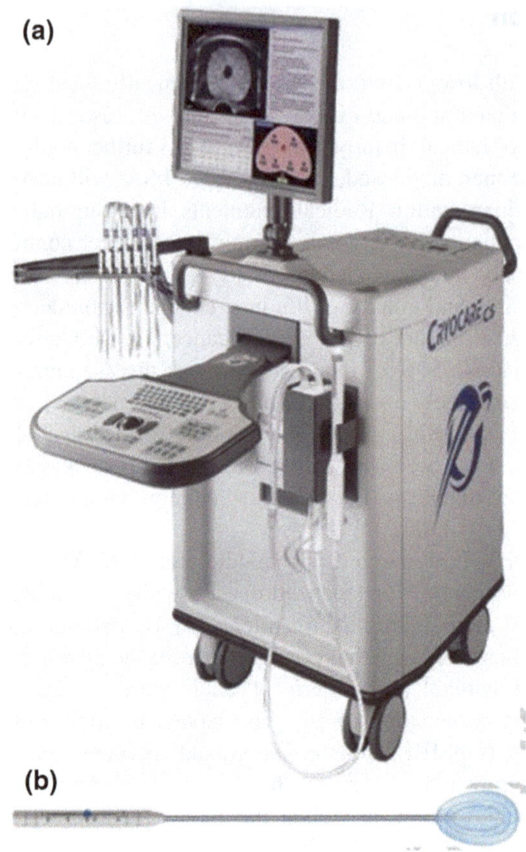

a Cryocare CS system and **b** adjustable Cryocare cryoprobe (used with permission of Endocare, Inc., a wholly owned subsidiary of HealthTronics, Inc.). Endocare Cryocare machine and adjustable cryoprobe (from Endocare of HealthTronics, Inc—http://www.radistribution.com/index.php/products-videos/cryoablation-endocare); also Fig. 13.1 (a and b) on page 166 of Interventional Urology, Springer, 2016

incidental, secondary lesions had a volume less than 0.5 cc [16]. In a more recent study, 96 prostate specimens from men who underwent cystoprostatectomy without clinically manifested prostate cancer were examined. It was shown that of the 215 PCa foci identified, 88% were clinically insignificant with a volume less than 0.5 cc and no grade 4 or 5 [14]. Taken together, these findings strongly support the hypothesis that satellite, low-grade lesions are clinically insignificant and natural history of disease is almost always driven by the largest, often highest grade tumor focus—known as the "index lesion" [17, 18].

Growing reliability of mpMRI with targeted and mapping biopsies is critical for the success of FT in appropriately selected patients. In addition to ruling out CS lesions with high accuracy, it is equally important to reliably detect index lesions, determine their extent, and accurately target them. Currently, the ideal candidate for FT is a matter of controversy. Karavitakis and colleagues defined criteria for focal ablation as organ-confined disease Gleason $\leq 3 + 4$; in the case of multifocal disease, secondary foci must be <0.5 cc in Gleason 6. On examining the histopathological characteristics of the index lesion in 100 whole-mount radical prostatectomy specimens, they found that 51% of men could have suitable for focal therapy on the basis of these criteria. Further, they showed that Gleason score, tumor volume, and the presence of extracapsular extension and/or seminal vesicle invasion were invariably determined by the index lesion, while secondary lesions were generally small and well differentiated [19]. The Prostate Cancer Randomized Controlled Trial Consensus Group proposed inclusion criteria for a randomized trial to best study men with CS localized PCa undergoing FT. Patients should have localized disease (stage $\leq$ cT2cN0M0), PSA < 15 ng/ml, and Gleason score of 4 + 3 or less. Less restrictive thresholds (PSA < 20 ng/ml, Gleason score up to 4 + 4, radiological stage $\leq$ cT3aN0M0) were proposed and deemed clinically acceptable, though not entirely supported by several of the more conservative contributors [20]. More recently, an international consensus meeting of FT experts agreed on a number of criteria to help guide patient eligibility in clinical practice and for inclusion in future trials. There was strong agreement that FT was best suited for patients with a life expectancy of greater than 10 years, good performance status, and Gleason 3 + 3 or 3 + 4 disease. Moreover, FT is acceptable in patients with multifocal disease leaving small, secondary lesions ≤ 5 mm of Gleason 3 + 3 untreated [21].

2 Cryotherapy

2.1 History

Cryotherapy is one of the most researched technologies for focal ablation of prostate cancer. The analgesia and anti-inflammatory properties of cold have been known for thousands of years, dating back to the Ancient Egyptians and Hippocrates. The first reported use of extreme cold for therapeutic tissue destruction was in the mid-nineteenth century. James Arnott used a salt-ice solution to freeze and reduce tumor size for palliation of pain associated with cancers of the breast and cervix [22]. Over the next 100 years, advancements in knowledge and technology fueled the development and growth of the field now known as cryotherapy. Major advances included the development of liquid nitrogen-cooled probes and temperature probes allowing for simultaneous measurement of surrounding tissue temperatures [23, 24]. The first experience of cryotherapy of the prostate was the transurethral treatment of benign prostatic hyperplasia [25]. This was shortly followed by both open perineal and transperineal cryoablation of prostate cancer tissue in the 1970s [26, 27]. Modern cryotherapy has been particularly influenced by more recent advances, including the use of thinner cryoprobes, multiple probes, argon gas and helium gas for freezing and thawing of tissue, respectively [28], and real-time transrectal ultrasound (TRUS) to monitor depth and shape of ice ball formation [29].

2.2 Technical Aspects

Cryotherapy (cryo) relies on extreme cold temperatures to induce cellular destruction through direct and indirect mechanisms. Rapid freezing and thawing of the targeted tissue creates a "cryolesion," noted by central necrosis and reactionary peripheral edema [30]. On a cellular level, freezing of water in the extracellular space leads to intracellular dehydration and osmotic stress. Meanwhile, rapid intracellular ice crystal formation produces shearing forces that disrupt cellular membranes, organelles, and cytoskeleton structures resulting in direct cell lysis. Microvascular damage has also been shown to indirectly contribute to tissue ablation. Freezing and subsequent thawing of tissues contributes to vascular hyperpermeability, edema, and ischemia by direct endothelial injury and stimulation of inflammatory cytokines. Subsequent reperfusion injury and oxidative stress from toxic-free radicals denatures cellular proteins and damages cell membranes [31]. Finally, persistent non-necrotic cells on the periphery of the cryolesion may be induced to undergo apoptosis, though the mechanism is not well understood [32].

The procedure is performed in the extended dorsal lithotomy position under anesthesia. Using ultrasound guidance, hollow cryoprobe needles are stereotactically inserted into the target prostate lesion transperineally. Argon and helium gases are then circulated through the cryoprobes allowing for freezing and thawing of the tissue, respectively. Control of ice ball formation relies on the Joule–Thomson effect, in which high-pressure gases undergo rapid, adiabatic expansion when flowing through a narrow, high-resistance system [33]. At the terminal tip of the needle within the target tissue, rapid expansion of the inflowing gas results in temperature change—decreased temperature for argon and increased for helium. Argon rapidly cools the cryoprobe tip to −187 °C for the freezing phase and then is rapidly exchanged with helium at 67 °C for an active thawing phase [34]. Two freeze-thaw cycles with separate ice ball formations are performed, as initially described by Onik and colleagues [29]. During the freezing phase, temperature probes monitor surrounding tissues for collateral damage and a urethral warming catheter protects the urethra from injury and concomitant complications.

2.3 Data

Prior to examining existing data on prostate cryotherapy, it is important to acknowledge the inherent limitations of their interpretation. The majority of studies are retrospective in design and reflect single-institution experiences. There is also notable diversity in the clinical experience with prostate cryoablation, including

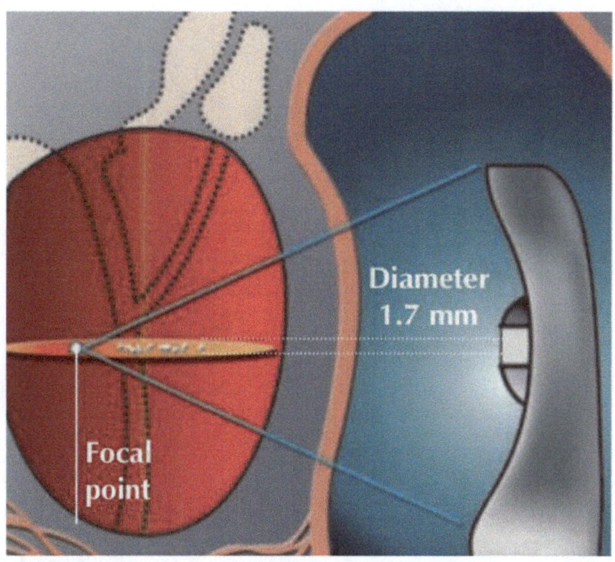

Schematic illustration of HIFU. Transrectal probe emits high-intensity ultrasound waves that are focused on the target prostate lesion. HIFU illustration (from Ablatherm, EDAP TMS)

whole-gland primary therapy, primary focal therapy, and post-radiation salvage therapy. Moreover, much of the contemporary data available is based on now outdated technology, including liquid nitrogen-based systems, which lacked the refinement and control of more modern argon/helium devices. Further, a lack of standardized outcome variables obscures the ability to draw concrete conclusions. There is currently no consensus definition of PSA failure following prostate cryotherapy. Many authors report biochemical recurrence (BCR) rates according to ASTRO or Phoenix criteria, both of which have been adapted from their intended use in post-radiation therapy monitoring and have not been formally studied in cryotherapy patients.

Cancer control outcomes may be further muddled by misinterpreting disease recurrence from missed treatment for cancer that was missed at the time of diagnosis. In a small prospective series of 25 patients undergoing cryosurgical hemi-ablation, Lambert et al. noted a 12% rate of BCR (defined as >50% PSA nadir reduction) after median follow-up of 28 months. Seven patients with suspicion for recurrence underwent repeat biopsy, of whom 3 had a positive rebiopsy. However, only one of these patients had evidence of recurrence on the ipsilateral side of cryoablation [35]. Truesdale and colleagues demonstrated a BCR of 27% (based on Phoenix criteria) with a 46% rate of biopsy-proven recurrence on repeat biopsy. Of note, the vast majority of these "recurrences" were found in the untreated contralateral lobe, raising suspicion for missed disease at initial diagnosis, as opposed to true recurrence from treatment failure [36].

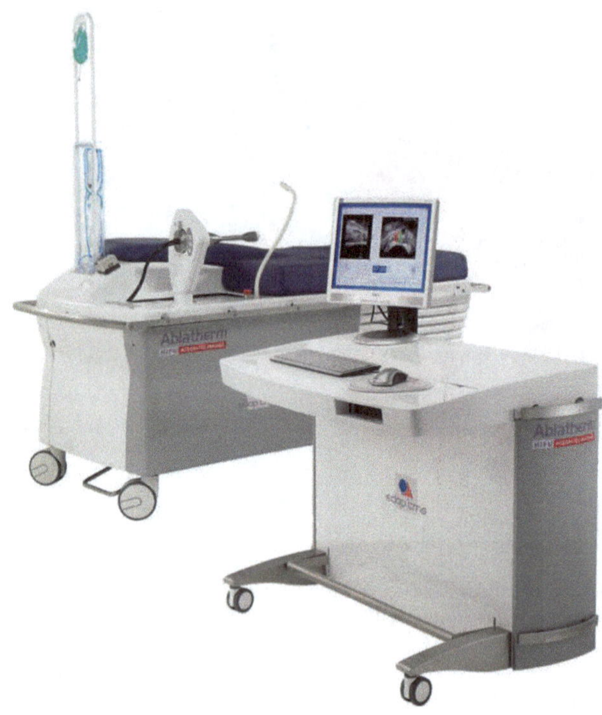

Ablatherm (R) HIFU device. Ablatherm machine (from EDAP TMS—http://www.edap-tms.com/en/products-services/prostate-cancer/ablatherm-hifu)

Since its inception, the Cryo On-Line Data (COLD) Registry has served as the largest prospectively maintained treatment registry for patients undergoing prostate cryotherapy. In the most recent update of registry data, it was shown that the use of primary focal cryoablation for PCa has dramatically risen since 1999. Ward and Jones went on to report that biochemical recurrence-free rate (based on ASTRO criteria) was 75.7% at 2 years post-treatment. Among those treated with suspicion for recurrence, 14.0% underwent a biopsy. Twenty-six percent of these biopsied men had evidence of recurrence, though this only represents 3.7% of the entire primary focal cryo cohort. With respect to morbidity, rectourethral fistulas were exceedingly rare, reported in just 1 of 1160 patients. Urinary incontinence and prolonged urinary retention (>30 days) both occurred infrequently, seen in 1.6 and 1.1% of patients, respectively. New onset erectile dysfunction (ED) was documented in ~40% of men treated. Of note, the incidences of all morbidities were considerably lower in the primary focal cryotherapy cohort as compared to those who underwent primary whole-gland or salvage cryotherapy [37].

Multiple prospective trials exist that evaluate the oncological efficacy and safety of primary whole-gland cryotherapy for more than 10 years of follow-up. Unfortunately, outcomes for men undergoing primary focal therapy are scarce and less robust, with shorter follow-ups, great variability in "focal" treatment template, and limited to participants with unilateral disease. Still, intermediate-term outcomes suggest good oncological control with minimal collateral damage in appropriately selected patients. Onik and colleagues reported on 48 men who received focal cryoablation with contralateral nerve sparing and at least 2 years follow-up (mean 4.5 years). The 24 patients with stable PSA (per ASTRO criteria) remained free of recurrence as demonstrated by negative routine follow-up biopsies. Of note, 4 of 6 men with a rising PSA had a positive biopsy. All 48 men remained continent and 90% (36/40) of men with preoperative potency were satisfied with their erectile function following treatment [38].

2.4 Summary

While it remains investigational, focal cryotherapy for localized prostate cancer appears to be a safe treatment with short- to medium-term oncological efficacy. Additionally, it appears to offer good preservation of urinary and sexual function in appropriately selected patients.

3 High-Intensity Focused Ultrasound (HIFU)

3.1 History

The origins of modern ultrasonography date back to 1880 with the discovery of the piezoelectric effect by Pierre and Jacques Curie. It wasn't until 1917, near the end of the First World War, that Langevin and colleagues used the piezoelectric properties of a quartz crystal to develop a sonar transducer in an attempt to detect enemy submarines [39]. The initial reports of high-intensity focused ultrasound (HIFU) for therapeutic medical purposes came in 1942 [40], but clinical applications HIFU in humans did not appear until William and Francis Fry investigated US for the treatment of neurologic disorders in 1960 [41]. Over the next 30 years, the field expanded with studies testing the use of HIFU for the treatment of Parkinson disease, brain tumors, and a number of ophthalmologic maladies, among others [42–44]. It wasn't until the 1990s that HIFU made its appearance in urology. Since that time, multiple investigations have been undertaken to examine its efficacy in benign prostatic hypertrophy (BPH) and later prostate cancer [45–49]. In 2015, the United States Food and Drug Administration (FDA) awarded HIFU approval for "prostate tissue ablation," though it did not specifically mention prostate cancer [50]. Similar to other FT modalities, HIFU did not gain major promise for clinical use until the recent advent of modern, advanced imaging modalities, such as mpMRI.

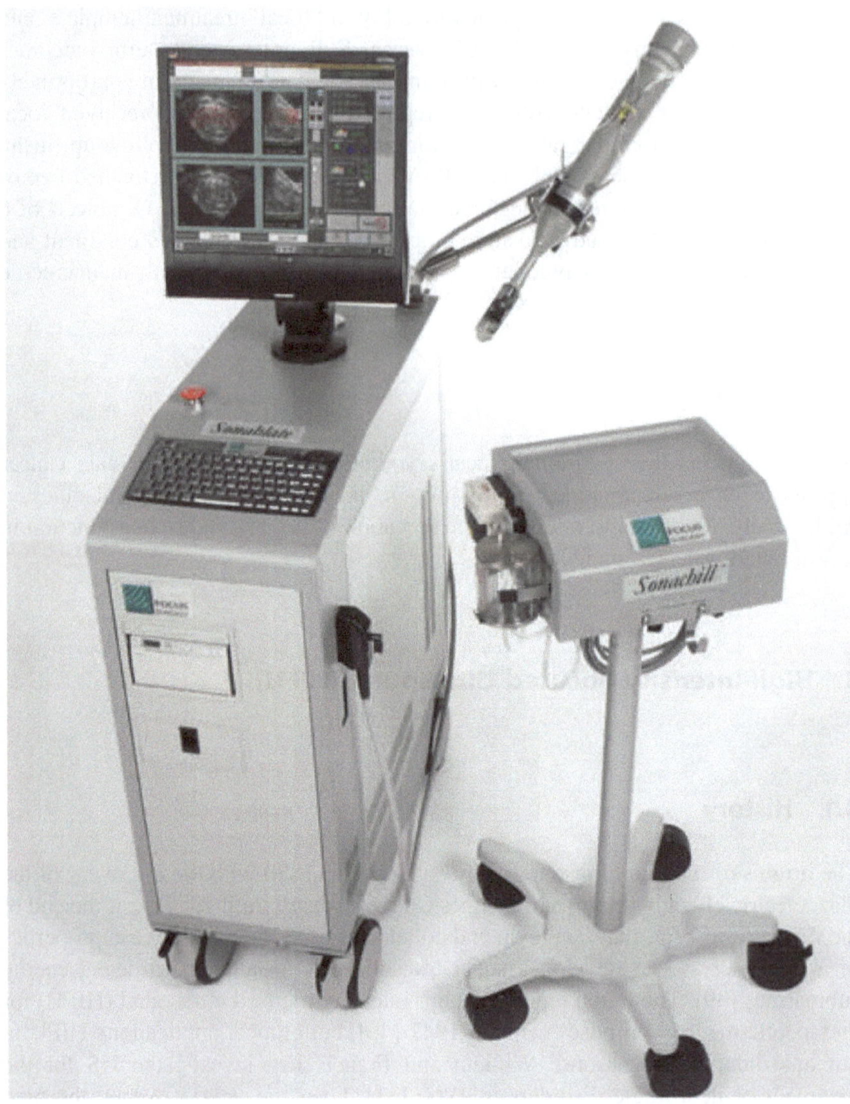

Sonablate (R) HIFU device. Sonablate machine (from SonaCare Medical, Charlotte, NC—http://www.sonacaremedical.com/)

3.2 Technical Aspects

HIFU utilizes this principle of focused US waves to induce coagulative necrosis of a targeted tissue through two mechanisms: thermal damage and acoustic cavitation. As ultrasound (US) waves propagate through tissue, fluctuations in pressure lead to microscopic shearing motion and deposition of frictional energy in the form of heat.

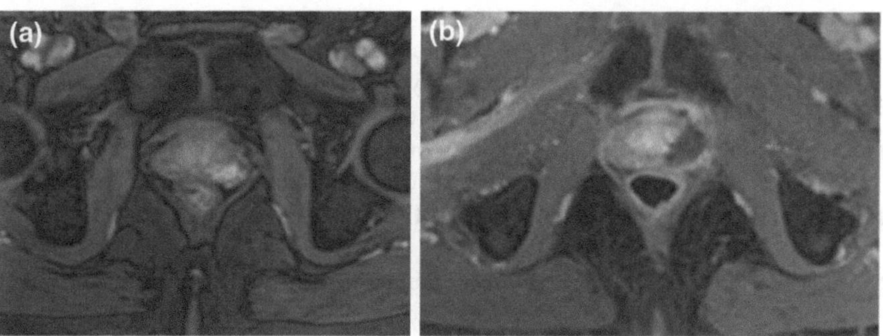

a T2-weighted image demonstrating a left peripheral zone lesion. **b** T2-weighted image following focal HIFU to the left posterior quadrant. page 146 (Chap. 10)—Fig. 10.4 of Interventional Urology, Springer, 2016

At lower intensities, the thermal and mechanical energy generated by US waves is insignificant. However, when focused on a single point at increased intensities, the energy produced at that point can cause tissue destruction. Specifically, an US transducer containing an acoustic lens creates a HIFU beam by concentrating multiple US waves on single convergence point. At this focal point, known as the elementary lesion (EL), the amount of thermal energy and heat generated is capable of inducing cellular damage via protein denaturation, vaporization, and apoptosis. Immediately outside the EL, the energy sharply drops thereby protecting surrounding tissues from incidental injury. At very high HIFU beam intensities (>3500 W/cm^3), cavitation phenomena can occur. Microbubbles of water vapor rapidly form due to extremely low static pressure within the sonicated tissue. These bubbles subsequently collapse and emit forceful pressure shocks that mechanically damage tissue and enhance ablation [51, 52].

The procedure is typically performed under spinal or general anesthesia with the patient lying in the right lateral recumbent position and knees brought up to the chest. Patients receive a pre-procedural enema and antibiotic prophylaxis. Insertion of a urinary catheter facilitates identification of the bladder neck on US. A transducer with a protective, active cooling mechanism is inserted into the rectum. The cooling system of circulated cool water also helps to minimize acoustic interference of the rectal wall. In general, size of the ablated lesion is dependent on the acoustic intensity, duration of exposure, on/off ratio, and the distance between ELs [51]. Lesions can be seen as hyperechoic areas on diagnostic US; however, MRI is the gold-standard modality for measuring the true extent of ablation and determining the efficacy of treatment.

Currently, there are two available devices on the market for prostate HIFU. Ablatherm® (EDAP-TMS SA, Vaulx en Velin, France) features two separate transducers, one for imaging (7.5 Hz) and the other for ablation (3 Hz), with a maximum focal point of 45 mm from the transducer. The system includes a treatment table, integrated imaging system for US-scanned reconstruction of the gland, external motion sensor, and inbuilt controls that correct or stop treatment based on probe distance from the rectal wall and patient movement. Collectively, the device allows the physician to safely perform and monitor ablation with real-time imaging and automatic safety mechanisms. Treatment pulses last 4–5 s, followed by an interval of 47 s to allow for tissue cooling [53].

The Sonablate® device (SonaCare Medical, Charlotte, NC, USA) consists of a console, a flat screen monitor, and two 4 MHz transducers, mounted back-to-back, operating at focal distances of 4.5, 4, or 3 cm. Each transducer features a central part that is used for real-time US imaging and a peripheral part used for treatment. Each pulse generally lasts for 3 s, followed by a 6-s gap for tissue cooling. The power intensity of each pulse is guided by the real-time US changes seen within the targeted area. Treatment is executed over two or three separate blocks. The anterior part of the gland is treated first, followed by the mid-zone and posterior part. The posterior gland is always treated using a focal length of 3 cm at lower energy levels to prevent rectal injury. Rectal cooling is achieved by pumping chilled degassed water through the endorectal probe [54].

Ideally, HIFU should not be performed in glands greater than 40 cc or in the presence of significant calcifications, which may interfere with HIFU wave transmission. Pre-procedural transurethral resection of prostate (TURP) prior to HIFU has been used for gland downsizing to improve treatment efficacy and reduce postoperative obstructive symptoms. This technique is particularly beneficial for decreasing the distance from anterior lesions, which can be technically difficult to reach [52].

3.3 Data

While early and intermediate results in terms of efficacy and safety have been promising, long-term outcomes are lacking. Moreover, the majority of investigations have tested HIFU as a whole-gland therapy and the limited contemporary data on focal therapy is largely based on investigations of hemiablation strategies for unilateral PCa.

In comparison with 70 patients undergoing whole-gland therapy, Muto et al. reported the results of 29 men with unilateral disease who underwent focal hemiablation HIFU with the Sonablate® 500 system. They noted comparable oncological and functional outcomes between the whole-gland and focal therapy at 12-month follow-up. Overall, 81.6% of men had a negative biopsy at 1 year. The 2-year disease-free survival (DFS) rates, stratified by low- and intermediate-risk disease, were similar as well. There was no significant difference in urinary morbidity [55]. El Fegoun and colleagues reported on 12 patients with Gleason $\leq 3 + 4$, localized, unilateral PCa who underwent hemiablation HIFU using the Ablatherm® device with 10-year median follow-up. Recurrence-free survival at 5 and 10 years was 90 and 38%, respectively. There were no cases of metastasis, although 5 patients underwent salvage therapy (4 with hormonal therapy and 1 with salvage HIFU). There was one case of urinary retention [56]. A phase I/II trial of 20 patients with unilateral disease reported by Ahmed et al. showed that 89% of participants had no histological evidence of ipsilateral disease and none had evidence of CS PCa (Gleason ≥ 7 and/or high volume disease) at 6-month follow-up. One year post-treatment, nearly 90% were pad-free, leak-free, and had erections sufficient for intercourse [57].

In the largest known series of truly focal therapy, Ahmed et al. performed focal HIFU on MRI-visible index lesions in 56 men of varying PCa risk level. The majority of patients had multifocal, bilateral disease, and 83.9% (47/56) had intermediate-risk cancer by NCCN categorization. At 12-month follow-up, 85.7% (48/56) men had histological or radiographic absence of PCa (biopsy and/or mpMRI) and 80.8% (42/52) had no histological evidence of CS disease. Of note, two (3.6%) patients had recurrence of CS disease, based on the presence of lesions in untreated areas not detected at baseline. Among those men with leak-free and pad-free continence with erections sufficient for penetration at baseline, 82.5% (33/40) had no significant change in their urinary or sexual function at 12 months post-ablation. This represents the largest series to date to demonstrate promising short-term outcomes of truly focal ablation of index lesions with HIFU with respect to oncological efficacy and safety [58].

3.4 Summary

The therapeutic potential for HIFU in the treatment of PCa has been known since the 1990s. Major advancements in imaging and US technology have allowed for investigations into the application of HIFU for focal therapy—initially hemiablation, and more recently targeted ablation of CS index lesions. The noninvasive nature of treatment and absence of ionizing radiation are apparent advantages compared to FT options. Ablation causes immediate necrosis with sharply demarcated boundaries on imaging, and there is no lifetime dose limit to preclude a patient from repeat sessions in the event of previous HIFU treatment failure. Therapy is, however, initially limited to smaller prostates (<40 mL) and can be technically challenging for anterior-located lesions. Though contemporary results are limited by few studies with small cohorts, variability in technique, and short-term follow-up, there is growing recognition of the potential of HIFU for FT of localized PCa. Widespread use hinges on the maturation of existing studies and better standardization of treatment and outcomes reporting to increase confidence in the long-term cancer control and patient safety of this treatment.

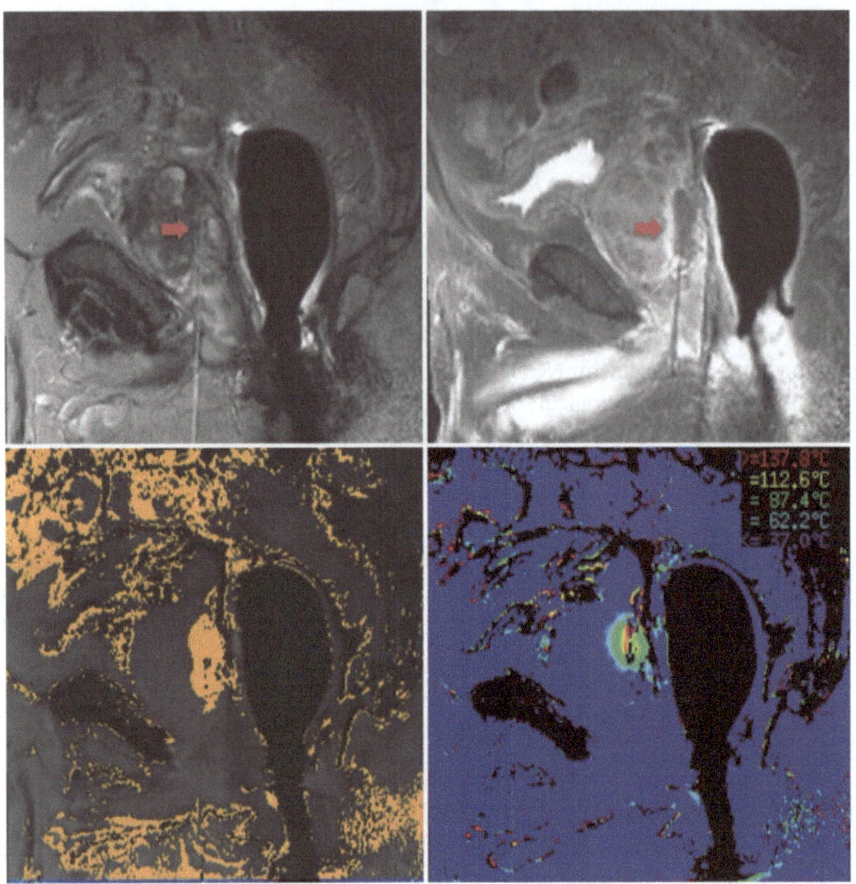

MRI images obtained before (*top left*) and after (*top right*) FLA with the tip of the laser fiber (*red arrow)* visualized within the target lesion. Destruction mapping (*bottom left*) and real-time thermometry (*bottom right*) of laser ablation. page 157 (Chap. 11)—Fig. 11.1 of Interventional Urology, Springer, 2016

4 Focal Laser Ablation (FLA)

4.1 History

The first description of laser ablation was by Bown in 1983. Using a 400-um glass fiber and a neodymium:yttrium-aluminum-garnet (Nd:YAG) laser system, he treated a metastatic skin lesion by necrosis of the target area [59]. Subsequent applications of FLA for tumors have included metastatic liver lesions [60] and inoperable hepatocellular carcinoma [61]. FLA for PCa treatment was first reported by Sander and Beisland in 1984. The authors cystoscopically treated PCa lesions with a Nd:YAG beam transmitted down a flexible quartz fiber [62].

Further investigation into FLA for PCa began to gain significant traction in the early 1990s [63, 64]. However, the technique was limited by the ability to accurately localize lesions, calculate appropriate dosimetry, and follow up treatment. Initially, treatment localization and monitoring relied on TRUS and contrast-enhanced ultrasonography (CEUS), respectively. Reduction in perfusion of the target region secondary to the ablation process could be detected by signal loss on CEUS [65]. More recently, in-bore MRI reconstruction and thermometry has improved the precision of laser localization and estimation of the extent of tissue ablation.

Other known names for this technology include laser interstitial tumor therapy, laser interstitial photocoagulation, and photothermal therapy.

4.2 Technical Aspects

FLA involves the thermal destruction of targeted prostate tissue by conversion of laser energy to heat. Rapid focal absorption of heat causes a rise in temperature to greater than 60 °C, inducing instantaneous protein denaturation and irreversible tissue damage by coagulative necrosis [66]. Thermal damage can also be achieved at lower temperatures, between 42 and 60 °C, though longer heating periods required to ensure lethality [67]. Further, there exists some evidence that laser energy may penetrate tumor cells more effectively than normal tissue allowing for larger and more selective tumor ablation [68]. The extent of the thermal ablation is determined by both the optical and thermal properties of the tissue, as well as the parameters of the laser—wavelength, power, and density. The optical and thermal properties of the tissue are based on its structure, water content, and vascularity. The prostate, in particular, is well suited for FLA due to its optical absorption rate and relatively low vascularity, which allow for accurate photothermal coagulation [69]. However, it is important to note that the laser energy does provide a homogenous zone of tissue ablation resulting in variability between the intended and actual areas of ablation. This is due in part to changes in the thermal conductivity of the tissue with rising temperatures, as well as potential charring of near-field tissue that can limit the penetration of photons. Limitations in thermal necrosis prediction are also related to the use of cooled applicators that prevent tissue charring or photovaporization during the heating phase [70].

The procedure is performed through either transperineal or transrectal placement of a laser fiber into the targeted lesion under real-time MRI. While the 1064-nm Nd:YAG laser has been classically used for PCa ablation, more portable and cost-effective diode lasers (800–980 nm) with greater potential power output have gained popularity [71]. On laser activation, an ellipsoid zone of ablation is created over several minutes, the size of which can be adjusted by manual advancement or retraction of the fiber [72, 73].

Accurate target ablation relies on real-time, three-dimensional MRI reconstruction and thermometry. In canine prostate models, Stafford and colleagues demonstrated that they could accurately position laser energy to a target site within a mean ±SD of 1.1 ± 0.7 mm with real-time, three-dimensional (3D) MRI. They also showed that the area of ablation seen post-contrast imaging correlated well with thermal damage predicted on MRI [74]. A number of other studies have further supported the accuracy of real-time MR thermometry in predicting the region of tissue destruction while minimizing collateral damage to surrounding tissue and neurovascular structures [75, 76].

4.3 Data

Similar to other FT modalities, data on treatment outcomes for FLA are limited. Currently, most information is based on several small non-randomized phase I studies with short-term follow-up.

The first reported case of FLA for treatment of PCa was by Amin and colleagues in 1993. The authors [63] achieved local disease control following failed EBRT with two attempts of FLA. Treatment was confirmed by demonstration of a non-enhancing, avascular region in the treatment region on follow-up CT, as well as confirmation of necrosis without residual disease on follow-up biopsies from the ablated area. The procedure was well tolerated, and there were no significant treatment-related complications reported.

In 2009, Lindner and colleagues reported on one of the first phase I studies to assess the feasibility and safety of CEUS-guided FLA. The study examined 12 men with biopsy-proven low-risk PCa (T1c or T2a, PSA < 10 ng/mL; Gleason score ≤ 6; only 1 of 12 cores exhibiting <30% cancer following TRUS-guided biopsy). The target zone of ablation was determined by mpMRI and subsequently fused with 3D-US imaging for laser guidance. The photothermal effect was monitored with CEUS, and temperature probes were used to monitor temperatures at the target borders and in surrounding tissues. The median treatment volume was 2.2 cm^3, based on post-FLA MRI. At 3- to 6-month follow-up, 6 patients (50%) were tumor-free on TRUS-guided 10 core biopsies and 2 targeted lesion biopsies. Two men (16.7%) had tumor on the untreated, contralateral side, and four men (33.3%) had residual disease in the targeted areas. Of these four, two were found to have minimal disease while the other two had >50% Gleason 6 PCa in two cores. In total, 67% were tumor-free in the zone of ablation and 50% were completely disease free. With respect to safety, adverse events were mild, including perineal discomfort (2/12), mild hematuria (2/12), hematospermia (2/12), and fatigue (1/12). There were no changes in mean urinary and sexual function scores up to 6 months postoperatively [77]. In a subsequent study, the same group also showed that the MRI-calculated ablated volume correlated well with the volume of necrosis seen on whole-mount radical prostatectomy histology (n = 4). These findings suggest that post-treatment MRI can be a useful modality for determining the extent of ablation [78].

Raz and colleagues later studied the use of real-time MRI guidance for FLA in two patients. Their experience highlighted many of the advantages now known of MRI guidance of FT. These include enhanced visualization of the target lesion, accurate guidance of laser fiber insertion, improved real-time control of the ablation zone and monitoring of surrounding tissues, and immediate confirmation of treatment by evidence of devascularization of the lesion on contrast-enhanced MRI [79].

Another phase I trial by Oto and colleagues sought to evaluate the oncologic efficacy and safety profile of MRI-guided FLA in 9 men with low-risk PCa. Eligibility criteria of participants included clinical stage T1c–T2a, PSA < 10 ng/ml, Gleason ≤ 7, 3 or fewer cores with cancer on minimum 12-core biopsy, no single biopsy with >50% tumor involvement, and a suspicious lesion visible on MRI corresponding to the biopsy site. At 6-month follow-up, MRI-guided biopsies of ablated areas revealed benign tissue in seven of nine patients (78%) and Gleason 6 cancer in the remaining two patients (22%). Retrospective review of the ablation images showed that the target lesion site was not completely covered by the zone of ablation for the two men with residual disease on follow-up biopsy. There were no statistically significant changes from baseline in urinary or sexual function at 6 months post-ablation, and no major complications or serious adverse events were reported [80].

Currently, there are a number of phase II clinical trials underway to further investigate the oncologic efficacy of FLA for localized PCa.

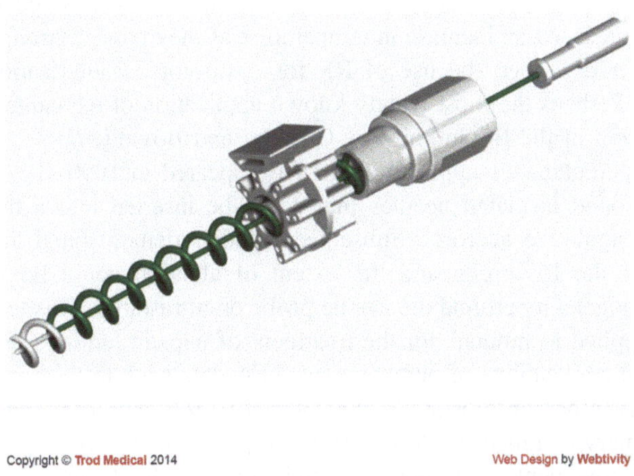

Trod Medical's Encage (TM) radiofrequency ablation device. Encage (TM) device (from Trod Medical US, LLC, St. Petersburg, FL—http://www.trodmedical.com/)

4.4 Summary

Like many other FT treatments, outcomes data for FLA are in their infancy and long-term demonstration of oncologic control and safety are needed. Despite these limitations, FLA appears a promising energy modality for FT of organ-confined prostate cancer. Advantages of the technology include the wide availability of lasers, relatively low cost compared to other investigational FT treatments, MR compatibility of lasers, and ability to easily monitor treatment and surrounding tissues with real-time MR and CEUS imaging. FLA is, however, not without its limitations. Notably, the reliance on MRI for instrumentation and thermometry presents challenges to accessing the patient for manipulation within the scanner bore.

5 Radiofrequency Ablation (RFA)

5.1 History

Radiofrequency ablation (RFA) is a form of thermal ablation shown to be effective and safe for a variety of indications across many disciplines of medicine. Applications include, but are not limited to, the treatment of hepatocellular carcinoma, pancreatic cancer, breast masses, and cardiac arrhythmias [81–84]. The basic technology of RFA dates back to 1891. D'Arsonval demonstrated that radiofrequency waves caused an increase in temperature as they passed through tissue [85]. In 1910, Beer described the use of RF for cystoscopic cauterization of bladder tumors [86]. Perhaps the most widely known application of RF came in 1928 with the introduction of the Bovie knife by Cushing and Bovie [87].

The first percutaneous applications of RF appeared in 1990. Two independent groups developed insulated needles that could be inserted into a tissue to cause interstitial coagulative necrosis. Subsequent studies demonstrated that the proper placement of the RF probe and the extent of ablation could be visualized by increased echogenicity around the needle probe on ultrasound. This technology was soon after applied to humans for the treatment of hepatic tumors [88–90].

Urological applications of percutaneous RFA date back to the early 1990s with investigations in benign prostatic hypertrophy [91, 92] and later the exploration of RFA for primary treatment of PCa in 1998 [93]. The success of this technology for the targeted treatment of tumors in other surgical fields in conjunction with advancements in prostate imaging and knowledge of PCa has fueled the renewed urological interest in focal RFA as a potential treatment of localized PCa.

5.2 Technical Aspects

RFA uses high-frequency (radiofrequency) alternating electrical current to cause thermal damage to tissue resulting in coagulative necrosis. Ionic agitation within the target tissue, secondary to current flow from a needle electrode, results in the generation of heat. The degree of tissue damage from RFA is dependent on the duration of ablation and the maximum temperature achieved within the target area. Irreversible injury and cell death occurrence have been shown to occur after 4–6 min at temperatures greater than 50 °C and almost immediately above 60 °C. Temperatures within the target can exceed 100 °C. Direct cytotoxic effects occur by protein denaturation and the disruption of cellular membranes. Secondary microvascular thrombosis and resultant ischemia potentiate cell death.

In practice, a radiofrequency probe is inserted into the ablation zone transperineally under image guidance. A computer-controlled generator provides the radiofrequency current. Based on the design of the device, the current can be delivered by monopolar or bipolar probe. The temperature within the tissue is based on the generator's power, heat conductivity, and the dissipation of heat through local vascular structures (e.g., heat sink effect). With monopolar probes, tissue impedance of the current is also an important determinant of temperature as it causes local tissue conversion of thermal energy to heat. The risk of excessive tissue hyperthermia in surrounding tissues is minimized with the use of bipolar RFA. The Encage™ device (Trod Medical, Leuven, Belgium) is the only device currently under investigation for PCa focal therapy and features a bipolar, helical ablation probe [93, 94].

5.3 Data

Only one stage I study evaluating primary focal RFA is currently available. In 1998, Zlotta and colleagues reported their experience using interstitial RFA in 15 patients with biopsy-proven localized PCa scheduled for radical prostatectomy. Needle electrodes were inserted transperineally with US guidance and placed in close proximity to the target lesion(s). Patients underwent 12 min of ablation with target region temperatures measured up to 105 °C. On histological examination of prostate specimens, there was extensive coagulative necrosis identified predictably in the tumor tissue, which correlated well with the predicted lesion size. There was residual tumor in all patients, though the primary purpose of the study was not to treat. Being a safety and feasibility study, there were no recorded oncological or functional outcomes. The procedure was well tolerated by all patients, and there were no reported complications [93].

Currently, there are three ongoing phase IIa prospective development trials evaluating primary focal ablation by RFA in men with low- or intermediate-risk, localized PCa (NCT02303054: "MRI-Targeted Focal Ablation of the Prostate in

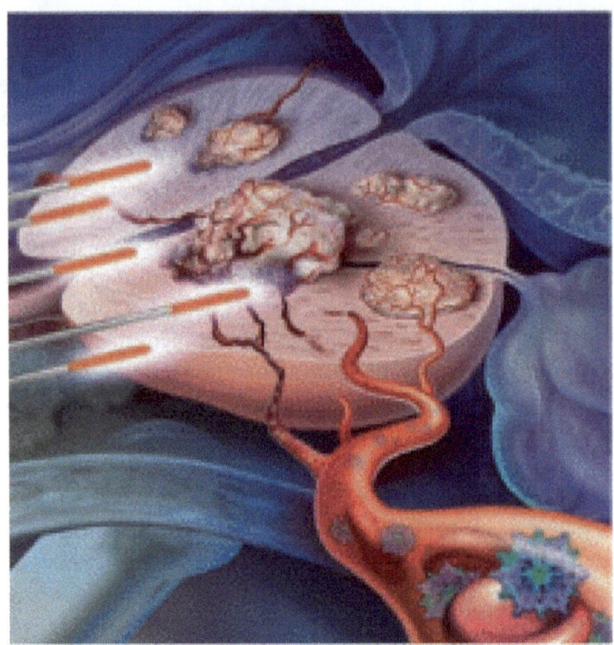

An intravenously administered photosensitizer is distributed throughout the body. Optic fibers are then positioned in the target lesion and deliver light energy of the appropriate wavelength to selectively activate the photosensitizing agent. Figure 1 from https://www.ncbi.nlm.nih.gov/pmc/articles/PMC2615102/ (Lepor H. Vascular targeted photodynamic therapy for localized prostate cancer. Rev Urol 2008: 10(4): 254–261.)

Men With Prostate Cancer"; NCT02328807: "Focal Prostate Radio-Frequency Ablation for the Treatment of Prostate Cancer"; NCT02294903: "Focal Prostate Radiofrequency Ablation").

5.4 Summary

RFA causes thermal ablation of a target tissue by the conversion of radiofrequency waves, generated by an alternating current, to heat. The utility of RFA for ablation of small renal masses and tumors in various organ systems is well documented; however, there has yet to be any significant data on its efficacy as a primary focal treatment for PCa. Ongoing investigations are needed to determine the future potential of this technique in the PCa space.

6 Photodynamic Therapy (PDT)

6.1 History

PDT ablation involves the local activation of a vascular photosensitizing agent within a target area by a light source, which results in the formation of cytotoxic reactive oxygen species (ROS) and subsequent cell death. Historically, a number of clinical trials have shown promise for PDT in treating malignancies and premalignant lesions in various organ systems, including esophagus, skin, and brain [95]. The first urological investigations of PDT were for the treatment of superficial bladder cancer [96]. Modest long-term response rates and risk of bladder contraction with the hematoporphyrin-derivative photosensitizer used for PDT in older studies limited widespread appeal of the technique. In 1990, Windahl and colleagues were the first to report their experience using PDT and hematoporphyrin for the treatment of two men with localized PCa [97]. Several other groups followed suit with similar small-scale studies, and more recently, PDT has been studies as a salvage therapy following failed external beam radiotherapy (EBRT) [98–100]. More recently, the development of novel photosensitizing agents with greater potency and safety profile, as well as portable light sources and more accurate treatment dosimetry, has led to increased interest in PDT for primary focal treatment of PCa [101].

6.2 Technical Aspects

The mechanism of ablation by PDT is based on the activation of a photosensitizing agent, or light-sensitive compound, within a target area. Intravenous administration of the photosensitizer generally precedes light delivery and activation by up to 48 h, though can be as quick as minutes before activation in the case of newer photosensitive drugs. The light is then delivered to the target area at a wavelength matched to the absorption maximum of the drug inciting a local photochemical reaction with formation of cytotoxic ROS. Specifically, cell death and tissue damage are mediated by ROS damage of endothelial cells leading to blood flow stasis, vascular leakage, and thrombosis. The resultant hypoxia eventuates in apoptosis and necrosis [101, 102]. At the same time, the release of inflammatory cytokines triggers an inflammatory cascade that recruits leukocytes and activates tumor-specific immunity, which may play a role in achieving long-term cancer control [103]. Ultimately, the selectivity and focality of PDT is based on differential accumulation of the photosensitive drug in the tumor versus normal tissue and site-specific activation of the compound by optic fibers coupled to an appropriate light source [101].

Several of the more novel photosensitizers under investigation for use in PDT of PCa are lutetium texaphyrin (LuTex), meso tetra hydroxy phenyl chlorin (mTHPC), WST-09 (TOOKAD®; STEBA Biotech N. V.) and its water-soluble sister molecule

WST-11 (TOOKAD® Soluble; STEBA Biotech N. V.). The latter two compounds are palladium bacteriopheophorbide molecules synthesized from the native bacteriochlorophyll a molecule of dark-growing bacteria. The majority of clinical studies reported to date in have utilized WST-09 (TOOKAD®). WST-09, WST-11, and similar molecules are strictly confined to the vasculature. Therefore, the primary mechanism of cell death with this photosensitizer is vascular occlusion mediated by the production of ROS limited to the vascular bed. When using these drugs, the therapeutic approach is sometimes referred to as *vascular-targeted photodynamic therapy* (VTP). Several apparent advantages of TOOKAD® and similar VTP agents have been identified, in comparison with older generation compounds. Being limited to the vasculature, the drug is rapidly cleared from the body within a few hours, rather than several weeks, thereby reducing skin photosensitivity and the need to avoid sunlight. Further, the optimal drug light interval is considerably short, such that light delivery for photoactivation can be initiated prior to completion of drug infusion [101, 104–109].

After intravenous instillation of the photosensitive agent, optic fibers are inserted transperineally into the target area under the guidance of real-time US imaging and a standard brachytherapy stabilizing frame and template with the patient in high lithotomy position. Light of the appropriate wavelength is then delivered to target via the optic fibers. WST-09 is activated by light with a wavelength of 763 nm, for example. The near-infrared wavelength of this agent allows for better penetration of the light source deep into the prostate for treatment [105].

6.3 Data

In 2006, Moore and colleagues reported the findings of their pilot phase I experience with PDT in men with organ-confined PCa, using mTHPC (main activation wavelength 650 nm) as a photosensitizing agent. In total, 10 PDT treatments were performed on six men (four patients received two treatments) with mean age of 66 years and Gleason 6 disease. Though outcomes were short term, there was no evidence of disease on follow-up biopsies of the treated areas at 1 to 2 months post-PDT. Similarly, early follow-up MRI demonstrated patchy necrosis edema, most of which had resolved by 2 to 3 months. A 67% fall in PSA level was noted, though the true oncologic significance of the outcomes remains unknown. The authors did acknowledge that prolonged skin photosensitivity was a significant disadvantage of using mTHPC for photosensitization as compared to VTP agents (e.g., TOOKAD®, which was still in early development at the time of this study) [99].

Two other prospective development studies evaluating focal PDT have been reported. A phase IIb study by Azzouzi et al., published in 2013, demonstrated promising short-term efficacy and safety of VTP with WST-11-TOOKAD® Soluble for the treatment of localized PCa. In all, 83 men underwent treatment with follow-up biopsy at 6 months and MRI at one week post-VTP. The study identified optimal treatment parameters: 4 mg/kg WST-11 intravenous infusion and 200 J/cm light. Using this regimen, 83% (38/46) of patients had no evidence of residual disease on biopsy at 6 months (95% CI 68.6–92.2%; $p < 0.001$). In total, approximately 75% (61/83) of all treated patients had a negative short-term follow-up biopsy. At least one adverse event requiring treatment was reported in 87% of patients, though most were mild or moderate in severity. Eight men (9.3%) had serious adverse events, none of which resulted in discontinuation of treatment. Moore et al. investigated the use of VTP with WST-11 in 39 patients with Gleason 6 PCa confirmed on transrectal or transperineal biopsy. Patients received a single dose of 2, 4, or 6 mg/kg WST-11 administered in a 10-minute infusion followed by photoactivation with 200 J/cm light at 753 nm. Ablation pattern was catered to each patient, including focal, hemiablation, and subtotal whole gland. Treatment effect was evaluated by MRI at 7 days post-VTP; patient follow-up occurred at 7 days, 1, 3, and 6 months with TRUS-guided prostate biopsy at 6 months. Among the 12 men who received the optimal VTP regimen (4 mg/kg WST-11, light dose of 200 J/cm), 83% (10/12) had a negative follow-up biopsy; a 45% (10/26) negative biopsy rate was observed in patients receiving alternative treatment parameters. There were no significant differences in urinary symptoms and erectile function between baseline and 6 months after VTP. There was no significant cancer reported in either of these two studies [110, 111].

In 2017, Azzouzi and colleagues published results of an open-label, phase III, randomized controlled trial that compared treatment with VTP to the standard of care, active surveillance (AS). In the study, 413 patients with low-risk, localized PCa without prior treatment were randomly assigned to treatment with padeliporfin (WST-11-TOOKAD® Soluble) VTP ($n = 206$) or active surveillance (AS) ($n = 207$). Patients in the treatment arm received 4 mg/kg padeliporfin intravenously over 10 min, followed by insertion of optical fibers into the prostate to cover the desired treatment zone with photoactivation by laser light 753 nm at a fixed power of 150 mW/cm for 22 min and 15 s.

Patients in the VTP arm were found to have a longer time to progression (28.3 vs. 14.1 months, $p < 0.0001$) and were less likely to progress at 24-month follow-up (28% of 206 vs. 58% of 207, adjusted hazard ratio 0.34, $p < 0.0001$). Progression was defined as advancement in the extent, grade, or stage of disease, increase in PSA concentration, or cancer-related death. At 2-year follow-up, 49% of men treated with PDT had a negative biopsy compared to 14% in the AS group (adjusted risk ratio 3.67, $p < 0.0001$). The authors reported a decreased use of radical surgery following trial enrollment among men in the treatment arm (6 *v* 29%, $p < 0.0001$). However, this finding could be accounted for by the fact that patients were not blinded to their treatment allocation and those who underwent PDT may have been less inclined to undergo subsequent radical treatment. In general, the procedure was well tolerated and few serious adverse events of PDT were reported, the most common of which was urinary retention in 15 patients, all of whom recovered by two months post-PDT [112].

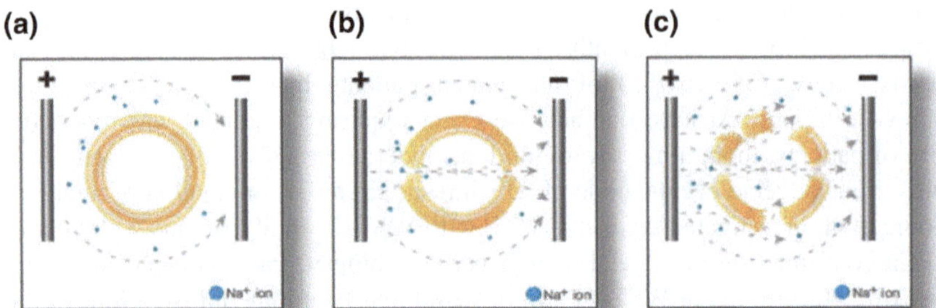

Schematic illustration of **a** no electroporation, **b** reversible electroporation (RE), and **c** irreversible electroporation (IRE). page 162 (Chap. 12)—Fig. 12.1 of Interventional Urology, Springer, 2016

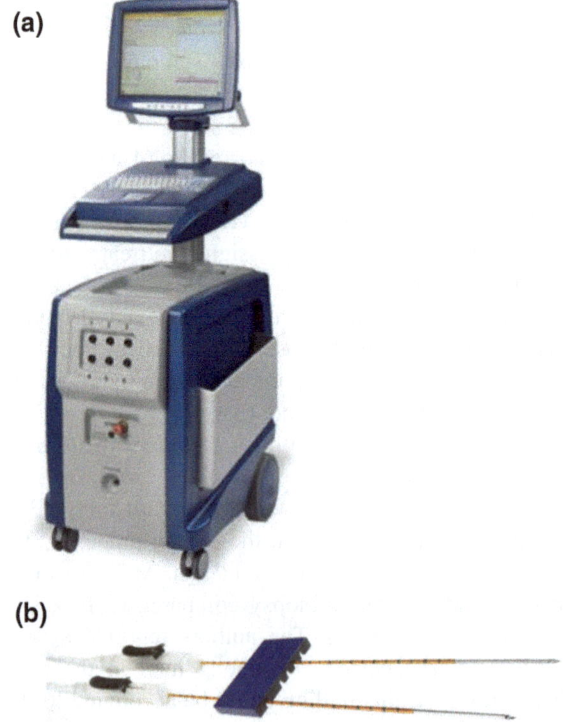

a NanoKnife (TM) IRE console and **b** 19G monopolar needle electrodes locked together with external spacers. NanoKnife system (from AngioDynamics, Latham, NY—http://www.angiodynamics.com/products/nanoknife)

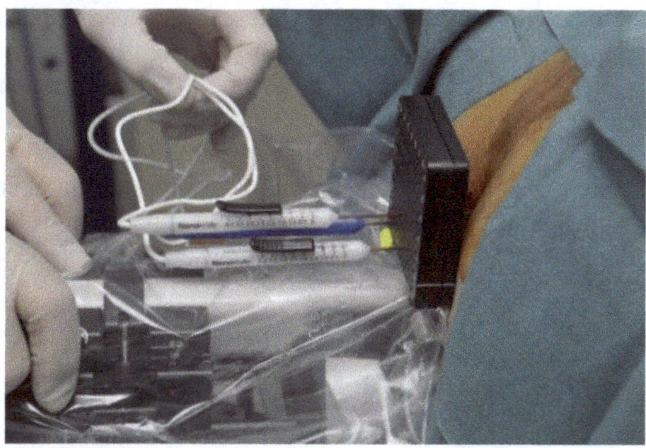

Unipolar electrode needles are inserted transperineally under real-time ultrasound guidance with the use of a brachytherapy grid. Page 163 (Chap. 12)—Fig. 12.3 of Interventional Urology, Springer, 2016

6.4 Summary

PDT involves the focal treatment of a target lesion by in situ activation of a photosensitizing agent with a light source. Advancements in photosensitive drugs have paved the way for investigations into the use of PDT for the treatment of localized PCa. Short-term histological results and patient-reported outcomes indicate PDT is a reasonably safe and promising modality for focal prostate ablation. However, contemporary data remains insufficient to definitively support the use of PDT over AS as the preferred management of men with low-risk disease. Looking forward, larger prospective studies with longer follow-up will be revealing.

7 Irreversible Electroporation (IRE)

7.1 History

Electroporation is a technique in which destabilizing electric pulses are used to create nanoscale defects in the cell membranes of biological tissues [113]. The process can be temporary with applications including gene transfection and electrochemotherapy (ECT), which optimizes chemotherapy by allowing cytotoxic medications to enter target cells at higher doses [114]. Above a certain threshold, the cell is unable to recover and these "nanopores" become irreversible, eventuating in cell death by impairing the ability to maintain homeostasis across the lipid bilayer [113, 115].

The use of electroporation to increase cell membrane permeability was introduced by Okino and Mohri in 1987. The study demonstrated that the antitumor effects of a cytotoxic drug were potentiated with reversible permeabilization of cell membranes using electric pulses as compared to standard treatment [116]. These findings were later corroborated by Mir et al. in 1991, examining the effects of bleomycin in mice, then termed electrochemotherapy [117]. Initially, the occurrence of IRE during reversible electroporate procedures was considered an unwanted side effect of treatment. More recently, the development of commercially available medical equipment has fostered attention to application of IRE for tumor ablation in various organ systems, including the lungs, liver, kidneys, pancreas, and prostate [118–121].

7.2 Technical Aspects

At the time of this publication, the only currently commercially available IRE system indicated for the surgical ablation of soft tissue is the NanoKnife™ (Angiodynamics Inc, Queensbury, NY, USA). The system consists of a low-energy direct current (LEDC) generator and needle electrodes, all of which is interfaced with a computer system and user-friendly treatment planning software [122]. The procedure is performed in the extended lithotomy position under general anesthesia and paralysis. TRUS with biplanar array is used to measure prostate volume and shape, both of which are entered into the treatment planning system, as well as to guide transperineal insertion of two or more unipolar electrode needles into the area of interest. By way of an electric potential across the electrodes, the computer-controlled LEDC generator delivers short-duration pulses of high-voltage direct current to the target lesion. The amount of voltage delivered ensures the irreversibility of cellular damage and is determined by the electric field strength and number of pulses. Importantly, electric pulses are synchronized to the patient's cardiac rate to minimize the risk of arrhythmias [123]. In comparison with thermal ablation techniques that often show a transitional zone of partially damaged tissue, IRE lesions show a sharp demarcation between ablated and non-ablated tissue [124].

7.3 Data

Given the novelty of the technology, contemporary data on IRE are limited with small sample sizes and reflect short-term outcomes. Neal and colleagues first reported their experience with IRE for focal ablation of PCa. Specifically, they examined the use of the non-thermal ablative technique on two men with organ-confined PCa planned for prostatectomy 3–4 weeks after the investigational IRE therapy. Each patient had a single tumor focus, Gleason 7 and 6, respectively. Their respective pretreatment PSA levels were 5.4 and 4.3 ng/ml. Both patients were discharged with a transurethral catheter for approximately one week. While both experienced mild hematuria in the immediate post-IRE period, they otherwise recovered without any serious adverse events. Histological examination of the two prostatectomy specimens revealed regions of necrosis surrounding the IRE electrodes with variable degrees of reactive stromal fibrosis and ductal epithelial lining regeneration beyond the margin of necrosis. The ablated regions for patients one and two were determined to be 1.14 and 2.46 cm^3 in total volume, respectively [121].

Valerio et al. reported findings of a prospective study in which 16 men with localized PCa underwent focal IRE. All men had an index lesion visible on MRI confirmed by transperineal targeted and template prostate mapping biopsies and a PSA level less than 15 ng/ml (median PSA 7.75 ng/ml). At 12-month follow-up, there were no serious adverse events recorded. All 16 patients were fully continent and erectile function among the cohort remained stable, based on IIEF scores. Median PSA had decreased to 1.71 ng/ml ($p = 0.001$). Of the 15 men who underwent repeat biopsy at 1 year, there was no evidence of residual disease in 11 patients (61.1%), clinically insignificant PCA in one patient (5.6%), and CS disease in six patients (33.3%) [125].

Ting et al. prospectively evaluated the short-term oncological and functional outcomes of IRE in 25 men with low- to intermediate-risk disease. At 6-month follow-up, median PSA level was 2.2 ng ml, from 6.0 ng/ml preoperatively. Within the treatment zone, there were no suspicious findings on MRI ($n = 24$) or biopsy ($n = 21$). Just outside the ablation area, 5 men (21%) had suspicious MRI findings on mpMRI, of which four (19%) were found to have CS disease on repeat biopsy. There was one patient (5%) with a biopsy-proven focus of significant disease in a region of the prostate distant from the treated lesion. There were no significant changes in urinary, sexual, and bowel function among the patients at 6 months. Most side effects were minor and low grade, including five patients who went into urinary retention and six patients reporting mild, intermittent hematuria in the

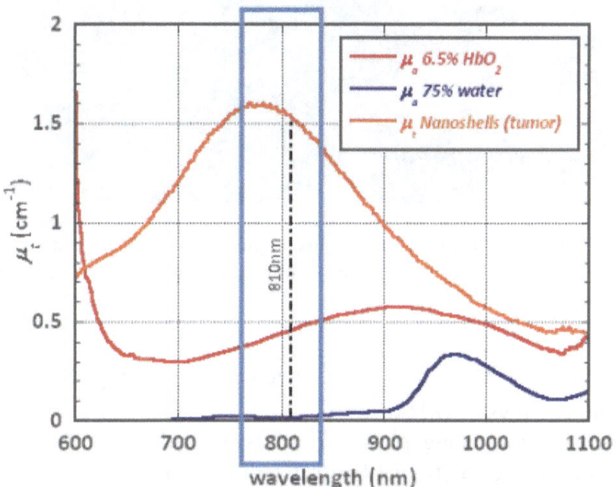

Near-infrared (NIR) peak absorption of GNP with minimal exogenous tissue absorption. Absorption graph (from Nanospectra Biosciences, Inc, Houston, TX)

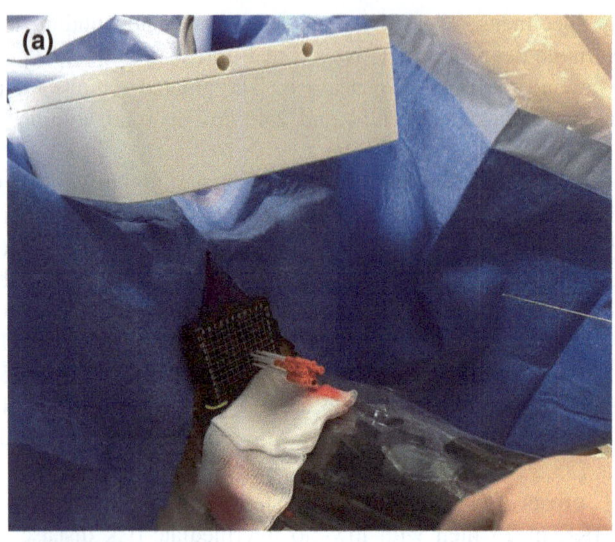

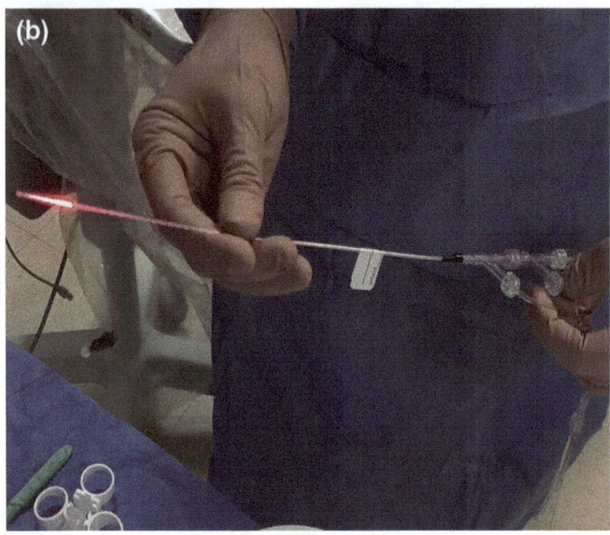

a Trocars placed into the lesion under MR/US fusion guidance. **b** 400 micron optical fiber, which is placed into trocars sequentially for GNP excitation and lesion ablation. Trocar placement and laser fiber (Dr Rastinehad's images)

post-procedure period. There was one Clavien grade 3 complication (non-ST elevation myocardial infarction) [126].

To date, several promising phase I/II trials have demonstrated the short-term oncological efficacy and safety of IRE for FT of PCa [126, 127]. Given the need of larger, randomized controlled trials evaluating the long-term oncological outcomes and morbidity of IRE in PCa, Scheltema and colleagues have designed and initiated

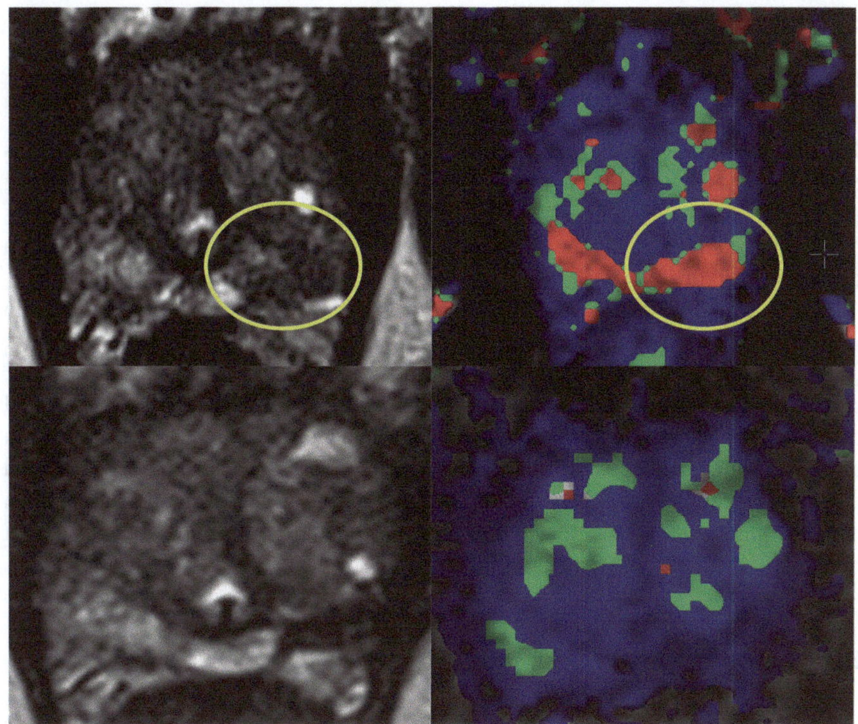

T2-weighted and dynamic contrast-enhanced (DCE) MR color map images from patient with solitary Gleason 3 + 4 lesion (*yellow circle*) in left apex peripheral zone before (*top*) and 3 months after (*bottom*) nanoparticle-directed laser ablation. Imaging (Dr Rastinehad's images)

enrollment for a trial that aims to recruit 200 men with treatment-naïve, unilateral low- to intermediate-risk PCa. Patients will be randomized to receive focal or extended IRE ablation with follow-up to 5 years. Outcomes measures will include urinary and sexual functional, quality of life, and oncological control with the use of standardized questionnaires, mpMRI, CEUS imaging if available, transperineal targeted and mapping biopsies, and serial PSA testing [128].

7.4 Summary

IRE is a promising focal therapy for the treatment of primary localized PCa. While its use remains investigational, it is an attractive FT modality for its non-thermal effect, precise demarcation on follow-up imaging, and tissue selectivity. The procedure can be both challenging and time-consuming to perform, and limited available data presents a gaping need for future investigations.

8 Gold Nanoparticle-Directed Ablation (GNP)

8.1 History

The use of tissue hyperthermia for tumor destruction has existed for some time, as evidenced by the urologic applications of focal laser ablation and HIFU, among others, for the management of localized PCa. Quite recently, gold nanoparticles (GNPs) have emerged as a novel agent with growing potential for targeted ablation of prostate tumors.

Based on their physical and electromagnetic properties, GNPs have been investigated for their use in a number of applications, including enhancement of drug delivery, bioimaging, and thermal ablation of tumors [129–133]. To date, several small trials have investigated the therapeutic safety and utility of nanoshell therapy for ablation of brain and head and neck tumor models [134, 135]. In urology, a number of preclinical studies have demonstrated the relative safety and potential efficacy of the treatment for PCa, including use of subcutaneous human prostate tumors (PC-3) inoculated into mice [136] and in other subcutaneous rodent models [133].

8.2 Technical Aspects

Gold nanoparticles are spherical gold-coated silica particles approximately 150 nm in diameter that maximally absorb near-infrared (NIR) energy, with peak absorption at about 800 nm. The particles are coated in polyethylene glycol to increase circulation time in the blood. Owing to their size and the leaky, fenestrated quality of tumor neovasculature, the particles selectively accumulate within the tumor, but do not extravasate into normal tissue. This phenomenon is explained by the "enhanced permeability and retention" (EPR) effect [137–140]. Based on preclinical studies, all circulating GNPs that have not accumulated within the tumor after 12–24 h are cleared from the blood by the liver and spleen, among other mechanisms of the reticuloendothelial system [133, 141]. Upon illumination with a NIR laser, the nanoparticles are maximally excited and release photothermal energy, which is converted to heat causing coagulative necrosis of the prostate tumor tissue. Importantly, the energy delivered by the laser is insufficient to reach ablative temperatures in normal tissues, which lack therapeutic concentrations of GNPs. Therefore, the extent of tissue ablation is defined by location of concentrated GNPs and not the positioning of the laser.

Preoperative planning and identification of the target lesion(s) is performed with transperineal MR/US fusion imaging. On day 0 of treatment, the patient receives an intravenous infusion of the nanoparticles with the goal of achieving a 15.2 ug/cc therapeutic concentration of GNPs in the tumor. Approximately 12–24 h following infusion, the patient returns for laser catheter insertion and application of laser energy for ablation. Under general anesthesia, the patient is prepped and draped in high lithotomy position in a similar setup to prostate brachytherapy seed implantation. Using MR/US fusion guidance, 14-gauge cannulas are inserted into the target lesion. The placement of these cannulas is based on pre-procedural planning and pattern recognition to ensure that all parts of the tumor are covered by the overlapping radii of ablation produced from each cannula site. The laser that will deliver energy through each cannula has an effective 4 mm radius of ablation. A thermocouple is commonly inserted if the lesion is in close proximity to the urethra or rectum.

The energy for ablation is delivered by a 400-um optical fiber, which is housed within a 16-gauge, liquid cooled catheter. Prior to initiating treatment, laser output power is measured by use of a calibrated integrating sphere optometer (Gigahertiz-Optik, GmbJ, Puccheim, Germany). It is important that the laser wavelength ($\sim$800 nm) falls within 1% of the peak of the broad GNP absorption region [142]. Within this therapeutic window, GNP absorption is maximized and endogenous absorption by oxy- and deoxyhemoglobin in surrounding vascularized tissues is minimized [143, 144]. The laser-containing catheter is sequentially inserted into each cannula to ensure that all areas of the lesion are ablated. Each "burn cycle" consists of continuous laser energy delivery for 3 min. Multiple burn cycles within a single cannula may be needed with pullback of the cannula and laser catheter to ensure that the entirety of the lesion along that path is ablated. In addition to continuous liquid cooling of the laser fiber, continuous bladder irrigation with cool irrigant is performed during the ablation procedure.

8.3 Data

Given the novelty of GNP, there is limited data on their use in humans. Preclinical safety of the particles has been previously established in both in vitro and in vivo animal studies [133, 141, 142, 145].

In 2015, Stern and colleagues reported their findings from an open-label, multicenter, pilot study of GNP therapy in men with resectable PCa for whom radical prostatectomy (RP) was indicated and scheduled. In total, 22 patients were enrolled and received an intravenous infusion of AuroShell (Nanospectra Biosciences, Inc, Houston, TX) particles. Subsequently, 7 men underwent RP the following day and 15 patients underwent laser activation and hemiablation of the prostate, followed by RP 3–7 days later. During laser ablation, anterior rectal wall temperature was monitored with a thermocouple. Follow-up consisted of regular exams, urinalyses, and standard blood and chemistry analyses at 9 time points over the 6 months following infusion and/or laser treatment. The study demonstrated an excellent safety profile for the GNP therapy. There were no recorded temperature rises >37 °C within the rectal wall and no significant, long-term hematologic or metabolic effects of the treatment. Of note, one patient had an allergic pruritus, which responded to intravenous antihistamines, and another patient reported a self-limited sensation of epigastric burning [146].

With clear demonstration of clinical safety in human subjects, there is currently an ongoing phase I, multicenter, open-label trial in the US that aims to determine the efficacy of using MRI/US fusion imaging technology to direct focal ablation of prostate tumors with GNP laser ablation (NCT02680535: “A Study of MRI/US Fusion Imaging and Biopsy in Combination with Nanoparticle-Directed Focal Therapy for Ablation of Prostate Tissue”). Specifically, the study treats men with low- to intermediate-risk localized PCa with a single infusion of GNPs 12–36 h prior to MR/US fusion-guided laser irradiation. All participants must have no more than two clinically significant lesions identifiable on mpMRI, confirmed by fusion-guided targeted biopsy. There must also be no evidence of disease in areas outside of MRI-visible lesions on systematic US-guided biopsy. Preliminary data from the trial was presented at the 2017 American Urological Association Annual Meeting. The investigators reported on the first 4 patients who underwent GNP treatment with 6-month follow-up. All 4 patients demonstrated ablation by coagulative necrosis on mpMRI at 48 h post-treatment, evidenced by the appearance of a “void.” On fusion-guided biopsy at 3 months, one patient had a microfocus of Gleason 3 + 3 disease and the remainder had no residual disease in the targeted area. The mean PSA at time of enrollment was 6.4 ng/ml with a mean reduction of 29.6% at 3 months following therapy. There were no reported serious events [147].

8.4 Summary

Gold nanoparticles are a novel, promising technology currently under investigation for their applications in focal therapy of localized PCa. Unlike other energy-based tissue ablation techniques, GNP does not rely on the components of normal tissue. Therefore, it can be viewed as a potentially “ultra-focal” treatment that more selectively targets the tumor, as opposed to a focal region in which the tumor is located. Further investigation into their safety and efficacy will determine what value, if any, they hold for the future of PCa treatment.

9 Conclusions

Concern for overdetection and subsequent overtreatment of prostate cancer in the PSA-era has bred life to alternative approaches to the management of low- to intermediate-risk, localized disease. Better understanding of the natural history of PCa has contributed to a rise in the number of patients enrolled into AS programs. However, there exist patients with low- to intermediate-risk disease who are confounded by the choice between AS and whole-gland radical treatment. Fueled in part by recent technological advances in mpMRI and targeted biopsy platforms, FT has emerged as a middle ground option with the potential to change how we approach localized PCa.

Concerns regarding FT are not unfounded given the limited, short-term evidence of safety and oncological efficacy. The long natural history of localized PCa warrants longer-term follow-up, and randomized clinical trials are needed to evaluate candidate selection criteria and core outcomes measures for post-treatment monitoring. The prospect of targeted cancer control with minimal collateral morbidity offers a promising outlook for the future of PCa treatment, but only time will tell whether FT is truly effective and practice-changing.

References

1. Potosky AL et al (2004) Five-year outcomes after prostatectomy or radiotherapy for prostate cancer: the prostate cancer outcomes study. J Natl Cancer Inst 96:1358–1367
2. Penson DF, Litwin MS (2003) The physical burden of prostate cancer. Urol Clin North Am 30:305–313
3. Klotz L (2005) Active surveillance for prostate cancer: for whom? J Clin Oncol 23:8165–8169
4. Hardie C et al (2005) Early outcomes of active surveillance for localized prostate cancer. BJU Int 95:956–960
5. Womble PR, Montie JE, Ye Z et al (2015) Michigan Urological Surgery Improvement Collaborative. Contemporary use of initial active surveillance among men in Michigan with low-risk prostate cancer. Eur Urol 67(1):44–50
6. Cooperberg MR, Carroll PR (2015) Trends in management for patients with localized prostate cancer, 1990-2013. JAMA 314(1):80–82
7. Klotz L, Zhang L, Lam A, Nam R, Mamedov A, Loblaw A (2010) Clinical results of long-term follow-up of a large, active surveillance cohort with localized prostate cancer. J Clin Oncol 28:126–131
8. Berglund RK, Masterson TA, Vora KC et al (2008) Pathological upgrading and up staging with immediate repeat biopsy in patients eligible for active surveillance. J Urol 180:1964–1968
9. Marshall S, Taneja S (2015) Focal therapy for prostate cancer: the current status. Prostate Int 3(2):35–41
10. Felker ER, Margolis DJ, Nassiri N, Marks LS (2016) Prostate cancer risk stratification with magnetic resonance imaging. Urol Oncol 34:311–319
11. Siddiqui MM, Rais-Bahrami S, Turkbey B et al (2015) Comparison of MR/ultrasound fusion-guided biopsy with ultrasound-guided biopsy for diagnosis of prostate cancer. JAMA 313:390
12. Rastinehad AR, Turkbey B, Salami SS et al (2014) Improving detection of clinically significant prostate cancer: magnetic resonance imaging/transrectal ultrasound fusion guided prostate biopsy. J Urol 191:1749
13. Wise AM, Stamey TA, McNeal JE, Clayton JL (2002) Morphologic and clinical significance of multifocal prostate cancers in radical prostatectomy specimens. Urology 60(2):264–269
14. Nevoux P, Ouzzane A, Ahmed HU et al (2012) Quantitative tissue analyses of prostate cancer foci in an unselected cystoprostatectomy series. BJU Int 110(4):517–523
15. Liu W, Laitinen S, Khan S et al (2009) Copy number analysis indicates monoclonal origin of lethal metastatic prostate cancer. Nat Med 15(5):559–565
16. Villers A, McNeal JE, Freiha FS, Stamey TA (1992) Multiple cancers in the prostate. Morphologic features of clinically recognized versus incidental tumors. Cancer 70:2313–2318

17. Stamey TA, McNeal JM, Wise AM, Clayton JL. Secondary cancers in the prostate do not determine PSA biochemical failure in untreated men undergoing radical retropubic prostatectomy. Eur Urol 39(Suppl. 4):22–23 (2001). (or Eur Urol 2001;39:Suppl 4:22–23)
18. Ahmed HU (2009) The index lesion and the origin of prostate cancer. N Engl J Med 361 (17):1704–1706
19. Karavitakis M, Winkler M, Abel P et al (2011) Histological characteristics of the index lesion in whole-mount radical prostatectomy specimen: implications for focal therapy. Prostate Cancer Prostatic Dis 14(1):46–52
20. Ahmed HU, Berge V, Bottomley D et al (2014) Can we deliver randomized trials of focal therapy in prostate cancer? Nat Rev Clin Oncol 11(8):482–491
21. Donaldson IA, Alonzi R, Barratt D et al (2015) Focal therapy: patients, interventions, and outcomes—a report from a consensus meeting. Eur Urol 67(4):771–777
22. Cooper SM, Dawber RPR (2001) The history of cryosurgery. J R Soc Med 94(4):196–201
23. Cooper IS (1963) Cryogenic surgery. A new method of destruction or extirpation of benign or malignant tissues. N Engl J Med 263:741–749
24. Bahn DK, Lee F, Badalament R et al (2002) Targeted cryoablation of the prostate: 7-year outcomes in the primary treatment of prostate cancer. Urology 60(suppl 2A):3–11
25. Gonder MJ, Soanes WA, Shulman S (1966) Cryosurgical treatment of the prostate. Invest Urol 3(4):372–378
26. Soanes WA, Gonder MJ (1968) Use of cryosurgery in prostatic cancer. J Urol 99(6):793–797
27. Megalli MR, Gursel EO, Veenema RJ (1974) Closed perineal cryosurgery in prostatic cancer. New Probe Technique. Urol 4(2):220–222
28. Lee F, Bahn DK, Badalament RA et al (1999) Cryosurgery for prostate cancer: improved ablation by use of 6–8 cryoprobes. Urology 54:135
29. Onik GM, Cohen JK, Reyes GD, Rubinsky B, Chang Z, Baust J (1993) Transrectal ultrasound-guided percutaneous radical cryosurgical ablation of the prostate. Cancer 72 (4):1291–1299
30. Ouzzane A, Betrouni N, Valerio M et al (2017) Focal therapy as primary treatment for localized prostate cancer: definition, needs, and future. Future Oncol 13(8):727–741
31. Mohammad A, Miller S, Douglas-Moore J et al (2014) Cryotherapy and its applications in the management of urologic malignancies: a review of its use in prostate and renal cancers. Urol Oncol 32:39
32. Hoffman NE, Bischof JC (2002) The cryobiology of cryosurgical injury. Urol suppl 60:40
33. Sprenkle PC, Mirabile G, Durak E et al (2010) The effect of argon gas pressure on ice ball size and rate of formation. J Endourol 24(9):1503–1507
34. De La Taille A, Benson MC, Bagiella E, Burchardt M, Shabsigh A, Olsson CA et al (2000) Cryoablation for clinically localized prostate cancer using an argon-based system: complication rates and biochemical recurrence. BJU Int 85(3):281–286
35. Lambert EH, Bolte K, Masson P, Katz AE (2007) Focal cryosurgery: encouraging health outcomes for unifocal prostate cancer. Urol 69:1117–1120
36. Truesdale MD, Cheetham PJ, Hruby GW (2010) An evaluation of patient selection criteria on predicting progression-free survival after primary focal unilateral nerve-sparing cryoablation for prostate cancer: recommendations for follow up. Cancer J 16:544–549
37. Ward JF, Jones JS (2012) Focal cryotherapy for localized prostate cancer: a report from the national cryo on-line database (COLD) registry. BJUI 109(11):1648–1654
38. Onik G, Vaughan D, Lotenfoe R et al (2008) The male lumpectomy: focal therapy for prostate cancer using cryoablation results in 48 patients with at least 2-year follow-up. Urol Oncol 26:500–505
39. Cordeiro ER, Cathelineau X, Thuroff S et al (2012) High-intensity focused ultrasound (HIFU) for definitive treatment of prostate cancer. BJUI 110(9):1228–1242
40. Lynn JG, Zwemer RL, Chick AJ, Miller AE (1942) A new method for the generation and use of focused ultrasound in experimental biology. J Gen Physiol 26:179–192

41. Fry WJ, Fry FJ (1960) Fundamental neurological research and human neurosurgery using intense ultrasound. IRE Trans Biomed Electron ME-7:166–181
42. Fry FJ, Johnson LK (1978) Tumour irradiation with intense ultrasound. Ultrasound Med Biol 4:337–341
43. Rosenberg RS, Purnell E (1967) Effects of ultrasonic radiation on the ciliary body. Am J Ophthalmol 63:403–409
44. Coleman DJ, Lizzi FL, Driller J, Rosado AL, Burgess SEP, Torpey JH, Smith ME, Silverman RH, Yablonski ME, Chang S et al (1985) Therapeutic ultrasound in the treatment of glaucoma—II clinical applications. Ophthalmol 92:347–353
45. Madersbacher S, Kratzik C, Susani M, Marberger M (1994) Tissue ablation in benign prostatic hyperplasia with high intensity focused ultrasound. J Urol 152:1956–1960
46. Gelet A, Chapelon JY, Margonari J et al (1993) High-intensity focused ultrasound experimentation on human benign prostatic hypertrophy. Eur Urol 23(Suppl. 1):44–47
47. Hegarty NJ, Fitzpatrick JM (1999) High intensity focused ultrasound in benign prostatic hyperplasia. Eur J Ultrasound 9:55–60
48. Chapelon JY, Margonari J, Vernier F, Gorry F, Ecochard R, Gelet A (1992) *In vivo* effects of high-intensity ultrasound on prostatic adenocarcinoma Dunning R3327. Cancer Res 52:6353–6357
49. Madersbacher S, Pedevilla M, Vingers L, Susani M, Marberger M (1995) Effect of high-intensity focused ultrasound on human prostate cancer in vivo. Cancer Res 55:3346–3351
50. Nelson R FDA approves first HIFU device for prostate tissue ablation. http://www.medscape.com/viewarticle/853120. [Accessed 2 March 2017]
51. Colombel M, Gelet A (2004) Principles and results of high-intensity focused ultrasound for localized prostate cancer. Prostate Cancer Prostatic Dis 7:289–294
52. Cordeiro ER, Cathelineau X, Thüroff S et al (2012) High-intensity focused ultrasound (HIFU) for definitive treatment of prostate cancer. BJU Int 110(9):1228–1242
53. Dickinson L et al (2013) Image-directed, tissue-preserving focal therapy of prostate cancer: a feasibility study of a novel deformable magnetic resonance-ultrasound (MR-US) registration system. BJU Int 112:594–601
54. Mearini L, Porena M (2010) Transrectal high-intensity focused ultrasound for the treatment of prostate cancer: past, present, and future. Indian J Urol 26(1):4–11
55. Muto S, Yoshii T, Saito K et al (2008) Focal therapy with high-intensity-focused ultrasound in the treatment of localized prostate cancer. Jpn J Clin Oncol 38(3):192–199
56. El Feguon AB, Barret E, Prapotnich D et al (2011) Focal therapy with high-intensity focused ultrasound for prostate cancer in the elderly. A feasibility study with 10 year follow-up. Int Braz J Urol 37(2):213–219
57. Ahmed HU, Freeman A, Kirkham A (2011) Focal therapy for localised prostate cancer: a phase I/II trial. J Urol 185:1246–1254
58. Ahmed HU, Dickinson L, Charman S et al (2015) Focal ablation targeted to the index lesion in multifocal localised prostate cancer: a prospective development study. Eur Urol 68:927–936
59. Bown SG (1983) Phototherapy in tumors. World J Surg 7:700–709
60. Vogl TJ, Straub R, Eichler K et al (2004) Colorectal carcinoma metastases in liver: Laser-induced interstitial thermotherapy—local tumor control rate and survival data. Radiology 230:450–458
61. Pacella CM, Francica G, Di Lascio FM et al (2009) Long-term outcome of cirrhotic patients with early hepatocellular carcinoma treated with ultrasound-guided percutaneous laser ablation: a retrospective analysis. J Clin Oncol 27:2615–2621
62. Sander S, Beisland HO (1984) Laser in the treatment of localized prostatic carcinoma. J Urol 132(2):280–281
63. Amin Z, Lees WR, Bown SG (1993) Technical note: interstitial laser photocoagulation for the treatment of prostatic cancer. Br J Radiol 66:1044–1047

64. Johnson DE, Cromeens DM, Price RE (1994) Interstitial laser prostatectomy. Lasers Surg Med 14:299–305
65. Atri M, Gertner MR, Haider MA, Weersink RA, Trachtenberg J (2009) Contrast-enhanced ultrasonography for real-time monitoring of interstitial laser thermal therapy in the focal treatment of prostate cancer. Can Urol Assoc J 3(2):125–130
66. Bomers JGR, Sedelaar JPM, Barentsz JO, Fütterer JJ (2012) MRI-guided interventions for the treatment of prostate cancer. AJR Am J Roentgenol 199(4):714–720
67. Heisterkamp J, van Hillegersberg R, Ijzermans JN (1999) Critical temperature and heating time for coagulation damage: implications for interstitial laser coagulation (ILC) of tumors. Lasers Surg Med 25:257–262
68. Germer CT, Roggan A, Ritz JP et al (1998) Optical properties of native and coagulated human liver tissue and liver metastases in the near infrared range. Lasers Surg Med 23:194–203
69. Lindner U, Lawrentschuk N, Trachtenberg J (2010) Focal laser ablation for localized prostate cancer. J Endourol 24:791–797
70. Colin P, Mordon S, Nevoux P et al (2012) Focal laser ablation of prostate cancer: definition, needs, and future. Adv Urol
71. Raz O, Haider MA, Davidson SRH et al (2010) Real-time magnetic resonance imaging-guided focal laser therapy in patients with low-risk prostate cancer. Eur Urol 58 (1):173–177
72. Marqa M-F, Colin P, Nevoux P et al (2011) Focal laser ablation of prostate cancer: numerical simulation of temperature and damage distribution. Biomed Eng Online 10:45
73. Lee T, Mendhiratta N, Sperling D et al (2014) Focal laser ablation for localized prostate cancer: principles, clinical trials, and our initial experience. Rev Urol 16(2):55–66
74. Stafford RJ, Shetty A, Elliott AM et al (2010) Magnetic resonance guided, focal laser induced interstitial thermal therapy in a canine prostate model. J Urol 184:1514–1520
75. Peters RD, Chan E, Trachtenberg J et al (2000) Magnetic resonance thermometry for predicting thermal damage: an application of interstitial laser coagulation in an in vivo canine prostate model. Magn Reson Med 44(6):873–883
76. Colin P, Nevoux P, Marqa M et al (2012) Focal laser interstitial thermotherapy (LITT) at 980 nm for prostate cancer: treatment feasibility in dunning R3327-AT2 rat prostate tumour. BJU Int 109(3):452–458
77. Lindner U, Weersink RA, Haider MA et al (2009) Image guided photothermal focal therapy for localized prostate cancer: phase I trial. J Urol 182:1371–1377
78. Lindner U, Lawrentschuk N, Weersink RA et al (2010) Focal laser ablation for prostate cancer followed by radical prostatectomy: validation of focal therapy and imaging accuracy. Eur Urol 57:1111–1114
79. Raz O, Haider MA, Davidson ST et al (2010) Real-time magnetic resonance imaging-guided focal laser therapy in patients with low-risk prostate cancer. Eur Urol 58:173–177
80. Oto A, Sethi I, Karczmar G et al (2013) MR imaging-guided focal laser ablation for prostate cancer: phase I trial. Radiology 267(3):932–940
81. Donadon M, Solbiati L, Dawson L et al (2016) Hepatocellular carcinoma: the role of interventional oncology. Liver Cancer 6(1):34–43
82. Song TJ, Seo DW, Lakhtakia S, et al (2016) Initial experience of EUS-guided radiofrequency ablation of unresectable pancreatic cancer. Gastrointest Endosc 83(2):440–443
83. Chen J, Zhang C, Li F et al (2016) A meta-analysis of clinical trials assessing the effect of radiofrequency ablation for breast cancer. Onco Targets Ther 9:1759–1766
84. Haghjoo M, Arya A, Emkanjoo Z et al (2004) Radiofrequency catheter ablation of idiopathic left ventricular tachycardia originating in both left posterior and anterior fascicles. J Interv Card Electrophysiol 11(3):217–220
85. D'Arsonval MA (1891) Action physiologique des courants alternatifs. C R Soc Biol 43:283–286

86. Beer E (1910) Removal of neoplasms of the urinary bladder: a new method employing high frequency (oudin) currents through a cauterizing cystoscope. JAMA 54:1768–1769
87. Cushing H, Bovie WT (1928) Electro-surgery as an aid to the removal of intracranial tumors. Surg Gynecol Obstet 47:751–784
88. McGahan JP, Browing PD, Brock JM, Tesluk H (1990) Hepatic ablation using radiofrequency electrocautery. Invest Radiol 25:267–270
89. Rossi S, Fornari F, Pathies C, Buscarini L (1990) Thermal lesions induced by 480 KHz localized current field in guinea pig and pig liver. Tumori 76:54–57
90. McGahan JP, Brock JM, Tesluk H et al (1992) Hepatic ablation with use of radiofrequency electro-cautery in the animal model. J Vasc Intervent Radiol 3:291–297
91. Schulman CC, Zlotta AR, Rasor J et al (1993) Transurethral needle ablation (TUNA): safety, feasibility, and tolerance of a new office procedure for treatment of benign prostatic hyperplasia. Eur Urol 24:415–423
92. Chen YY, Hossack T, Woo H (2011) Long-term results of bipolar radiofrequency needle ablation of the prostate for lower urinary tract symptoms. J Endourol 25(5):837–840
93. Zlotta AR, Djavan B, Matos C et al (1998) Percutaneous transperineal radiofrequency ablation of prostate tumour: safety, feasibility and pathological effects on human prostate cancer. Br J Urol 81:265–275
94. Corwin TS, Lindberg G, Traxer O et al (2001) Laparoscopic radiofrequency thermal ablation of renal tissue with and without hilar occlusion. J Urol 166(1):281–284
95. Dougherty TJ, Gomer CJ, Henderson BW et al (1998) Photodynamic therapy. J Natl Cancer Inst 90:889
96. Kelly JF, Snell ME (1976) Hematoporphyrin derivative: a possible aid in the diagnosis and therapy of carcinoma of the bladder. J Urol 115:150
97. Windahl T, Andersson SO, Lofgren L (1990) Photodynamic therapy of localized prostatic cancer. Lancet 336:1139
98. Du KL, Mick R, Busch T et al (2006) Preliminary results of interstitial motexafin lutetium-mediated PDT for prostate cancer. Lasers Surg Med 38:427–434
99. Moore CM, Nathan TR, Lees WR et al (2006) Photodynamic therapy using meso tetra hydroxy phenyl chlorin (mTHPC) in early prostate cancer. Lasers Surg Med 38:356–363
100. Nathan TR, Whitelaw DE, Chang SC et al (2002) Photodynamic therapy for prostate cancer recurrence after radiotherapy: a phase I study. J Urol 168:1427–1432
101. Pinthus JH, Bogaards A, Weersink R et al (2006) Photodynamic therapy for urological malignancies: past to current approaches. J Urol 175:1201–1207
102. Oleinick NL, Evans HH (1998) The photobiology of photodynamic therapy: cellular targets and mechanisms. Radiat Res 150:S146
103. Korbelik M, Cecic I (1999) Contribution of myeloid and lymphoid host cells to the curative outcome of mouse sarcoma treatment by photodynamic therapy. Cancer Lett 137:91
104. Hsi RA, Kapatkin A, Strandberg J et al (2001) Photodynamic therapy in the canine prostate using motexafin lutetium. Clin Cancer Res 7:651
105. Lepor H (2008) Vascular targeted photodynamic therapy for localized prostate cancer. Rev Urol 10:254–261
106. Mazor O, Brandis A, Plaks V et al (2005) WST11, a novel water-soluble bacteriochlorophyll derivative; cellular uptake pharmacokinetics, biodistribution, and vascular targeted photodynamic activity using melanoma tumors as a model. Photochem Photobiol 81:342–351
107. Madar-Balakirski N, Tempel-Brami C, Kalchenko V et al (2010) Permanent occlusion of feeding arteries and draining veins in solid mouse tumors by vascular targeted photodynamic therapy (vtp) with tookad. PLoS ONE 5:e10282
108. Chen Q, Huang Z, Luck D et al (2002) Preclinical studies in normal canine prostate of a novel palladium-bacteriopheophorbide (WST09) photosensitizer for photodynamic therapy of prostate cancers. Photochem Photobiol 76(4):438–445
109. Eggener SE, Coleman JA (2008) Focal treatment of prostate cancer with vascular-target photodynamic therapy. Sci World J 8:963–973

110. Azzouzi AR, Barret E, Moore CM et al (2013) TOOKAD Soluble vascular targeted photodynamic (VTP) therapy: Determination of optimal treatment conditions and assessment of effects in patients with localised prostate cancer. BJU Int 112:766–774
111. Moore CM, Azzouzi AR, Barret E et al (2015) Determination of optimal drug dose and light dose index to achieve minimally invasive focal ablation of localised prostate cancer using WST11-vascular-targeted photodynamic (VTP) therapy. BJU Int 116:888–896
112. Azzouzi AR, Vincendeau S, Barret E et al (2017) Padeliporfin vascular-targeted photodynamic therapy versus active surveillance in men with low-risk prostate cancer (CLIN1001 PCM301): an open-label, phase 3, randomised controlled trial. Lancet Oncol 18 (2):181–191
113. Lee EW, Wong D, Prikhodko SV et al (2012) Electron microscopic demonstration and evaluation of irreversible electroporation-induced nanopores on hepatocyte membranes. J Vasc Interv Radiol 23:107–113
114. Miklavcic D, Mali B, Kos B, Heller R, Sersa G (2014) Electrochemotherapy: from the drawing board into medical practice. Biomed Eng Online 13:29
115. Davalos RV, Mir LM, Rubinsky B (2005) Tissue ablation with irreversible electroporation. Ann Biomed Eng 33:223–231
116. Okino M, Mohri H (1987) Effects of a high-voltage electrical impulse and an anticancer drug on in vivo growing tumors. Jpn J Cancer Res 78:1319–1321
117. Mir LM, Orlowski S, Belehradek J Jr, Paoletti C (1991) Electrochemotherapy potentiation of antitumour effect of bleomycin by local electric pulses. Eur J Cancer 27(1):68–72
118. Bertacchini C, Margotti PM, Bergamini E, Lodi A, Ronchetti M, Cadossi R (2007) Design of an irreversible electroporation system for clinical use. Technol Cancer Res Treat 6 (4):313–320
119. Thomson KR, Cheung W, Ellis SJ et al (2011) Investigation of the safety of irreversible electroporation in humans. J Vasc Interv Radiol 22(5):611–621
120. Narayanan G, Hosein PJ, Arora G et al (2012) Percutaneous irreversible electroporation for downstaging and control of unresectable pancreatic adenocarcinoma. J Vasc Intervent Radiol 23:1613–1621
121. Neal RE, Milar JL, Kavnoudias H et al (2014) In vivo characterization and numerical simulation of prostate properties for non-thermal irreversible electroporation ablation. Prostate 74(5):458–468
122. Lee EW, Loh CT, Kee ST (2007) Imaging guided percutaneous irreversible electroporation: ultrasound and immunohistological correlation. Technol Cancer Res Treat 6:287–294
123. Valerio M, Ahmed HU, Emberton M (2015) Focal therapy of prostate cancer using irreversible electroporation. Tech Vasc Interv Radiol 18(3):147–152
124. Edd JF, Horowitz L, Davalos RV, Mir LM, Rubinsky B (2006) In vivo results of a new focal tissue ablation technique: irreversible electroporation. IEEE Trans Biomed Eng 53(7):1409–1415
125. Valerio M, Dickinson L, Ali A et al (2017) Nanoknife electroporation ablation trial: A prospective development study investigating focal irreversible electroporation for localized prostate cancer. J Urol 197(3):647–654
126. Ting F, Tran M, Bohm M et al (2016) Focal irreversible electroporation for prostate cancer: functional outcomes and short-term oncological control. Prostate Cancer Prostatic Dis 19:46–52
127. Valerio M, Stricker PD, Ahmed HU et al (2014) Initial assessment of safety and clinical feasibility of irreversible electroporation in the focal treatment of prostate cancer. Prostate Cancer Prostatic Dis 17:343–347
128. Scheltema MJ, van den Bos W, de Bruin DM, et al Focal versus extended ablation in localized prostate cancer with irreversible electroporation; a multi-center randomized controlled trial. https://www.ncbi.nlm.nih.gov/pubmed/27150293 [Accessed 15 March 2017]

129. Jain S, Hirst DG, O'Sullivan JM (1010) Gold nanoparticles as novel agents for cancer therapy. Br J Radiol 2012(85):101–113
130. Alric C, Taleb J, Duc GL et al (2008) Gadolinium chelate coated gold nanoparticles as contrast agents for both X-ray computed tomography and magnetic resonance imaging. J Am Chem Soc 130(18):5908–5915
131. Brown SD, Nativo P, Smith JA et al (2010) Gold nanoparticles for the improved anticancer drug delivery of the active component of oxaliplatin. J Am Chem Soc 132(13):4678–4684
132. Cheng YC, Samia A, Meyers JD et al (2008) Highly efficient drug delivery with gold nanoparticle vectors for in vivo photodynamic therapy of cancer. J Am Chem Soc 130 (32):10643–10647
133. O'Neal DP, Hirsch LR, Halas NJ et al (2004) Photo-thermal tumor ablation in mice using near infrared-absorbing nanoparticles. Cancer Lett 209(2):171–176
134. Bernardi RJ, Lowery AR, Thompson PA, et al (2008) Immunonanoshells for targeted photothermal ablation in medulloblastoma and glioma: an in vitro evaluation using human cell lines. J Neurooncol 86(2):1 65–172
135. Popovtzer A, Mizrachi A, Motiei M et al (2016) Actively targeted gold nanoparticles as novel radiosensitizer agents: an in vivo head and neck cancer model. Nanoscale 8:2678–2685
136. Stern JM, Stanfield J, Kabbani W et al (2008) Selective prostate cancer thermal ablation with laser activated gold nanoshells. J Urol 179(2):748–753
137. Maeda H, Fang J, Inutsuka T, Kitamoto Y (2003) Vascular permeability enhancement in solid tumor: various factors, mechanisms involved and its implications. Int Immunopharmacol 3(3):319–328
138. Maeda H, Sawa T, Konno T (2001) Mechanism of tumor-targeted delivery of macromolecular drugs, including the EPR effect in solid tumor and clinical overview of the prototype polymeric drug SMANCS. J Control Release 74(1–3):47–61
139. Ishida O, Maruyama K, Sasaki K et al (1999) Size-dependent extravasation and interstitial localization of polyethyleneglycol liposomes in solid tumor-bearing mice. Int J Pharm 190 (1):49–56
140. Maeda H (2001) The enhanced permeability and retention (EPR) effect in tumor vasculature: the key role of tumor-selective macromolecular drug targeting. Adv Enzyme Regul 41:189–207
141. James WD, Hirsch LR, West JL et al (2007) Application of INAA to the build-up and clearance of gold nanoshells in clinical studies in mice. J Radioanal Nuclear Chem 271 (2):455–459
142. Schwartz JA, Price RE, Gill-Sharp KL et al (2011) Selective nanoparticle-directed ablation of the canine prostate. Lasers Surg Med 43:213–220
143. Oldenburg SJ, Averitt RD (1998) Westcott SL, etc. Nanoengineering of optical resonances. Chem Phys Lett 288:243–247
144. Oldenburg SJ, Jackson JB, Westcott SL et al (1999) Infrared extinction properties of gold nanoshells. Appl Phys Lett 75(19):2897–2899
145. Gad SC, Sharp KL, Montgomery C et al (2012) Evaluation of the toxicity of intravenous delivery of auroshell particles (gold-silica nanoshells). Int J Toxicol 31(6):584–594
146. Stern JM, Solomonov V, Sazykina E et al (2016) Initial evaluation of the safety of nanoshell-directed photothermal therapy in the treatment of prostate disease. Int J Toxicol 35 (1):38–46
147. Winoker JS, Shukla PA, Carrick MA, et al (2017) Gold nano-particle directed focal laser ablation for prostate tumors using US and MR fusion technology. Poster session presented at: American Urological Association Annual Meeting, Boston, MA, pp 12–16

Prostate Cancer Markers

Adam J. Gadzinski and Matthew R. Cooperberg

Contents

Abstract

Diagnostic biomarkers derived from blood, urine, or prostate tissue provide additional information beyond clinical calculators to determine the risk of

A. J. Gadzinski · M. R. Cooperberg (✉)
Department of Urology, University of California—San Francisco, San Francisco, CA, USA
e-mail: Matthew.Cooperberg@ucsf.edu

S. Daneshmand and K. G. Chan (eds.), *Genitourinary Cancers*, Cancer Treatment and Research 175, https://doi.org/10.1007/978-3-319-93339-9_3

detecting high-grade prostate cancer. Once diagnosed, multiple markers leverage prostate cancer biopsy tissue to prognosticate clinical outcomes, including adverse pathology at radical prostatectomy, disease recurrence, and prostate cancer mortality; however the clinical utility of some outcomes to patient decision making is unclear. Markers using tissue from radical prostatectomy specimens provide additional information about the risk of biochemical recurrence, development of metastatic disease, and subsequent mortality beyond existing multivariable clinical calculators (the use of a marker to simply sub-stratify risk groups such as the NCCN groups is of minimal value). No biomarkers currently available for prostate cancer have been prospectively validated to be predict an improved clinical outcome for a specific therapy based on the test result; however, further research and development of these tests may produce a truly predictive biomarker for prostate cancer treatment.

Keywords
4Kscore · Analytic validity · Biomarkers · CLIA-LDT · Clinical validity
Decipher · MolDX · Phi · Predictive biomarker · Prolaris · ProMark
Prostate-specific antigen · Risk calculators · Serum markers · Urinary markers

1 Introduction

1.1 Biomarkers

The past decade has seen a rapid discovery and development of numerous biomarkers for prostate cancer (PCa). These markers have implications for nearly all phases of care from disease detection through both initial and subsequent treatments. The type of markers reported for PCa spans the spectrum from DNA alterations and epigenetic changes (e.g., methylation of DNA regulating gene expression) to changes in gene mRNA expression and either single or multiplexed protein markers. The patient biomaterial source of these markers includes urine, blood, and prostate tissue. In many respects, moreover, emerging imaging tests, particularly those based on specific genetic or metabolic changes, function very much as biomarkers and need to meet the same standards for validity and clinical utility.

1.2 Diagnostic, Prognostic, and Predictive Biomarkers

Diagnostic biomarkers are those used in determining the probability of the disease being present. Some diagnostic markers in PCa also offer additional insight into the probability of the patient having high-grade (HG) disease or clinically significant disease (frequently defined as any Gleason pattern 4 or 5 disease). Indeed, to the extent that cancers with Gleason pattern ≤ 3 (grade group 1) [1] are increasingly recognized to have minimal metastatic potential [2] and are most often over diagnosed, most contemporary markers are developed and validated specifically with the goal of identifying HG disease (grade group ≥ 2). *Prognostic* biomarkers are associated with a clinical time-to-event outcome such as cancer-specific survival (CSS) or recurrence-free survival (RFS) [3]. In the clinical context, these markers are helpful in providing guidance on how aggressive a patient's disease is and whether they should pursue treatment. *Predictive* biomarkers provide information on the potential to benefit from a specific treatment, e.g., whether patients with a specific mutation may benefit from a new treatment modality [3]. Prognostic markers therefore correlate tumor and/or patient characteristics to outcome, whereas predictive markers correlate the effects of treatment on outcome. A common pitfall in terminology occurs from predictive statistical models in which an independent variable (e.g., the biomarker) is found to be statistically associated with the measured outcome (e.g., CSS). These statistically significant biomarkers are frequently referred to as "predictive"; however, this does not make it a true *predictive biomarker*, because proving that a cancer has more aggressive biology does not necessarily mean it is more or less suitable for a given management approach [4].

An example of a predictive biomarker is human epidermal growth factor 2 (HER2) overexpression in women with breast cancer [5]. Women with HER2 overexpression benefit from the use of the targeted therapy trastuzumab (Herceptin®), while those without HER2 overexpression gain no benefit from the therapy [6]. An analogous biomarker as clearly predictive for prostate cancer has yet to be discovered and prospectively validated. The currently available biomarkers for PCa are therefore diagnostic or prognostic, though some are moving closer to meeting the predictive standard.

1.3 Regulation and Oversight

Few of the biomarkers available for prostate cancer have undergone the approval process to evaluate clinical validity through the US Food and Drug Administration (FDA). Most biomarkers are provided by commercial laboratories that are regulated and approved under Clinical Laboratory Improvement Amendments (CLIA) under the auspices of the Centers for Medicare and Medicaid Services (CMS). These non-FDA-approved PCa biomarkers are deemed Laboratory Developed Tests (LDTs), under which designation CLIA prohibits the release the results of laboratories tests until the specific laboratory has demonstrated *analytic* validity of the test (i.e., the results are accurate and reliable only in terms of measuring the analytes claimed to be measured) [7]. CLIA does not address nor regulate the *clinical* validity of any LDT [7]. Thus, CLIA-LDTs have accurate and repeatable results, but there is no government regulatory oversight over the clinical relevance and use of the test. The FDA has recently considered more involvement in oversight of LDTs by evaluating their clinical validity, specifically citing commercially available prostate cancer markers as an area of concern [8], but ultimately no decision was made to begin FDA oversight of these tests [9].

The FDA has, however, already made decisions regarding some of the earlier blood and urine-based markers. Payment for these tests is not associated with FDA decisions; instead, the Molecular Diagnostic Services Program (MolDX®) makes recommendations to state-specific Medicare Administrative Contractors about which tests should be covered for reimbursement under the Medicare program [10]. MolDX is part of a private corporation, though it uses an evaluation process derived from both the FDA and the Centers for Disease Control and Prevention to assess and advise payment for tests based on analytical validity, clinical validity, and clinical utility [11]. Independent of payment decisions, patients and clinicians must utilize the published scientific literature to determine the clinical usefulness of non-FDA-approved prostate cancer biomarkers available as CLIA-LDTs in the USA.

1.4 Assessing Clinical Utility

The means to evaluate the usefulness of a particular biomarker depends on the specific markers intended contribution to clinical care. In the case of delineating a specific clinical outcome or endpoint, such as prostate cancer detected on biopsy, standard statistical properties such as sensitivity, specificity, positive predictive value (PPV), and negative predictive value (NPV) are utilized. A frequently utilized metric to assess the level of association with an outcome is the area under the receiver operator characteristic curve (AUC) [12]. The AUC ranges from 0.5 to 1.0; a result of 0.5 means the test is no better than a coin flip at delineating the outcome of interest, whereas a test with an AUC of 1.0 has perfect association with the outcome of interest (e.g., the test is always positive when prostate cancer is present on biopsy, and always negative in a benign biopsy). There is no standardization for what defines an "excellent" AUC, but in general it is helpful in comparing models, with the higher AUC suggesting better overall accuracy.

The actual clinical utility of a new biomarker, however, is not completely dependent on its accuracy and favorable performance statistics in validation studies—there are other factors involved [13, 14]. First, there should be a magnitude of improvement relative to current multivariable clinical predictors such as the Prostate Cancer Prevention Trial risk calculator (PCPTRC) [15], Cancer of the Prostate Risk Assessment (CAPRA) score [16, 17], or post-radical prostatectomy (RP) nomograms [18, 19]. Simply sub-stratifying standard risk groups (e.g., American Urological Association (AUA) [20] or National Comprehensive Cancer Network (NCCN) [21]) is *not* sufficient as this can already be done with clinical tools and no additional effort or expense. Second, the biomarker should improve outcomes in real-world situations across a broad range of probabilities (i.e., a test with a very restricted range of accuracy is unlikely to provide much clinical benefit) [13]. Third, there should be clinical treatments or interventions that are facilitated by biomarkers results (e.g., undergo a prostate biopsy, elect to undergo active surveillance, or chose to pursue adjuvant radiation). Lastly, economic impacts of a biomarker must not be ignored—if the economic burden of a test is excessive, then its clinical utility may be limited.

One statistical method developed to help estimate if a new test conveys meaningful clinical utility is the decision curve analysis (DCA) [22]. These analyses provide a graphical assessment of a test's net benefit (*y*-axis) in making a clinical decision across a range of threshold probabilities for intervention (*x*-axis) [22–24]. DCA allows for evaluation of a new biomarker and relative comparison to other decision tools in a multitude of clinical scenarios to see if the marker has an impact. Of note, in situations where a clinical decision will almost assuredly be made regardless of the markers value, the decision curve typically demonstrates that there is minimal clinical benefit to the marker. Thus, DCA provides a critical statistical method of assessing the clinical utility of biomarkers as they emerge.

1.5 Clinical Situations

The biomarkers discussed here will be separated by their clinical uses: (1) detection of prostate cancer, (2) initial treatment decision, and (3) post-radical prostatectomy prognosis. Table 1 outlines these markers, their source biomaterial, clinical use, if they have been implemented in any clinical guidelines, and government oversight in the USA.

2 Detection of Prostate Cancer

Since the advent of prostate-specific antigen (PSA) screening, a large majority of men diagnosed with prostate cancer present with localized disease [25]. The markers discussed aim to provide additional information beyond PSA and clinical factors that allow patients and clinicians to estimate the probability of finding cancer on biopsy. Some biomarkers provide additional estimates of finding clinical significant or HG cancer in an attempt to decrease detection of clinically indolent disease unlikely to impact the patient's health. Some markers have also been evaluated for clinical utility for active surveillance patient selection.

2.1 Serum Markers

Prostate Health Index (phi) (Beckman Coulter, Indianapolis, Indiana)

An FDA-approved serum test combines total PSA (tPSA), free PSA (fPSA), and the [-2]proPSA isoform to calculate a score that provides men with a risk of having PCa and HG PCa (Gleason score ≥ 7) [26]. The FDA approval covers men aged >50

Table 1 Prostate cancer biomarkers

Biomarker	Source biomaterial	Clinical requirements	Marker measurement	Biomarker class	Reported outcome	Guidelines	FDA approved	CLIA-LDT
Pre-diagnosis								
phi	Blood	Age > 50, PSA 4–10, negative DRE	Protein (PSA, fPSA, p2PSA)	Diagnostic	Any and high-grade cancer	EUA, NCCN	Yes	N/A
4Kscore	Blood	Age 40–80, no DRE within 96 h, no 5-alpha-reductase inhibitors in prior 6 months, no prostate procedure in past 6 months	Protein (PSA, fPSA, iPSA, hK2)	Diagnostic	High-grade cancer	EUA, NCCN	No	Yes
PCA3	Post-DRE urine	Prior negative biopsy, no ASAP	mRNA (PCA3/PSA ratio)	Diagnostic	Any and high-grade cancer	EUA, NCCN	Yes	N/A
MiPS	Blood and urine	None	Protein (PSA serum), mRNA (PCA3, TMPRSS2:ERG urine)	Diagnostic	Any and high-grade cancer		No	Yes
SelectMDx	Post-DRE urine	None	mRNA(HOXC6, DLX1, KLK3)	Diagnostic	Any and high-grade cancer		No	Yes
ExoDx prostate IntelliScore	Urine (No DRE)	Age > 50, PSA 2–10, no prior biopsy	Exosomal RNA (ERG, PCA3, SPDEF)	Diagnostic	High-grade cancer		No	Yes
ConfirmMDx	Negative biopsy tissue	Prior negative biopsy, no ASAP	DNA methylation (GSTP1, APC, RASSF1, ACTB)	Diagnostic	Any cancer	NCCN	No	Yes
Post-diagnosis								
Oncotype Dx GPS	Positive biopsy tissue	Gleason 3+3 or 3+4, NCCN very low to intermediate risk	RNA (17 gene expression: AZGP1, FAM13C, KLK2, SRD5A2, FLNC, GSN,	Prognostic	Risk stratification, adverse pathology at RP (Gleason > 4+3	NCCN	No	Yes

(continued)

Table 1 (continued)

Biomarker	Source biomaterial	Clinical requirements	Marker measurement	Biomarker class	Reported outcome	Guidelines	FDA approved	CLIA-LDT
			GSTM2, TPM2, BGN, COL1A1, SFRP4, TPX2, ARF1, ATP5E, CLTC, GPS1, PGK1)		or $\geq$ pT3a), 10-year metastasis after RP, 10-year CSS after RP			
ProMark	Positive biopsy tissue	Gleason 3+3 or 3+4	Protein (DERL1, CUL2, SMAD4, PDSS2, HSPA9, FUS, pS6, YBOX1)	Prognostic	Risk of unfavorable pathology at RP (Gleason > 3+4 or $\geq$ pT3a), pN1, pM1	NCCN	No	Yes
Prolaris	Positive biopsy tissue or RP	None	RNA (46 gene expression: 31 cell cycle progression genes, 15 housekeeping genes)	Prognostic	Risk stratification, 10-year CSS with conservative management, 10-year metastatic risk with definitive treatment	NCCN	No	Yes
Decipher	Positive biopsy tissue or RP	None	RNA (22 gene expression: NFIB, NUSAP1, ZWILCH, ANO7, PCAT-32, UBE2C, CAMK2N1, MYBPC1, PBX1, THBS2, EPPK1, IQGAP3, LASP1, PCDH7, RABGAP1, GLYATL1P4, S1PR4, TNFRSF19, TSBP, 3 RNA markers not associated with genes)	Prognostic	Risk stratification, high-grade disease at RP (primary Gleason 4 or 5), 5-year metastasis after RP, 10-year CSS after RP	NCCN	No	Yes

Table modified in part from Hendriks et al. [23]

ASAP Atypical small acinar proliferation, *AUA* American Urological Association, *CLIA-LDT* Clinical Laboratory Improvement Amendments-Laboratory Developed Test, *CSS* Cancer-specific survival, DRE: Digital rectal Examination, *EUA* European Urological Association, *FDA* Federal Food and Drug Administration, *NCCN* National Comprehensive Cancer Network, *RP* Radical prostatectomy years, no known diagnosis of PCa, a total serum PSA 4–10 ng/mL, and benign digital rectal examination (DRE) [27]. The formula was refined in a retrospective study of stored serum samples from European Study of Screening for Prostate Cancer and PCa screening trial at the University of Innsbruck [28]. The test and formula have been validated in multicenter prospective trials from Europe and North America [26, 27, 29, 30]. Catalona et al. in a study of 892 men undergoing biopsy with PSA 2.0–10.0 ng/mL found that the AUC of phi was 0.703 for any PCa and 0.724 for detecting $\geq$ Gleason 4+3 PCa, both of which were superior to fPSA ratio [26]. A subsequent analysis of this cohort limiting the pre-biopsy PSA to 4.0–10.0 ng/mL (the FDA-approved range) found that the AUC of phi alone improved to 0.708 for any cancer and 0.707 for Gleason $\geq$ 3+4. [27] These authors also reported that a cutoff phi value of 28.6 would have spared approximately 30% of men in the cohort from an unnecessary biopsy (i.e., a biopsy that was benign or found clinically insignificant disease), compared to only 22% using %fPSA. Thus, phi provides additional information beyond fPSA and PSA.

More recent studies have compared the additional information provided by phi to the previously established clinical risk calculators from PCPT and European Randomized study of Screening for Prostate Cancer (ERSPC) risk calculator [31–33]. Loeb et al. [31] found that the AUC for high-grade prostate cancer significantly improved with the addition of phi to both PCPT and ERSPC risk calculators; they also proposed a new nomogram to specifically predict aggressive disease using clinical data and phi. On DCA, the new nomogram revealed net benefit relative to an all-or-none biopsy protocol, but it was not directly compared to the other studied risk calculators. Foley et al. did show that addition of phi to the ERSPC risk calculator did provide a net benefit on DCA compared to the risk calculator alone [33]. Overall, the data to date suggest that phi provides clinical utility over standard risk calculators for men contemplating biopsy for an elevated PSA.

Of note, phi has also been investigated in both active surveillance settings and in predicting adverse pathology (Gleason score $\geq$ 7 or $\geq$ pT3a) at RP. Regarding active surveillance, retrospective studies have reported that increased baseline phi was associated with biopsy reclassification on subsequent surveillance biopsies; however, no prospective studies have assessed or validated such findings [34, 35]. Studies assessing phi in predicting adverse surgical pathology at the time of RP in general did not provide strong support for its use [36, 37]. Guiazzoni et al. [36] showed net benefit on DCA of adding phi to the clinical variables of age, Gleason score, PSA, free PSA, and clinical stage. However, in a multicenter study, Fossati et al. [37] showed that with the addition of percent of positive biopsy cores to the collection of clinical variables, the net benefit of phi on DCA was no longer present for predicting adverse pathology. Thus, phi has clinical utility for men contemplating biopsy, but provides minimal clinical value once the diagnosis is made.

4Kscore® (OPKO, Elmwood Park, New Jersey)

The 4-kallikrein (4K) panel comprises of four serum markers: tPSA, fPSA, intact PSA (iPSA), and human kallikrein 2 (HK2). Like phi, it is intended to be used in men with elevated PSA contemplating biopsy. Vickers et al. in 2008 utilized the Göteborg screening trial cohort to assess the 4K panel in the frozen serum of 740 men who previously underwent biopsy for PSA $\geq$ 3.0 ng/mL [38]. The levels of the 4K panel were then added to both a predictive laboratory model (patient age and PSA) and a clinical model (age, PSA, and DRE findings). The addition of the 4K laboratory values significantly increased the AUC of each model to 0.84 (95% CI: 0.81–0.88) for any PCa and 0.90 (95% CI: 0.86–0.96) for high-grade PCa (Gleason score $\geq$ 7). DCA showed a notable net benefit with the addition of 4K panel results. This model was then modified, independently validated, and shown to provide net benefit in subsequent retrospective studies of men from ERSPC who had (1) initially screened positive [39, 40], (2) had subsequent elevated PSA after initial screening PSA < 3.0 ng/ml [41], and (3) those with prior negative biopsy [42]. A modification of the model was also developed using data retrospective data from 6129 men who underwent biopsy in the Prostate Testing for Cancer and Treatment (ProtecT) study in the UK, again showing accurate prediction and clinical benefit on DCA [43].

These 4K panel models combined with patient age, DRE, and prior biopsy facilitated development of the 4Kscore which provides a patient with their percent probability of having high-grade cancer on biopsy. The 4Kscore was then prospectively validated in a multi-institutional cohort of 1012 men undergoing biopsy in the USA and found to demonstrate high discrimination with a AUC of 0.82 (95% CI: 0.79–0.85) for high-grade cancer at biopsy [44]. Based on the results, had men with a 4Kscore < 6% not undergone biopsy, then 30% of all biopsies could have been avoided with only missing 13 high-grade cases (5.6% of HG Ca, 1.3% of studied men). The authors also performed a DCA comparing 4Kscore to the PCPTRC and found a notable net benefit to 4Kscore relative to the PCPTRC, clearly demonstrating its clinical utility.

Thus, the 4Kscore and phi in separate studies both demonstrated clinical utility beyond standard clinical factors in predicting which men are more likely to have high-grade PCa. In the one head-to-head study reported, Nordström et al. compared phi to 4Kscore in the same cohort of 531 men undergoing first-time biopsy for a PSA 3–15 ng/mL in Sweden from 2010 to 2012 [45]. The main limitations of the study included (1) DRE information was not available (phi is intended for men with benign DRE), (2) the PSA range extended beyond phi's approved range of 4–10 ng/mL, and (3) the base clinical model for comparison only contained age and PSA. These limitations seemed to put phi at a slight disadvantage a priori, as this population extended beyond the scope of its intended use. However, this cohort does likely represent a more "real-world" population of patients presenting to an urologist. The authors found that phi and 4K panel had AUCs of 0.71 (95% CI: 0.66–0.76) and 0.72 (95% CI: 0.67–0.78), respectively. In DCA, both appeared to provide a slight net benefit relative to the clinical model for detecting high-grade PCa. Lastly, using a cutoff of 39 for phi and 10% for 4K, both tests would have spared 30% of biopsies, while missing 9.8–10.5% of high-grade cancers (2.6–2.8% of studied men). Despite the limitations of the study, both phi and 4K performed similarly and either could be used in men with elevated PSA who are contemplating biopsy.

The 4K panel has also been studied in the areas of predicting surgical pathology at RP and active surveillance. Carlsson et al. assessed whether the 4K panel provided clinical benefit for predicting aggressive PCa on surgical pathology at RP (Gleason score $\geq$ 7, tumor volume $\geq$ 0.5 cm^3, or $\geq$ pT3a). The authors retrospectively examined the preoperative blood levels of the 4K panel in 392 men of the ERSPC screening arm who were treated with RP between 1994 and 2004 [46]. They found that the 4K panel did provide clinical benefit above a clinical model to predict aggressive disease. This study contrasts with the multicenter prospective study for phi by Fossati et al. which found no significant clinical benefit to phi. To emphasize some key study differences, Fossati et al. were a contemporary cohort with all RPs performed between 2011 and 2012 and the classification of adverse pathology was limited to either Gleason score $\geq$ 7 or $\geq$ pT3a; tumor volume was not included [37]. While both studies had approximately 2/3 of the patients classified as "pathologically aggressive" disease following prostatectomy, in the study using phi 69% of patients had Gleason $\geq$ 7 versus only 36% in the 4K study. Thus, given these differences in patient cohort and outcome assessment, one definitely cannot conclude that the 4K panel has clinical utility for predicting adverse pathology and phi does not. A trial prospectively assessing both markers on a contemporary cohort measuring the same outcome would be best situated to critically assess their relative clinical utility in this situation.

Finally, in the active surveillance setting, Lin et al. evaluated the 4K panel's discriminatory capacity for biopsy reclassification from Gleason 6 on diagnosis to Gleason $\geq$ 7 at surveillance biopsy [47]. Among 718 men placed on active surveillance in the Canary Prostate Active Surveillance Study, they found that while the 4K panel helped discriminate high-grade cancer on the initial biopsy, 4K offered no benefit over clinical and pathological factors in predicting subsequent surveillance biopsy reclassification. Thus, very similar to phi, the 4K panel offers limited clinical benefit once the diagnosis of prostate cancer is made.

2.2 Urinary Markers

Prostate Cancer Antigen 3 (PCA3) (Progensa® Hologic, Inc., Marlborough, Massachusetts)

The PCA3 gene is significantly overexpressed by prostate cancer cells [48]; an FDA-approved assay measures voided mRNA copies of PCA3 following a DRE and reports a ratio of PCA3:PSA mRNA in the urine [49]. Based on studies validating predictive accuracy [50–52], it was approved by the FDA for men with a prior negative biopsy and no evidence of atypical small acinar proliferation (ASAP) to help clinicians and patients decide whether to forego a repeat biopsy based on a threshold result of 25 [53]. In a recent prospective study, Wei et al. [54] examined the use of PCA3 in men undergoing either initial ($N = 562$) or repeat ($N = 297$) biopsy. They found that adding PCA3 to the PCPTRC improved the prediction model beyond the PCPTRC alone for both any and HG cancer in the initial and repeat biopsy settings. The study showed that a PCA3 threshold of 20 would result in avoiding 41% of initial biopsies while missing 31 high-grade cancers (20.1% of HG PCa, 5.5% of studied men). In the repeat biopsy setting, 46% of biopsies would be avoided with four high-grade cancers missed (15.4% of HG PCa, 1.3% of studied men). Similar initial biopsy performance was reported by Crawford et al., who evaluated 1962 biopsy naïve men with PSA > 2.5 ng/mL, and found that a PCA3 cutoff of 10 would prevent 20% of biopsies while missing 53 high-grade cancers (the exact percent of all HG Ca not discussed, but this comprised 2.7% of studied men) [53]. On the other hand, Gittelman et al. studied 466 men undergoing repeat biopsy and reported that a PCA3 cutoff of 25 would have prevented 48% of biopsies and missed 8 high-grade cancers (30.7% of HG PCa, 1.7% of studied men) [55]. Thus, PCA3 appears less effective in biopsy naïve men at a single threshold level. These studies, and in particular Wei et al. [54], highlight the fact that PCA3, like most other prostate cancer tests, does not function well as a binary test, for the simple reason that PCa presents a continuum of risk—men cannot be dichotomized as "low" and "high" risk either before or after diagnosis. Just as 4.0 ng/mL was never a good "one size fits all" threshold for PSA, PCA3 does not work well with a single threshold. The concept of a high NPV *below* a given threshold and a high PPV *above* a second threshold, with a gray zone in between, are much more reflective of the reality of prostate cancer biology.

PCA3 was also compared to newer biomarkers to evaluate its continued role on PCa care. Scattoni et al. compared PCA3 to phi prospectively in men undergoing initial ($N = 116$) or repeat ($N = 95$) biopsy [56]. Relative to their clinical model (PSA, fPSA:PSA ratio, and prostate volume), the addition of phi increased the predictive accuracy for any cancer in both the initial and repeat biopsy cohort, though the difference was not statistically significant. The addition of PCA3 to both the clinical model alone and the clinical model with phi did not improve accuracy. A DCA showed a slight net benefit when phi was added to the clinical model for the initial and repeat biopsy group. However, it is important to note that this study's outcome was *any* prostate cancer; the authors did not perform a separate analysis for HG cancers. Furthermore, the samples sizes for each cohort were modest, and the clinical model did not include age, DRE findings, or family history (factors present in the PCPTRC). In a similar study, Perdona et al. measured PCA3 and phi prior to the first biopsy in 160 men with benign DRE and PSA 2-20 ng/mL; both biomarkers were added to the clinical model (age, PSA density, and fPSA:PSA ratio) to assess improved accuracy in detecting any cancer [57]. In their final predictive model and DCA, the addition of both PCA3 and phi to the clinical model produced the greatest net benefit to patients; however, the authors concluded the addition of PCA3 was modest and did not warrant widespread use in screening men for biopsy. A similar conclusion was reached by Seisen et al. who found that phi had greater accuracy for predicting clinically significant PCa (Gleason $\geq$ 7, positive biopsy cores >3, or >50% cancer involvement in any core) at biopsy compared to PCA3 in 138 biopsy naïve men with elevated PSA or positive DRE [58].

Of note, the authors did not construct a base clinical model for comparison; thus, the clinical implications are limited.

PCA3 as a standalone marker has usefulness in the population; it was initially intended for men with a negative biopsy who are contemplating a repeat biopsy. At this decision point, a very low PCA3 score would allow a portion of these men to forego biopsy with a low chance of missing a high-grade cancer.

Transmembrane Protease Serine 2:ERG Fusion (TMPRSS2:ERG)

The gene fusion of TMPRSS2:ERG occurs frequently in PCa carcinogenesis [59]. TMPRSS2 expression is regulated by androgens, and the gene fusion creates androgen-driven overexpression of the ERG oncogene [60]. Transcripts from this fusion are quantifiable measured in urine following DRE, and this result has been combined with PCA3 to predict PCa and HG PCa at the time of initial biopsy [61, 62]. In 443 men undergoing biopsy for PSA $\geq$ 3 ng/mL, Leyten et al. found that adding TMPRSS2:ERG and PCA3 to the ERSPC risk calculator increased the predictive accuracy for any cancer [62]. They also demonstrated that the combination cutoffs of PCA3 <25 and TMPRSS2:ERG <10 would have avoided 35% of biopsies while missing 11 cases of high-grade cancer (9.6% of HG PCa, 2.4% of studied men). Tomlins et al. confirmed this finding and validated a predictive model combining TMPRSS2:ERG, PCA3, and the PCPTRC in 1244 men presenting for biopsy [61]. Their predictive model, the Michigan Prostate Score (MiPS, University of Michigan Labs, Ann Arbor, Michigan), showed superior predictive accuracy compared to the PCPTRC for any and high-grade PCa (AUC for high-grade PCa 0.779 versus 0.707, $p < 0.001$). On DCA, there was a clear net benefit of MiPS relative PCPTRC for detection of any and HG PCa. A MiPS threshold of <15% would have avoided 36% of biopsies while missing 19 high-grade cancers (8.5% of HG PCa, 1.6% of studied men). These studies demonstrate the additional value of TMPRSS2:ERG and that when it is combined with PCA3 there is a notable clinical utility in reducing biopsies without missing a large number of HG PCa cases.

The clinical utility of MiPS appears similar to that of phi and the 4Kscore; however, a head-to-head comparison of MiPS to these serum markers does not exist. Stephan et al. did perform a study that assessed the predictive accuracy for any prostate cancer of TMPRSS2:ERG, PCA3, and phi in 246 men undergoing biopsy for PSA 0.5–20 ng/mL or suspicious clinical findings; of note, 45% of men had a prior biopsy [63]. They reported that TMPRSS2:ERG only added additional predictive value relative to phi and PCA3 in the repeat biopsy cohort. In DCA, they found that the addition of PCA3 and phi to their clinical model (age, PSA, fPSA/PSA ratio, prostate volume, and DRE) provided net benefit over the clinical model. While this study assessed all three biomarkers, it did not assess the predictive accuracy for HG cancers nor compare their model to an established clinical predictive model (e.g., PCPT or ESPRC); thus, the implications are limited. Overall, the available data demonstrate that a large number of men can avoid a biopsy when TMPRSS2:ERG is used in combination with PCA3 without missing many HG cancers.

Lin et al. also used the Canary Prostate Active Surveillance Study cohort to investigate PCA3 and TMPRSS2:ERG utility in active surveillance [64]. The authors assessed the accuracy of PCA3 and TMPRSS2:ERG to predict HG disease on subsequent surveillance biopsy. While there were increasing urine levels of both PCA3 and TMPRSS2:ERG in men with HG disease, the predictive model for HG disease showed no significant difference between a model with PSA (AUC 0.68) and combining PSA, PCA3, and TMPRSS2:ERG (AUC 0.70, $p = 0.08$). Thus, like 4K and phi, there is minimal clinical value of these urinary markers once a diagnosis of prostate cancer has been made.

ExoDx™ Prostate IntelliScore (Exosome Diagnostics, Inc., Waltham, Massachusetts)

A novel test that measures the exosomal RNA of ERG and PCA3 normalized to SPDEF in voided urine *without* a prior DRE [65, 66]. Exosomes are small nanovesicles secreted by both normal and cancerous cells into both blood and urine [49, 65]. In 195 men with PSA 2–10 ng/mL and no prior biopsy, Donovan et al. retrospectively developed a model including the urinary exosomal levels of ERG and PCA3 that provided additional predictive accuracy above a clinical model (PSA, age, race, and family history) to predict HG PCa (AUC 0.80, 95% CI: 0.73–88) [65]. With a binary cutoff of 10 on their Exo106 model, the authors reported that 39% of biopsies would have been avoided in their population with 2 HG cancers missed (4.8% of HG PCa, 1.1% of studied men). In a prospective trial, McKiernan et al. re-evaluated this model on a training cohort ($N = 255$) and then applied it to a validation cohort ($N = 519$) of men with PSA 2–10 ng/mL and no prior biopsy. The gene expression model (ExoDx Prostate IntelliScore) combined with clinical variables (PSA, age, race, and family history) had greater predictive accuracy than PCPTRC for HG cancer, with AUCs of 0.73 (95% CI:0.68–0.77) versus 0.62 (95% CI: 0.57–0.67), respectively. The authors performed a DCA comparing the IntelliScore alone to their clinical model, showing net benefit of the IntelliScore, though PCPTRC was not included in the DCA. With a cutoff IntelliScore cutoff of 15.6, the assay would have prevented 27% of biopsies while missing 12 cases of HG cancer (8% of HG PCa, 2.3% of studied men). These initial results suggest that the IntelliScore can also markedly decrease the number of biopsies performed, but validation on an independent cohort and comparative studies are needed.

SelectMDx (MDxHealth, Irvine, California)

The mRNA transcripts from a set of three genes (HOX6, TDRD1, and DLX1) in post-DRE urine were first reported by Leyten et al. to have high predictive accuracy for high-grade PCa in 358 men undergoing biopsy [67]. Van Neste et al. [68] then developed and validated a model to predict high-grade cancer at biopsy involving levels of HOX6 and DLX1 normalized to KLK3 (the gene that encodes PSA) along with clinical factors (age, PSA density, DRE, prior biopsy, PSA, and family history). Interestingly, they found that excluding DRE findings from the model produced greater accuracy (AUC 0.90, 95% CI: 0.85–0.95), which they attributed to interobserver variability of DRE. They then performed a DCA that clearly demonstrated that their model provided greater net benefit that the both PCPTRC and the combination of PCPTRC with PCA3 results. If the cutoff for biopsy was set to a rigorous NPV of 98%, then 42% of biopsies in their cohort could have been avoided. However, these impressive values remain to be demonstrated in an independent cohort and compared to other biomarkers.

2.3 Negative Biopsy Tissue

ConfirmMDx (MDxHealth, Irvine, California)

An assay is developed that utilizes negative prostate biopsy tissue to examine promoter region methylation levels of three genes associated with PCa: GSTP1, APC, and RASSF1 relative to the methylation of the ACTB gene [69]. The test is developed on the finding of methylation field effect in that gene expression changes are detectable in benign tissue adjacent to cancerous regions [70]. The utility of predicting cancer on subsequent biopsies after an initial negative biopsy has been assessed in two retrospective patient cohorts: (1) initial development in the Methylation Analysis to Locate Occult Cancer (MATLOC) [69] in the UK and Belgium which assessed 483 subjects and (2) the Detection Of Cancer Using Methylated Events in Negative Tissue (DOCUMENT) [71] validation cohort of 320 subjects from 5 centers in the USA. In the MATLOC study, a model was generated with the methylation levels of the three genes of interest and clinical factors (age, PSA, DRE, pathology of first biopsy). The combined model resulted in a NPV of 90% (95% CI: 87–93%) for any prostate cancer on repeat biopsy [69]. A similar finding was found in the validation DOCUMENT cohort where the multivariable model with the methylation markers had a NPV of 88% (95% CI: 85–91%) [71]. These two cohorts were then combined by Van Neste et al. to assess the predictive accuracy of the assay (EpiScore) for HG PCa when combined with a clinical model (age, PSA, DRE, and pathology of first biopsy) [72]. The AUC of the EpiScore and the clinical model combined was 0.76 (95% CI: 0.68–0.84). A DCA revealed the EpiScore added to plus the clinical model demonstrated a notable net benefit over the PCPTRC. The authors estimated that 30% of repeat biopsies could be avoided, though they did not explicitly discuss how many HG cancers would be avoided at this threshold. Thus, the ConfirmMDx does provide benefit over PCPTRC based on initial studies. However, additional prospective validation studies have yet to be performed for this assay; moreover, its performance has yet to be directly compared to other markers in men with a prior negative biopsy.

3 Summary Points—Detection of Prostate Cancer

(1) The blood tests phi and the 4Kscore provide similar benefit in men contemplating biopsy prior to the diagnosis of PCa and can be used to forego biopsy.
(2) PCA3 as a standalone urinary marker is suitable for use in men with prior negative biopsy who are contemplating a repeat biopsy. The combination of PCA3 and TMPRSS2:ERG can be used for men contemplating either an initial or repeat biopsy.
(3) SelectMDx and ExoDx are novel urinary markers that remain to be and compared to other markers; however, early results suggest that a large number of men can be spared a biopsy with few high-grade cancers missed.
(4) ConfirmMDx appears to provide clinical benefit for men with a prior negative biopsy, based on a high NPV for men with a negative test.
(5) Few of these studies have been prospective, and very few have compared tests head-to-head. Moreover, the optimal timing and use of these markers relative to each other and in the setting of multiparametric MRI remain incompletely defined.

4 Initial Treatment Decision

Following the diagnosis of prostate cancer, multiple instruments have been designed to assess gene or protein expression changes in the cancerous biopsy tissue that allow for further prognostic risk stratification. This additional prognostic information can be used to help patients and provider make decisions in terms of pursuing definitive treatment. It is important to emphasize that while many of these markers have increased statistical predictive accuracy for a clinical outcome, to date, none of them has been prospectively validated as a truly *predictive* biomarker which can identify a particular treatment that would provide benefit to a specific patient. Furthermore, no direct comparisons of these biomarkers have been reported to date; thus, we are left to compare the utility of each outcome assessed by a specific marker, and whether providing additional prognostic information *for that outcome* provides assistance to patients making a treatment decision. Finally, clinicians must exercise caution in making radical treatment recommendations based solely on the findings of these markers, particularly since a recent report found significant heterogeneity of gene expression levels associated with these markers both within the same tumor and within different tumors of the same patient [73]. Nonetheless, these markers can provide assistance for patients in clinical situations that do not have a clear treatment recommendation.

Oncotype Dx Genomic Prostate Score® (GPS) (Genomic Health, Inc., Redwood City, California)

The Oncotype GPS score drives from a genomic panel that measures the gene expression at the RNA level of 12 genes associated with aggressive prostate cancer relative to 5 housekeeping genes [13, 74]. The panel was developed from 732 candidate genes tested in RP specimens and prostate biopsy cores [75, 76]. Klein et al. [75] initially examined 441 RP specimens and assessed gene expression correlation with clinical recurrence, prostate cancer death, and RP adverse pathology (defined as (1) Gleason primary pattern ≥ 4 or (2) stage $\geq$ pT3a). They then used separate cohort of 167 biopsy specimens from patients who subsequently underwent RP to derive the final 12 genes associated with adverse pathology at RP (plus the 5 housekeeping genes) to arrive at the final 17 gene panel. The panel was then validated for predicting adverse RP pathology on a new cohort of 395 biopsy specimens from men with (1) CAPRA score < 5, (2) Gleason $\leq$ 3+4, and (3) $\leq$ cT2 disease [75]. On multivariable analysis in models that included clinical variables (age, PSA, clinical stage, and biopsy Gleason) and CAPRA score, the GPS remained a significant predictor of adverse pathology at RP [75]. The AUC of the adverse pathology predictive model was 0.67 when combining CAPRA and GPS versus 0.63 with CAPRA alone. Lastly, a DCA revealed that there was a net benefit adding the GPS to CAPRA compared with CAPRA alone. Thus, as a prognostic score for adverse RP pathology, the GPS added information beyond a patient's clinical variable and biopsy pathology results.

To further validate the GPS on a separate, more racially diverse, RP cohort, Cullen et al. assessed the correlation of biopsy specimen GPS with (1) adverse pathology at RP, (2) biochemical recurrence (BCR), and (3) metastatic recurrence for 431 men with very low to intermediate NCCN risk disease and Gleason $\leq$ 7 on biopsy [77]. They found that in a model including NCCN risk group and GPS that GPS remained a statistically significant predictor of BCR and adverse pathology at RP [77]. Multivariable analysis for metastatic recurrence was unable to be modeled due to a low number of events. For predictive models, the AUC of NCCN risk category (a relatively inferior, and not truly multivariable, baseline comparator) for adverse pathology was 0.63, but increased to 0.72 with the addition of GPS. In the BCR outcome, the c-index (analogous to the AUC, but used for time-dependent survival outcomes) of NCCN risk category alone was 0.59 and increased to 0.68 with the addition of GPS. Thus, this study suggests that may be a prognostic association with the GPS for BCR in addition to adverse pathology at the time of RP. However, the authors did not perform a DCA for these outcomes with NCCN risk categories alone versus with the addition of GPS, and as noted above, improving predictions based on the NCCN risk categories can be done for free with better, readily available clinical models.

Most recently, Van Den Eden et al. [78] found that higher GPS from biopsy tissue is prognostic of post-RP outcomes. In a retrospective cohort study of 279 men treated with RP from 1995 to 2010 for localized PCa spanning low to high NCCN risk groups, the authors found that the GPS score was independently associated with BCR, PCa metastasis, and PCa death after adjusting for CAPRA score and NCCN risk category. The c-index for the PCa metastasis at 10 years rose from 0.65 for CAPRA alone to 0.73 with the addition of GPS. For PCa death, a similar increase of 0.78–0.84 was observed with the addition of GPS to CAPRA [78]. While this association is noteworthy, it is unclear what impact these data have on clinical decisions, particularly since models were not adjusted for receipt of any adjuvant therapies post-RP.

The GPS score provides clinicians and patients with additional information regarding their overall disease prognosis and their likelihood of having adverse pathological features if they were to undergo immediate RP. However, it is unclear how GPS scores correlates with disease progression should they chose active surveillance, or if they chose primary radiation therapy. Also, the GPS report makes reference to risk group reclassification based on thresholds which are arbitrary and not statistically validated. Thus, the GPS provides additional risk stratification for patients, but is likely best reserved for patients whose clinical risk does not indicate a clear clinical recommendation for or against treatment.

ProMark® (Metamark Genetics, Inc., Waltham, Massachusetts)

It is a test that uses quantitative tissue proteomics [79] to generate a risk score from the levels of 8 target proteins for men with Gleason 3+3 and 3+4 cancer on biopsy. The score provides patients and providers with the probability of having adverse pathology at the time of prostatectomy, again defined as (1) Gleason $\geq$ 4+3, (2) stage $\geq$pT3a, or (3) N1/M1 disease. The protein panel was derived from a candidate biomarker study [80]. A clinical prognostic risk model was developed in 381 patients with biopsy and RP specimens and then validated in a new cohort of 276 RP patients comparing their proteomic panel risk to NCCN risk category and D'Amico classification [81]. In the validation cohort, the authors report that the AUC of predicting unfavorable pathology for the proteomic panel alone was 0.68 (CI 0.61–0.74) compared to the NCCN model of 0.69 (CI 0.62–0.75) and D'Amico 0.65 (CI 0.59–0.71). However, there were increases in AUC with the addition of the proteomic panel to the NCCN model to 0.75 (CI 0.69–0.81) and for the D'Amico model to 0.75 (CI 0.69–0.81). Additionally, when the authors utilized clinical cutoffs for the protein panel combined with NCCN risk categories, they reported that the favorable pathology PPV was 82% for NCCN intermediate risk, 82% for low risk, and 95% for NCCN very low risk. Using just the NCCN categories, the PPVs for intermediate, low, and very low risk were 41, 64, and 80%, respectively. Conversely, an *unfavorable* protein panel score resulted in a PPV for *unfavorable* pathology in 85% of NCCN intermediate-risk patients, 50% of low, and 75% of very low cases (n = 4 for the very low category). The authors did perform a DCA that demonstrated a net benefit with the addition of the protein panel for patients in the NCCN intermediate and high-risk groups. Thus, particularly for patients in the intermediate-risk category, the addition of the protein panel information could alter a treatment recommendation. However, for patients with lower clinical risk, the ProMark is more adept to offer reassurance that they are in fact low risk. However, it has not been demonstrated that ProMark improved on any bona fide multivariable clinical risk score. Moreover, it is important to recall that the outcomes predicted by the ProMark panel are specific to unfavorable pathology at the time of RP. While unfavorable pathology is associated with a less favorable prognosis, there is no study to date that shows an unfavorable ProMark score to either predict or have a direct correlation with decreased survival or post-surgical disease recurrence.

Prolaris® (Myriad Genetics, Inc., Salt Lake City, Utah)

It is a panel that measures the RNA expression levels of 31 genes involved in cell cycle progression (CCP) relative to the expression of 15 housekeeping genes in cancerous tissue [82]. The primary clinical outcome prognosticated by the test is 10-year prostate cancer mortality with conservative management [74]. The genes were initially selected, and the model was developed using cohorts of patients who underwent radical prostatectomy and those with prostate cancer found during transurethral resection of the prostate (TURP) [82]. Higher CCP scores were associated with BCR in the RP cohort and prostate cancer death in the TURP cohort [82]. The prostate cancer mortality prognostic finding was then validated in a cohort of conservatively managed patients undergoing transrectal prostate biopsy, which demonstrated that the CCP was associated with prostate cancer death in a multivariable analysis including clinical variables [83]. Of note, the CCP was not initially compared with existing multi-component clinical prognostic risk calculators (e.g., CAPRA score). Such a comparison was done by Cuzick et al. in a subsequent study of 585 men diagnosed with needle biopsy and then managed conservatively [84]. They assessed the 10-year prostate cancer mortality by CAPRA score, CCP score, and a combination of the two designated the cell cycle risk (CCR). In the predictive model, the c-index for CAPRA alone was 0.74 and increased modestly to 0.78 for the CCR model (CAPRA and CCP). The authors also discussed that the CCP score facilitated stratification of risk within each CAPRA score [84]. However, from a clinical perspective, this stratification would likely be relevant to only low- and intermediate-risk patients (i.e., stratification of high risk is unlikely to modify treatment recommendation).

In addition to assessing mortality in conservatively managed men, the CCP score has been assessed on the biopsy specimens of men who later underwent definitive local therapy. Bishoff et al. [85] calculated CCP scores on the biopsy specimens of 582 men who subsequently were treated with RP. They found that elevated biopsy CCP scores were significantly associated with BCR on multivariable analysis. The authors also reported a significant association with metastasis; however, only 12 of the 582 patients (2%) experienced this outcome. The CCP score was not significantly associated with clinical variables in any models, suggesting that it provides additional predictive information beyond clinical data. However, the prognostic value of the CCP was not directly compared to any established clinical calculators. In a subsequent study using this same cohort of patients, Tosioan et al. found that for men with clinically NCCN low-risk disease (Gleason score ≤ 6, $\leq$cT2a, PSA < 10 ng/mL), the CCP score from the biopsy was able to provide additional prognostic value for biochemical recurrence after RP beyond the CAPRA score [86]. They reported that 35% of men with a high CCP score had BCR at 5-years, and the c-index was 0.56 for the CAPRA score alone and 0.66 for CAPRA combined with CCP score. Furthermore, the authors assessed clinical utility with a DCA, which revealed the CCP score provided net benefit beyond CAPRA [86]. Thus, using only pre-treatment data, the CCP score does allow for prognostic stratification within the low-risk category, and this information could be used in making active surveillance vs local treatment decisions with certain patients.

A similar finding for radiation treatment was found by Freedland et al. [87] who studied the CCP score of biopsy tissue in 141 men who underwent definitive local treatment with external beam radiation therapy (EBRT). They found that higher CCP scores were associated with biochemical failure using the Phoenix criteria [88]; however, in their multivariable model the c-index increased slightly from 0.78 to 0.80 with the addition of the CCP score to standard clinical variables [87]. Nonetheless, for a given clinical risk, the CCP did further stratify the risk for experiencing biochemical failure, and this information could potentially be used in men contemplating radiation therapy vs active surveillance.

In higher-risk clinical categories, the CCP may provide less assistance. In a small study of 52 patients who underwent RP, Oderda et al. used pre-RP clinical variables and biopsy CCP score to prognosticate changes in European Urology Association (EUA) risk categories based on final RP pathology and subsequent BCR [89]. The risk categories of the patients in the study included those from low, intermediate, and high pre-RP clinical risk. The authors found that there was modest improvement in predictive models for high-risk disease at RP based on EAU post-op classification. The AUC of the biopsy-based EUA risk classification rose from 0.79 to 0.88 with the addition of CCP [89]. However, there are questions as to whether or not classifying a clinically high-risk patient with "more aggressive" disease is of clinical value. Similarly, would a "less aggressive" CCP score in a clinically high-risk patient change a recommendation for treatment? Furthermore, the CCP was not a statistically significant predictor of BCR in models that included pre-RP EUA risk categories, CAPRA score, or in a model involving post-surgical EAU risk score based off of pathological variables. Thus, particularly for patients who have intermediate- or high-risk disease, the usefulness of the CCP score relatively to standard clinical risk predictors is not as clear, and its use may not change treatment recommendations or add additional predictive information for post-treatment recurrences.

Multiple studies have also utilized questionnaires completed by treating urologists to track changes in treatment recommendations both before and after CCP results are known [90–92]. Shore et al. described that in 294 newly diagnosed patients with localized disease, surveyed urologists reported that the CCP score revealed lower than expected risk in 47% of patients and higher than expected risk in 8% [92]. Notably, however, the measure of "expected risk" before the CCP score was left to the judgment of the urologist (i.e., no standardized risk calculators were used). These risk changes resulted in a different treatment recommendation for 32% of patients [92]. Similarly, in the preliminary analysis of a large CCP registry, Crawford et al. reported urologist survey results for 305 men with newly diagnosed PCa and found that the CCP score changed the treatment recommendation in 31%

of men [90]. In the follow-up report from this registry that involved 1206 men, it was noted that after patients and providers knew the CCP score, 24.2% of patients initially favoring a non-interventional approach switched to more aggressive therapy compared to 14.2% who changed from an interventional therapy to a non-interventional management strategy. These studies suggest that clinicians and patients took CCP results into consideration when selecting management. However, these results must be interpreted with caution as the study design used the clinical decision change as the measured outcome, and a change in decision is not always in the correct direction. Furthermore, neither urologists nor patients were randomized to use the test or not, and there are substantial opportunities for bias in this type of study, both in the pretest and post-test recorded decisions.

The CCP score provides patients and providers with an overall stratification within their clinical risk group and an estimated mortality risk should they chose a non-interventional management strategy. This information is most likely to help patients who do not have a definitive or clear decision based on their clinical risk estimates.

Decipher® (GenomeDx Biosciences, Inc., Vancouver, British Columbia)

The Decipher genomic classifier (GC) is comprised of RNA expression levels of 22 genomic markers that were initially selected from 1.4 million candidate RNA probes from a whole transcriptome microarray (including both protein-coding and non-coding RNA) [13, 74, 93]. The GC was derived and validated to predict metastasis based on a cohort of 545 patients who underwent RP at the Mayo clinic of which 213 experienced subsequent metastasis [93]. While the actual GC report provided to clinicians and patients is comprised only of the validated 22 markers, the clinical assay is based not on real-time PCR, but rather on a full transcriptome microarray, the full data from which are held to develop further genomic expression profiles that may have additional prognostic—and possibly predictive—characteristics for specific responses to radiation [94] or hormone therapy [95]. The initial focus of the GC was on post-RP prognostication and treatment decisions; however, the GC can now be performed on biopsy specimens, and results can be factored into the initial treatment decision.

The GC score ranges from 0 to 1 and then divided into low (0.0–0.44), average (0.45–0.59), and high (0.60–1.0) genomic risk based on the 22 markers. The biopsy report provides estimates of high-grade disease (primary Gleason $\geq$ 4) at RP, 5-year metastasis rate after RP, and 10-year prostate cancer mortality after RP. The model used to estimate the 10-year prostate cancer mortality is extrapolated from the GC scores of RP specimens [96, 97]. The models used to estimate the high-grade Gleason at RP and 5-year metastasis after RP were evaluated by Klein et al., who assessed the GC score on 57 biopsy specimens from men who subsequently had RP [98]. They found that in the model for high-grade Gleason at RP, the AUC for the GC was 0.71 (95% CI 0.56–0.86). For 5-year metastasis, the c-index for the GC was 0.87 (95% CI 0.76–0.97); however, only 5 men in the cohort developed this outcome [98]. Also, the authors assessed the GC on the RP specimens for all of these patients and found GC risk group (low, intermediate, high) concordance of 64% (95% CI 50–77%) between the biopsy and RP GC score. This GC risk concordance rate is similar to the 75% found in a study of 33 patients who had both GC biopsy and RP specimens [99]. In the same study, the authors found that the actual GC score correlation between biopsy and RP had $R = 0.7$ ($p < 0.001$) and that many of the discordant risk group cases had scores at the borders of the risk group cutoffs [99]. Thus, the biopsy-based GC score does provide patients and physicians with estimates of clinical outcomes, but it is important to note that all men underwent treatment with RP in deriving these estimates.

A recent study is proposed combining the GC score and NCCN risk classification system to better prognosticate the risk of distant metastasis at 10 years using novel clinical-genomic risk groups [100]. The authors proposed both a 3-tier (low, intermediate, and high) and 6-tier (very low, low, favorable intermediate, unfavorable intermediate, high, and very high) clinical-genomic risk groups that were derived by combining the 4-tier NCCN risk groups with the GC risk group. Again, this is a suboptimal strategy since the NCCN risk groups do not fully or adequately represent the prognostic information derivable from standard clinical parameters. The authors leveraged multicenter cohorts with a total of 991 patients to first develop the new clinical-genomic risk groups on pre-treatment clinical data and GC scores from RP specimens ($N = 756$) and then validated the risk groups using biopsy GC scores ($N = 235$) in patients who then underwent RP or radiation therapy as primary treatment. In the development cohort, the 10-year distant metastasis c-index for the NCCN 4 tiers was 0.68 (95% CI 0.64–0.72), CAPRA was 0.68 (95% CI 0.62–0.74), and for the 6-tier clinical-genomic risk was 0.77 (0.72–0.81). In the validation cohort, the c-index for the 6-tier clinical-genomic risk was 0.84 (95% CI 0.61–0.93). This combination the NCCN risk and GC risk overall improved the prognostication of determining metastatic disease at 10 years after primary therapy based on pre-treatment clinical factors and GC score from the biopsy specimen. These results could be helpful for (1) patients contemplating primary treatment who may pursue active surveillance if they have very low clinical-genomic risk and (2) identifying patients with very aggressive disease who may require multimodal therapy and treatment escalations.

Lastly, there is some evidence supporting the use of the GC score on biopsy tissue in men contemplating radiation therapy. Nguyen et al. assessed the GC score of biopsy tissue to predict post-treatment distant metastasis in 100 patients with NCCN intermediate- or high-risk disease who underwent primary radiation and androgen deprivation therapy (ADT) following biopsy [101]. The authors found that the GC was the only significant predictor of distant metastasis in multivariable analysis for different models that included clinical variables, CAPRA, or NCCN risk category [101]. For the model to predict 5-year metastasis following radiation, the c-index for the GC was 0.76 (95% CI 0.57–0.89), compared to CAPRA 0.45 (95% CI 0.27–0.64), and NCCN 0.63 (95% CI 0.40–0.78). On DCA, the GC score showed a net clinical benefit across the spectrum of threshold probabilities [101].

Thus, this study demonstrated the ability of the GC score from biopsy tissue to predict which men may have a high risk of developing metastatic disease despite radiation and ADT. These men could potentially select longer ADT courses, chemotherapy, or clinical trials.

The GC score from biopsy specimens allows for prognostication of disease progression in men undergoing treatment with radiation and ADT or RP. However, as with the other tests discussed above, there remain no data on GC scores in men who were actually followed with active surveillance. Thus, low GC scores prognosticate clinically less aggressive disease in patients who elect local therapy. This information can be incorporated into clinical risk factors to assist patients with their decision to pursue local therapy.

4.1 Summary Points—Initial Treatment Decision

(1) Oncotype GPS and ProMark provide additional risk stratification for having adverse pathology for patients with Gleason 3+3 or 3+4 disease on biopsy and with overall low or intermediate clinical risk. There is also some correlation of GPS with biochemical recurrence, metastasis, and cancer death following radical prostatectomy; however, it is unclear how this information should be factored into the initial clinical decision for treatment.

(2) The Prolaris CCP score adds prognostic value to clinical variables regarding the mortality risks of conservative management and of recurrence following treatment. While sub-stratification within some risk categories may prove to be less valuable, the ability to estimate outcomes in men not pursuing local therapy may be useful to patients.

(3) The Decipher GC provides prognostic information regarding the risk of disease progression or recurrence following local therapy and can be used to identify patients with less aggressive disease that may be amendable to surveillance. It may also be used to identify high-risk patients that might benefit from escalations in treatment, though it has not been validated to predict better responses to escalated treatment. There is not yet long-term evidence reporting the use of any biomarker in the setting of active surveillance.

5 Post-radical Prostatectomy Prognosis and Adjuvant Treatment Decisions

Patients who have undergone RP as definitive local treatment are faced with a series of decisions around adjuvant or salvage radiation, ADT, or continued surveillance in the setting of a slowly rising PSA. The ability for biomarkers to contribute additional prognostic value beyond clinical and pathological characteristics can assist with these decisions. There is also the potential for a truly *predictive* biomarker to be developed in this area that could predict which patients would benefit from additional radiation or hormone therapies. However, no marker has been proven to be predictive in this context. Indeed, for the adjuvant radiation discussion, the decision thresholds may well prove trifurcated rather than bifurcated: Men with relatively low-risk disease may not need adjuvant treatment and those with very high-risk disease may not benefit. The men in an optimal middle-risk zone presumably will benefit from early radiation, but no score has yet been studied or validated along these lines. The two biomarkers discussed below were explained in the prior section on biopsy tissue, but both panels can also be performed on RP specimens. The evidence for their use in post-RP treatment decisions using the RP specimen as a substrate will be discussed herein.

Prolaris®

Cooperberg et al. [102] focused on the CCP score derived from RP tissue to prognosticate and stratify the risk of BCR. In the study of 413 men who underwent RP, 20% had BCR. The authors found that the CCP score was able to effectively sub-stratify patients within CAPRA-S [17] risk groups. They also reported that regardless of CAPRA-S risk group, men with a very low CCP score never recurred within 5 years of RP, but that among those with a high CCP, nearly 50% experienced a recurrence. In the overall recurrence predictive model, the c-index of CAPRA-S alone was 0.73 and increased to 0.77 with the addition of the CCP score. In DCA, the combination of CAPRA-S and CCP score provided a greater net benefit across the broad range of risk than either test independently [102]. Thus, the CCP score provides additional prognostic information—beyond pathologic factors—on the risk of BCR following RP. This additional information could assist men with deciding on adjuvant treatments. If a patient had adverse pathologic features, but a low CCP score, they could forego adjuvant radiation. Importantly, this study did not report on outcomes of metastasis or PCa death; thus, the data provided should be reserved for counseling patients about the risk of BCR.

Decipher®

After being initially developed and validated to be an independent predictor of metastasis after RP [93], multiple other studies have confirmed this finding and shown the GC to improve prognostication of clinical outcomes following RP. Ross et al. showed that the GC had greater predictive discrimination of metastatic progression in a cohort of 85 men who developed BCR following RP [103]. They found that the GC had a c-index of 0.82 (95% CI 0.76–0.86) compared to 0.56 (95% CI 0.49–0.75) for CAPRA-S and 0.75 (95% CI 0.69–0.81) for the Stephenson nomogram [18]. A DCA showed a net benefit of GC relative to the clinical models. In a larger patient cohort of 260 men with intermediate- and high-risk disease at the time of RP who received no adjuvant therapy, Ross et al. found that the GC added additional prognostic accuracy to the CAPRA-S for estimating metastatic disease at

10 years post-RP [96]. The c-index of GC alone was 0.76 (95% CI 0.65–0.84) and CAPRA-S was 0.77 (95% CI 0.69–0.85); however, when the GC and CAPRA-S were combined, the c-index improved to 0.87 (95% CI 0.77–0.94). The greater net benefit of the combination was confirmed on DCA. Klein et al. also found the strong prognostication and clinical benefit of the GC for metastasis at 5 years after RP in a cohort of 169 high-risk men [104].

In addition to the ability of the GC to prognosticate metastasis after RP, Cooperberg et al. found that the combination of CAPRA-S and GC also predicted PCa death at 5 years after RP in 185 men with high-risk disease [97]. The combination of CAPRA-S and GC had greater clinical benefit on DCA than either the one alone [97]. Notably, this finding was less true for biochemical recurrence alone, and the role of GC may be greatest in distinguishing purely biochemical PSA failures vs those likely to progress to clinically apparent recurrence. Supporting this finding, Karnes et al. recently published a multicenter cohort of 561 men with adverse pathologic features at RP (pT3, pN1, positive surgical margins, or Gleason score > 7), showing that combination of GC and CAPRA-S was able to prognosticate 10-year PCa death following RP [105]. They report a c-index for CAPRA-S and GC of 0.76 (95% CI 0.71–0.82) compared to CAPRA-S alone of 0.73 (95% CI 0.68–0.78) and GC alone of 0.73 (95% CI 0.67–0.78). The DCA performed by the authors also confirmed the net benefit of GC combined with CAPRA-S for 10-year PCa mortality [105]. These studies in combination demonstrate that the GC has significant prognostic value for both metastatic disease and PCa mortality following local therapy with RP. This prognostic aspect alone can assist patients and providers in making treatment decisions for adjuvant therapy—if a patient's GC risk for metastasis and PCa death is low, he could potentially forego adjuvant treatments even if his pathological characteristics are less favorable.

Multiple studies have investigated if the GC can discern which patients are likely to benefit from post-RP radiation therapy (RT) either in the adjuvant setting (ART, PSA ≤ 0.2) or salvage setting (SRT, PSA > 0.2). Den et al. assessed the GC's association with metastasis in 188 men who underwent RT following RP. In the predictive model for metastasis at 5 years following RT, the c-index for CAPRA-S was 0.66 (95% CI 0.56–0.78), GC alone was 0.83 (95% CI 0.72–0.89), and the combination of CAPRA-S and GC was 0.85 (0.79–0.93) [106]. The DCA showed a relative net benefit for the GC and CAPRA-S model. Moreover, the authors then compared patients who underwent ART vs SRT based on their GC score. They found no difference between time to metastasis for men with GC < 0.4 between ART and SRT ($p = 0.788$); however, for men with GC > 0.40, there was a significant difference ($p < 0.008$) with men who received ART having lower cumulative incidence of metastasis following RT [106]. This retrospective study therefore suggests that men with low GC scores may derive little benefit from ART, whereas those with higher GC may derive greater benefit from ART than SRT. In a larger cohort of 422 men with pT3 disease or positive surgical margins at RP, Ross et al. assessed the association of GC with metastasis in men who received ART (PSA $<$ 0.2 at RT), minimal residual disease (MRD) SRT (PSA 0.2–0.49), SRT (PSA 0.50), and no-RT [107]. The authors found in multivariable analysis that Decipher remained a statistically significant predictor of metastasis ($p = 0.01$) in models including CAPRA-S and the type of post-op RT. They also found that at higher GC scores, there was improved metastasis-free survival in the ART and MRD SRT groups compared to the SRT and no-RT groups after adjusting for CAPRA-S [107]. This study therefore suggests that men with high GC scores may derive benefit from earlier RT. Thus, the decision to pursue ART may be aided by GC scores.

In addition to these retrospective studies on patient outcomes, a prospective study on clinician treatment recommendations before and after the ascertainment of GC score found that clinicians do change their recommendations for ART and SRT based on GC scores [108]. In patients who were candidates for ART, 18% received a changed treatment recommendation from their urologist after the GC score was known. For patients that were candidates for SRT, 37% received a changed treatment recommendation. Patients with higher-risk GC scores were more likely to receive a recommendation for ART or SRT, while those with lower GC scores were more likely to be recommended observation [108]. Whether or not patients pursue the recommended therapy and if they have improved clinical outcomes remains to be determined.

Lastly, the technology of the GC microarray allows for assessment of additional RNA genomic biomarker panels. Zhao et al. reported a new 24 biomarker panel that is intended to predict the effectiveness of post-RP RT based on the panel results [94]. The authors utilized the same training and validation patient cohorts as Decipher to develop the Post-Operative Radiation Therapy Outcomes Score (PORTOS) that was focused on assessing metastasis and receipt of RT after RP. The authors found in the validation cohort that for patients with a high PORTOS, the 10-year metastasis rate was 4% for patients who received RT versus 35% for those who had no-RT ($p = 0.002$) [94]. Conversely, for patients with a low PORTOS, the 10-year metastasis rate was 32% in patients who both did and did not receive post-RP RT ($p = 0.76$). Finally, the authors demonstrated that CAPRA-S, Decipher, and the microarray version of the Prolaris CCP did not predict the response to RT [94]. These results are promising, but they have not been validated in a prospective cohort, and thus, while PORTOS appears to have significant predictive characteristics, it cannot yet be considered a true *predictive biomarker.*

5.1 Summary Points—Post-radical Prostatectomy

(1) The Prolaris CCP score provides additional prognostic value for BCR beyond clinical variables and can be used to further stratify a patient's risk of experiencing BCR.

(2) The Decipher GC provides prognostic information for metastasis and PCa death following RP. This additional information can be helpful to characterize a patient's overall risk and facilitate adjuvant therapy treatment decisions. Future development of similar biomarker panels may ultimately provide predictive information on whether patients derive any benefit from a specific therapy.

6 Conclusions and Future Directions

The last decade has brought rapid development of numerous biomarkers for use in detection and treatment of prostate cancer. At present, these markers offer additional risk stratification and disease prognosis—information that may be helpful for men with clinical factors that do not heavily favor biopsy versus no biopsy or treatment versus surveillance. Thus, prudent ordering of these tests in the correct patients may be warranted. Prospective trials are still needed to validate whether any markers can actually improve (not just predict) outcomes such as metastasis and survival. Furthermore, comparisons between markers are required to determine whether a superior test exists. While much more research is required, these biomarkers point to an optimistic future with the ideal goal of only detecting cancers that pose a threat to a patient's life and then tailoring therapy to a given cancer's individual risk profile and treatment sensitivity.

References

1. Epstein JI, Zelefsky MJ, Sjoberg DD et al (2016) A contemporary prostate cancer grading system: a validated alternative to the Gleason score. Eur Urol 69(3):428–435. https://doi.org/10.1016/j.eururo.2015.06.046
2. Moschini M, Carroll PR, Eggener SE et al (2017) Low-risk prostate cancer: identification, management, and outcomes. Eur Urol 72(2):238–249. https://doi.org/10.1016/j.eururo.2017.03.009
3. McShane LM, Altman DG, Sauerbrei W, Taube SE, Gion M, Clark GM (2005) Reporting recommendations for tumor marker prognostic studies. J Clin Oncol 23(36):9067–9072. https://doi.org/10.1200/JCO.2004.01.0454
4. Ballman KV (2015) Biomarker: predictive or prognostic? J Clin Oncol 33(33):3968–3971. https://doi.org/10.1200/JCO.2015.63.3651
5. Duffy MJ, O'Donovan N, McDermott E, Crown J (2016) Validated biomarkers: the key to precision treatment in patients with breast cancer. Breast 29:192–201. https://doi.org/10.1016/j.breast.2016.07.009
6. Denduluri N, Somerfield MR, Eisen A et al (2016) Selection of optimal adjuvant chemotherapy regimens for human epidermal growth factor receptor 2 (HER2) -negative and adjuvant targeted therapy for HER2-Positive Breast Cancers. J Clin Oncol (An American Society of Clinical Oncology Guideline Adaptation of the Cancer C) 34(20):2416–2427. https://doi.org/10.1200/JCO.2016.67.0182
7. Centers for Medicare & Medicaid Services. Clinical Laboratory Improvement Amendments. https://www.cms.gov/Regulations-and-Guidance/Legislation/CLIA/Downloads/LDT-and-CLIA_FAQs.pdf. Published 2013. Accessed 1 Jan 2017
8. Office of Public Health Strategy and Analysis—Food and Drug Administration (2015) The public health evidence for FDA oversight of laboratory developed tests: 20 case studies. Silver Spring, MD. https://www.fda.gov/AboutFDA/ReportsManualsForms/Reports/ucm472773.htm
9. Food and Drug Administration (2017) Discussion paper of laboratory developed tests. Silver Spring, MD. https://www.fda.gov/medicaldevices/productsandmedicalprocedures/invitrodiagnostics/laboratorydevelopedtests/default.htm
10. Palmetto GBA (2018) Molecular diagnostic services program manual. Columbia, SC. https://www.palmettogba.com/Palmetto/moldx.Nsf/files/MolDX_Manual.pdf/$File/MolDX_Manual.pdf?Open&. Accessed 20 Jan 2018

11. Palmetto GBA (2015) MolDX clinical test evaluation process. Columbia, SC. https://www.palmettogba.com/Palmetto/Moldx.Nsf/files/MolDX_Clinical_Test_Evaluation_Process_(CTEP)_M00096.pdf/$File/MolDX_Clinical_Test_Evaluation_Process_(CTEP)_M00096.pdf. Accessed 20 Jan 2018
12. Fawcett T (2006) An introduction to ROC analysis. Pattern Recogn Lett 27(8):861–874. https://doi.org/10.1016/j.patrec.2005.10.010
13. Leapman MS, Nguyen HG, Cooperberg MR (2016) Clinical utility of biomarkers in localized prostate cancer. Curr Oncol Rep 18(5):30. https://doi.org/10.1007/s11912-016-0513-1
14. Nguyen CT, Kattan MW (2011) How to tell if a new marker improves prediction. Eur Urol 60(2):226–230. https://doi.org/10.1016/j.eururo.2011.04.029
15. Ankerst DP, Hoefler J, Bock S et al (2014) Prostate cancer prevention trial risk calculator 2.0 for the prediction of low- vs high-grade prostate cancer. Urology 83(6):1362–1367. https://doi.org/10.1016/j.urology.2014.02.035
16. Cooperberg MR, Broering JM, Carroll PR (2009) Risk assessment for prostate cancer metastasis and mortality at the time of diagnosis. J Natl Cancer Inst 101(12):878–887. https://doi.org/10.1093/jnci/djp122
17. Cooperberg MR, Hilton JF, Carroll PR (2011) The CAPRA-S score: a straightforward tool for improved prediction of outcomes after radical prostatectomy. Cancer 117(22):5039–5046. https://doi.org/10.1002/cncr.26169
18. Stephenson AJ, Scardino PT, Eastham JA et al (2005) Postoperative nomogram predicting the 10-year probability of prostate cancer recurrence after radical prostatectomy. J Clin Oncol 23(28):7005–7012. https://doi.org/10.1200/JCO.2005.01.867
19. Eggener SE, Scardino PT, Walsh PC et al (2011) Predicting 15-year prostate cancer specific mortality after radical prostatectomy. J Urol 185(3):869–875. https://doi.org/10.1016/j.juro.2010.10.057
20. Sanda MG, Cadeddu JA, Kirkby E et al (2017) Clinically localized prostate cancer: AUA/ASTRO/SUO guideline. Part I: risk stratification, shared decision making, and care options. J Urol. https://doi.org/10.1016/j.juro.2017.11.095
21. Mohler JL, Antonarakis ES, Armstrong AJ et al (2017) NCCN clinical practice guidelines in oncology—prostate cancer. Version 2. https://www.nccn.org/professionals/physician_gls/pdf/prostate.pdf. Published 2017. Accessed 3 Oct 2017
22. Vickers AJ, Elkin EB (2006) Decision curve analysis: a novel method for evaluating prediction models. Med Decis Mak 26(6):565–574. https://doi.org/10.1177/0272989X06295361
23. Vickers AJ, Cronin AM, Elkin EB, Gonen M (2008) Extensions to decision curve analysis, a novel method for evaluating diagnostic tests, prediction models and molecular markers. BMC Med Inform Decis Mak 8:53. https://doi.org/10.1186/1472-6947-8-53
24. Fitzgerald M, Saville BR, Lewis RJ (2015) Decision curve analysis. JAMA 313(4):409–410. https://doi.org/10.1001/jama.2015.37
25. Lee DJ, Mallin K, Graves AJ et al (2017) Recent changes in prostate cancer screening practices and epidemiology. J Urol. https://doi.org/10.1016/j.juro.2017.05.074
26. Catalona WJ, Partin AW, Sanda MG et al (2011) A multicenter study of [-2]pro-prostate specific antigen combined with prostate specific antigen and free prostate specific antigen for prostate cancer detection in the 2.0 to 10.0 ng/ml prostate specific antigen range. J Urol 185 (5):1650–1655. https://doi.org/10.1016/j.juro.2010.12.032
27. Loeb S, Sanda MG, Broyles DL et al (2015) The prostate health index selectively identifies clinically significant prostate cancer. J Urol 193(4):1163–1169. https://doi.org/10.1016/j.juro.2014.10.121
28. Jansen FH, van Schaik RHN, Kurstjens J et al (2010) Prostate-specific antigen (PSA) isoform p2PSA in combination with total PSA and free PSA improves diagnostic accuracy in prostate cancer detection. Eur Urol 57(6):921–927. https://doi.org/10.1016/j.eururo.2010.02.003

29. de la Calle C, Patil D, Wei JT et al (2015) Multicenter evaluation of the prostate health index to detect aggressive prostate cancer in biopsy naive men. J Urol 194(1):65–72. https://doi.org/10.1016/j.juro.2015.01.091
30. Boegemann M, Stephan C, Cammann H et al (2016) The percentage of prostate-specific antigen (PSA) isoform [-2]proPSA and the prostate health index improve the diagnostic accuracy for clinically relevant prostate cancer at initial and repeat biopsy compared with total PSA and percentage free PSA in men. BJU Int 117(1):72–79. https://doi.org/10.1111/bju.13139
31. Loeb S, Shin SS, Broyles DL et al (2017) Prostate health Index improves multivariable risk prediction of aggressive prostate cancer. BJU Int 120(1):61–68. https://doi.org/10.1111/bju.13676
32. Foley RW, Gorman L, Sharifi N et al (2016) Improving multivariable prostate cancer risk assessment using the prostate health index. BJU Int 117(3):409–417. https://doi.org/10.1111/bju.13143
33. Foley RW, Maweni RM, Gorman L et al (2016) European randomised study of screening for prostate cancer (ERSPC) risk calculators significantly outperform the prostate cancer prevention trial (PCPT) 2.0 in the prediction of prostate cancer: a multi-institutional study. BJU Int 118(5):706–713. https://doi.org/10.1111/bju.13437
34. Hirama H, Sugimoto M, Ito K, Shiraishi T, Kakehi Y (2014) The impact of baseline [-2] proPSA-related indices on the prediction of pathological reclassification at 1 year during active surveillance for low-risk prostate cancer: the Japanese multicenter study cohort. J Cancer Res Clin Oncol 140(2):257–263. https://doi.org/10.1007/s00432-013-1566-2
35. Tosoian JJ, Loeb S, Feng Z et al (2012) Association of [-2]proPSA with biopsy reclassification during active surveillance for prostate cancer. J Urol 188(4):1131–1136. https://doi.org/10.1016/j.juro.2012.06.009
36. Guazzoni G, Lazzeri M, Nava L et al (2012) Preoperative prostate-specific antigen isoform p2PSA and its derivatives, %p2PSA and prostate health index, predict pathologic outcomes in patients undergoing radical prostatectomy for prostate cancer. Eur Urol 61(3):455–466. https://doi.org/10.1016/j.eururo.2011.10.038
37. Fossati N, Buffi NM, Haese A et al (2015) Preoperative prostate-specific antigen isoform p2PSA and its derivatives, %p2PSA and prostate health index, predict pathologic outcomes in patients undergoing radical prostatectomy for prostate cancer: results from a multicentric European prospective Stud. Eur Urol 68(1):132–138. https://doi.org/10.1016/j.eururo.2014.07.034
38. Vickers AJ, Cronin AM, Aus G et al (2008) A panel of kallikrein markers can reduce unnecessary biopsy for prostate cancer: data from the European randomized study of prostate cancer screening in Goteborg, Sweden. BMC Med 6:19. https://doi.org/10.1186/1741-7015-6-19
39. Vickers A, Cronin A, Roobol M et al (2010) Reducing unnecessary biopsy during prostate cancer screening using a four-kallikrein panel: an independent replication. J Clin Oncol 28(15):2493–2498. https://doi.org/10.1200/JCO.2009.24.1968
40. Benchikh A, Savage C, Cronin A et al (2010) A panel of kallikrein markers can predict outcome of prostate biopsy following clinical work-up: an independent validation study from the European randomized study of prostate cancer screening, France. BMC Cancer 10:635. https://doi.org/10.1186/1471-2407-10-635
41. Vickers AJ, Cronin AM, Roobol MJ et al (2010) A four-kallikrein panel predicts prostate cancer in men with recent screening: data from the European randomized study of screening for prostate cancer, Rotterdam. Clin Cancer Res 16(12):3232–3239. https://doi.org/10.1158/1078-0432.CCR-10-0122
42. Gupta A, Roobol MJ, Savage CJ et al (2010) A four-kallikrein panel for the prediction of repeat prostate biopsy: data from the European randomized study of prostate cancer screening in Rotterdam, Netherlands. Br J Cancer 103(5):708–714. https://doi.org/10.1038/sj.bjc.6605815

43. Bryant RJ, Sjoberg DD, Vickers AJ et al (2015) Predicting high-grade cancer at ten-core prostate biopsy using four kallikrein markers measured in blood in the ProtecT study. J Natl Cancer Inst 107(7). https://doi.org/10.1093/jnci/djv095
44. Parekh DJ, Punnen S, Sjoberg DD et al (2015) A multi-institutional prospective trial in the USA confirms that the 4K score accurately identifies men with high-grade prostate cancer. Eur Urol 68(3):464–470. https://doi.org/10.1016/j.eururo.2014.10.021
45. Nordstrom T, Vickers A, Assel M, Lilja H, Gronberg H, Eklund M (2015) Comparison between the four-kallikrein panel and prostate health index for predicting prostate cancer. Eur Urol 68(1):139–146. https://doi.org/10.1016/j.eururo.2014.08.010
46. Carlsson S, Maschino A, Schroder F et al (2013) Predictive value of four kallikrein markers for pathologically insignificant compared with aggressive prostate cancer in radical prostatectomy specimens: results from the European randomized study of screening for prostate cancer section Rotterdam. Eur Urol 64(5):693–699. https://doi.org/10.1016/j.eururo.2013.04.040
47. Lin DW, Newcomb LF, Brown MD et al (2017) Evaluating the four Kallikrein panel of the 4Kscore for prediction of high-grade prostate cancer in men in the canary prostate active surveillance study. Eur Urol 72(3):448–454. https://doi.org/10.1016/j.eururo.2016.11.017
48. Bussemakers MJ, van Bokhoven A, Verhaegh GW et al (1999) DD3: a new prostate-specific gene, highly overexpressed in prostate cancer. Cancer Res 59(23):5975–5979
49. Tosoian JJ, Ross AE, Sokoll LJ, Partin AW, Pavlovich CP (2016) Urinary biomarkers for prostate cancer. Urol Clin North Am 43(1):17–38. https://doi.org/10.1016/j.ucl.2015.08.003
50. Marks LS, Fradet Y, Deras IL et al (2007) PCA3 molecular urine assay for prostate cancer in men undergoing repeat biopsy. Urology 69(3):532–535. https://doi.org/10.1016/j.urology.2006.12.014
51. Haese A, de la Taille A, van Poppel H et al (2008) Clinical utility of the PCA3 urine assay in European men scheduled for repeat biopsy. Eur Urol 54(5):1081–1088. https://doi.org/10.1016/j.eururo.2008.06.071
52. Auprich M, Haese A, Walz J et al (2010) External validation of urinary PCA3-based nomograms to individually predict prostate biopsy outcome. Eur Urol 58(5):727–732. https://doi.org/10.1016/j.eururo.2010.06.038
53. Crawford ED, Rove KO, Trabulsi EJ et al (2012) Diagnostic performance of PCA3 to detect prostate cancer in men with increased prostate specific antigen: a prospective study of 1,962 cases. J Urol 188(5):1726–1731. https://doi.org/10.1016/j.juro.2012.07.023
54. Wei JT, Feng Z, Partin AW et al (2014) Can urinary PCA3 supplement PSA in the early detection of prostate cancer? J Clin Oncol 32(36):4066–4072. https://doi.org/10.1200/JCO.2013.52.8505
55. Gittelman MC, Hertzman B, Bailen J et al (2013) PCA3 molecular urine test as a predictor of repeat prostate biopsy outcome in men with previous negative biopsies: a prospective multicenter clinical study. J Urol 190(1):64–69. https://doi.org/10.1016/j.juro.2013.02.018
56. Scattoni V, Lazzeri M, Lughezzani G et al (2013) Head-to-head comparison of prostate health index and urinary PCA3 for predicting cancer at initial or repeat biopsy. J Urol 190(2):496–501. https://doi.org/10.1016/j.juro.2013.02.3184
57. Perdona S, Bruzzese D, Ferro M et al (2013) Prostate health index (phi) and prostate cancer antigen 3 (PCA3) significantly improve diagnostic accuracy in patients undergoing prostate biopsy. Prostate 73(3):227–235. https://doi.org/10.1002/pros.22561
58. Seisen T, Roupret M, Brault D et al (2015) Accuracy of the prostate health index versus the urinary prostate cancer antigen 3 score to predict overall and significant prostate cancer at initial biopsy. Prostate 75(1):103–111. https://doi.org/10.1002/pros.22898
59. Tomlins SA, Rhodes DR, Perner S et al (2005) Recurrent fusion of TMPRSS2 and ETS transcription factor genes in prostate cancer. Science 310(5748):644–648. https://doi.org/10.1126/science.1117679
60. Tomlins SA, Bjartell A, Chinnaiyan AM et al (2009) ETS gene fusions in prostate cancer: from discovery to daily clinical practice. Eur Urol 56(2):275–286. https://doi.org/10.1016/j.eururo.2009.04.036

61. Tomlins SA, Day JR, Lonigro RJ et al (2016) Urine TMPRSS2:ERG Plus PCA3 for Individualized prostate cancer risk assessment. Eur Urol 70(1):45–53. https://doi.org/10.1016/j.eururo.2015.04.039
62. Leyten GHJM, Hessels D, Jannink SA et al (2014) Prospective multicentre evaluation of PCA3 and TMPRSS2-ERG gene fusions as diagnostic and prognostic urinary biomarkers for prostate cancer. Eur Urol 65(3):534–542. https://doi.org/10.1016/j.eururo.2012.11.014
63. Stephan C, Jung K, Semjonow A et al (2013) Comparative assessment of urinary prostate cancer antigen 3 and TMPRSS2:ERG gene fusion with the serum [-2]proprostate-specific antigen-based prostate health index for detection of prostate cancer. Clin Chem 59(1):280–288. https://doi.org/10.1373/clinchem.2012.195560
64. Lin DW, Newcomb LF, Brown EC et al (2013) Urinary TMPRSS2:ERG and PCA3 in an active surveillance cohort: results from a baseline analysis in the canary prostate active surveillance study. Clin Cancer Res 19(9):2442–2450. https://doi.org/10.1158/1078-0432.CCR-12-3283
65. Donovan MJ, Noerholm M, Bentink S et al (2015) A molecular signature of PCA3 and ERG exosomal RNA from non-DRE urine is predictive of initial prostate biopsy result. Prostate Cancer Prostatic Dis 18(4):370–375. https://doi.org/10.1038/pcan.2015.40
66. McKiernan J, Donovan MJ, O'Neill V et al (2016) A novel urine exosome gene expression assay to predict high-grade prostate cancer at initial biopsy. JAMA Oncol 2(7):882–889. https://doi.org/10.1001/jamaoncol.2016.0097
67. Leyten GHJM, Hessels D, Smit FP et al (2015) Identification of a candidate gene panel for the early diagnosis of prostate cancer. Clin Cancer Res 21(13):3061–3070. https://doi.org/10.1158/1078-0432.CCR-14-3334
68. Van Neste L, Hendriks RJ, Dijkstra S et al (2016) Detection of high-grade prostate cancer using a urinary molecular biomarker-based risk score. Eur Urol 70(5):740–748. https://doi.org/10.1016/j.eururo.2016.04.012
69. Stewart GD, Van Neste L, Delvenne P et al (2013) Clinical utility of an epigenetic assay to detect occult prostate cancer in histopathologically negative biopsies: results of the MATLOC study. J Urol 189(3):1110–1116. https://doi.org/10.1016/j.juro.2012.08.219
70. Chai H, Brown RE (2009) Field effect in cancer-an update. Ann Clin Lab Sci 39(4):331–337
71. Partin AW, Van Neste L, Klein EA et al (2014) Clinical validation of an epigenetic assay to predict negative histopathological results in repeat prostate biopsies. J Urol 192(4):1081–1087. https://doi.org/10.1016/j.juro.2014.04.013
72. Van Neste L, Partin AW, Stewart GD, Epstein JI, Harrison DJ, Van Criekinge W (2016) Risk score predicts high-grade prostate cancer in DNA-methylation positive, histopathologically negative biopsies. Prostate 76(12):1078–1087. https://doi.org/10.1002/pros.23191
73. Wei L, Wang J, Lampert E et al (2017) Intratumoral and intertumoral genomic heterogeneity of multifocal localized prostate cancer impacts molecular classifications and genomic prognosticators. Eur Urol 71(2):183–192. https://doi.org/10.1016/j.eururo.2016.07.008
74. Loeb S, Ross AE (2017) Genomic testing for localized prostate cancer: where do we go from here? Curr Opin Urol 27(5):495–499. https://doi.org/10.1097/MOU.0000000000000419
75. Klein EA, Cooperberg MR, Magi-Galluzzi C et al (2014) A 17-gene assay to predict prostate cancer aggressiveness in the context of Gleason grade heterogeneity, tumor multifocality, and biopsy undersampling. Eur Urol 66(3):550–560. https://doi.org/10.1016/j.eururo.2014.05.004
76. Knezevic D, Goddard AD, Natraj N et al (2013) Analytical validation of the oncotype DX prostate cancer assay—a clinical RT-PCR assay optimized for prostate needle biopsies. BMC Genom 14:690. https://doi.org/10.1186/1471-2164-14-690
77. Cullen J, Rosner IL, Brand TC et al (2015) A Biopsy-based 17-gene genomic prostate score predicts recurrence after radical prostatectomy and adverse surgical pathology in a racially diverse population of men with clinically low- and intermediate-risk prostate cancer. Eur Urol 68(1):123–131. https://doi.org/10.1016/j.eururo.2014.11.030
78. Van Den Eeden SK, Lu R, Zhang N et al (2018) A biopsy-based 17-gene genomic prostate score as a predictor of metastases and prostate cancer death in surgically treated men with clinically localized disease. Eur Urol 73(1):129–138. https://doi.org/10.1016/j.eururo.2017.09.013

79. Shipitsin M, Small C, Giladi E et al (2014) Automated quantitative multiplex immunofluorescence in situ imaging identifies phospho-S6 and phospho-PRAS40 as predictive protein biomarkers for prostate cancer lethality. Proteome Sci 12:40. https://doi.org/10.1186/1477-5956-12-40
80. Shipitsin M, Small C, Choudhury S et al (2014) Identification of proteomic biomarkers predicting prostate cancer aggressiveness and lethality despite biopsy-sampling error. Br J Cancer 111(6):1201–1212. https://doi.org/10.1038/bjc.2014.396
81. Blume-Jensen P, Berman DM, Rimm DL et al (2015) Development and clinical validation of an in situ biopsy-based multimarker assay for risk stratification in prostate cancer. Clin Cancer Res 21(11):2591–2600. https://doi.org/10.1158/1078-0432.CCR-14-2603
82. Cuzick J, Swanson GP, Fisher G et al (2011) Prognostic value of an RNA expression signature derived from cell cycle proliferation genes in patients with prostate cancer: a retrospective study. Lancet Oncol 12(3):245–255. https://doi.org/10.1016/S1470-2045(10)70295-3
83. Cuzick J, Berney DM, Fisher G et al (2012) Prognostic value of a cell cycle progression signature for prostate cancer death in a conservatively managed needle biopsy cohort. Br J Cancer 106(6):1095–1099. https://doi.org/10.1038/bjc.2012.39
84. Cuzick J, Stone S, Fisher G et al (2015) Validation of an RNA cell cycle progression score for predicting death from prostate cancer in a conservatively managed needle biopsy cohort. Br J Cancer 113(3):382–389. https://doi.org/10.1038/bjc.2015.223
85. Bishoff JT, Freedland SJ, Gerber L et al (2014) Prognostic utility of the cell cycle progression score generated from biopsy in men treated with prostatectomy. J Urol 192(2):409–414. https://doi.org/10.1016/j.juro.2014.02.003
86. Tosoian JJ, Chappidi MR, Bishoff JT et al (2017) Prognostic utility of biopsy-derived cell cycle progression score in patients with national comprehensive cancer network low-risk prostate cancer undergoing radical prostatectomy: implications for treatment guidance. BJU Int. https://doi.org/10.1111/bju.13911
87. Freedland SJ, Gerber L, Reid J et al (2013) Prognostic utility of cell cycle progression score in men with prostate cancer after primary external beam radiation therapy. Int J Radiat Oncol Biol Phys 86(5):848–853. https://doi.org/10.1016/j.ijrobp.2013.04.043
88. Roach M 3rd, Hanks G, Thames HJ et al (2006) Defining biochemical failure following radiotherapy with or without hormonal therapy in men with clinically localized prostate cancer: recommendations of the RTOG-ASTRO Phoenix Consensus conference. Int J Radiat Oncol Biol Phys 65(4):965–974. https://doi.org/10.1016/j.ijrobp.2006.04.029
89. Oderda M, Cozzi G, Daniele L et al (2017) Cell-cycle progression-score might improve the current risk assessment in newly diagnosed prostate cancer patients. Urology 102:73–78. https://doi.org/10.1016/j.urology.2016.11.038
90. Crawford ED, Scholz MC, Kar AJ et al (2014) Cell cycle progression score and treatment decisions in prostate cancer: results from an ongoing registry. Curr Med Res Opin 30(6):1025–1031. https://doi.org/10.1185/03007995.2014.899208
91. Shore ND, Kella N, Moran B et al (2016) Impact of the cell cycle progression test on physician and patient treatment selection for localized prostate cancer. J Urol 195(3):612–618. https://doi.org/10.1016/j.juro.2015.09.072
92. Shore N, Concepcion R, Saltzstein D et al (2014) Clinical utility of a biopsy-based cell cycle gene expression assay in localized prostate cancer. Curr Med Res Opin 30(4):547–553. https://doi.org/10.1185/03007995.2013.873398
93. Erho N, Crisan A, Vergara IA et al (2013) Discovery and validation of a prostate cancer genomic classifier that predicts early metastasis following radical prostatectomy. PLoS ONE 8(6):e66855. https://doi.org/10.1371/journal.pone.0066855
94. Zhao SG, Chang SL, Spratt DE et al (2016) Development and validation of a 24-gene predictor of response to postoperative radiotherapy in prostate cancer: a matched, retrospective analysis. Lancet Oncol 17(11):1612–1620. https://doi.org/10.1016/S1470-2045(16)30491-0

95. Zhao SG, Chang SL, Erho N et al (2017) Associations of luminal and basal subtyping of prostate cancer with prognosis and response to androgen deprivation therapy. JAMA Oncol. https://doi.org/10.1001/jamaoncol.2017.0751
96. Ross AE, Johnson MH, Yousefi K et al (2016) Tissue-based genomics augments post-prostatectomy risk stratification in a natural history cohort of intermediate- and high-risk men. Eur Urol 69(1):157–165. https://doi.org/10.1016/j.eururo.2015.05.042
97. Cooperberg MR, Davicioni E, Crisan A, Jenkins RB, Ghadessi M, Karnes RJ (2015) Combined value of validated clinical and genomic risk stratification tools for predicting prostate cancer mortality in a high-risk prostatectomy cohort. Eur Urol 67(2):326–333. https://doi.org/10.1016/j.eururo.2014.05.039
98. Klein EA, Haddad Z, Yousefi K et al (2016) Decipher genomic classifier measured on prostate biopsy predicts metastasis risk. Urology 90:148–152. https://doi.org/10.1016/j.urology.2016.01.012
99. Knudsen BS, Kim HL, Erho N et al (2016) Application of a clinical whole-transcriptome assay for staging and prognosis of prostate cancer diagnosed in needle core biopsy specimens. J Mol Diagn 18(3):395–406. https://doi.org/10.1016/j.jmoldx.2015.12.006
100. Spratt DE, Zhang J, Santiago-Jimenez M, et al (2017) Development and validation of a novel integrated clinical-genomic risk group classification for localized prostate cancer. J Clin Oncol November JCO2017742940. https://doi.org/10.1200/jco.2017.74.2940
101. Nguyen PL, Martin NE, Choeurng V et al (2017) Utilization of biopsy-based genomic classifier to predict distant metastasis after definitive radiation and short-course ADT for intermediate and high-risk prostate cancer. Prostate Cancer Prostatic Dis 20(2):186–192. https://doi.org/10.1038/pcan.2016.58
102. Cooperberg MR, Simko JP, Cowan JE et al (2013) Validation of a cell-cycle progression gene panel to improve risk stratification in a contemporary prostatectomy cohort. J Clin Oncol 31(11):1428–1434. https://doi.org/10.1200/JCO.2012.46.4396
103. Ross AE, Feng FY, Ghadessi M et al (2014) A genomic classifier predicting metastatic disease progression in men with biochemical recurrence after prostatectomy. Prostate Cancer Prostatic Dis 17(1):64–69. https://doi.org/10.1038/pcan.2013.49
104. Klein EA, Yousefi K, Haddad Z et al (2015) A genomic classifier improves prediction of metastatic disease within 5 years after surgery in node-negative high-risk prostate cancer patients managed by radical prostatectomy without adjuvant therapy. Eur Urol 67(4):778–786. https://doi.org/10.1016/j.eururo.2014.10.036
105. Karnes RJ, Choeurng V, Ross AE et al (2017) Validation of a genomic risk classifier to predict prostate cancer-specific mortality in men with adverse pathologic features. Eur Urol. https://doi.org/10.1016/j.eururo.2017.03.036
106. Den RB, Yousefi K, Trabulsi EJ et al (2015) Genomic classifier identifies men with adverse pathology after radical prostatectomy who benefit from adjuvant radiation therapy. J Clin Oncol 33(8):944–951. https://doi.org/10.1200/JCO.2014.59.0026
107. Ross AE, Den RB, Yousefi K et al (2016) Efficacy of post-operative radiation in a prostatectomy cohort adjusted for clinical and genomic risk. Prostate Cancer Prostatic Dis 19 (3):277–282. https://doi.org/10.1038/pcan.2016.15
108. Gore JL, du Plessis M, Santiago-Jimenez M et al (2017) Decipher test impacts decision making among patients considering adjuvant and salvage treatment after radical prostatectomy: interim results from the multicenter prospective PRO-IMPACT study. Cancer 123 (15):2850–2859. https://doi.org/10.1002/cncr.30665

Liquid Biopsy in Prostate Cancer: Circulating Tumor Cells and Beyond

Daniel Zainfeld and Amir Goldkorn

Contents

Abstract

Prostate cancer is a common malignancy impacting countless men without curative options in the advanced state. Numerous therapies have been introduced

D. Zainfeld · A. Goldkorn (✉)
USC Keck/Norris Comprehensive Cancer Center, Los Angeles, CA, USA
e-mail: agoldkor@med.usc.edu

S. Daneshmand and K. G. Chan (eds.), *Genitourinary Cancers*, Cancer Treatment and Research 175, https://doi.org/10.1007/978-3-319-93339-9_4

in recent years improving survival and symptom control, yet optimal methods for predicting or monitoring response have not been developed. In the era of precision medicine, characterization of individual cancers is necessary to inform treatment decisions. Liquid biopsies, through evaluation of various blood-based analytes, provide a method of patient evaluation with potential applications in virtually all disease states. In this review, we will describe current approaches with a particular focus on demonstrated clinical utility in the evaluation and management of prostate cancer.

Keywords
Prostate cancer · Liquid biopsy · CTCs · cfDNA · Extracellular vesicles
Biomarker

1 Introduction

Prostate cancer is the most common solid malignancy among men worldwide [1]. The prevalence of prostate cancer in combination with a relatively protracted clinical course creates significant need for biomarkers to inform management decisions. Localized prostate cancer treatment options, including active surveillance, surgical excision, or targeted radiation, are made based on individual risk stratification including pathologic characteristics from prostate biopsy, prostate-specific antigen (PSA) level, imaging, and other patient factors [2, 3]. Despite increasing use of advanced imaging modalities, improved biopsy techniques, and development of novel systemic therapies, prostate-specific antigen (PSA) remains the dominant biomarker in clinical use for prostate cancer monitoring. Though controversial in its application for population-based screening due to concerns regarding overtreatment of otherwise indolent cancers, PSA is utilized for monitoring prostate cancer at all stages. Unfortunately, PSA levels often fail to accurately reflect disease burden or activity [4], and multiple therapies impact patient survival and symptoms without corresponding changes in serum PSA levels [5, 6]. As such, an urgent need exists for improved biomarkers that reflect therapy response; as importantly, tumor heterogeneity necessitates effective molecular profiling techniques to guide appropriate therapy selection. “Liquid biopsies” comprised of analytes from a peripheral blood draw offer an appealing modality for comprehensive cancer analysis. These techniques are simple, safe, and easily repeatable throughout disease course and can serve as prognostic and predictive biomarkers as well as ready tissue sources for molecular profiling. Findings from liquid biopsy have capacity to inform treatment decisions at all phases of cancer care from screening to advanced disease states. Liquid biopsy analytes including circulating tumor cells (CTCs), plasma cell-free genetic materials such as cell-free

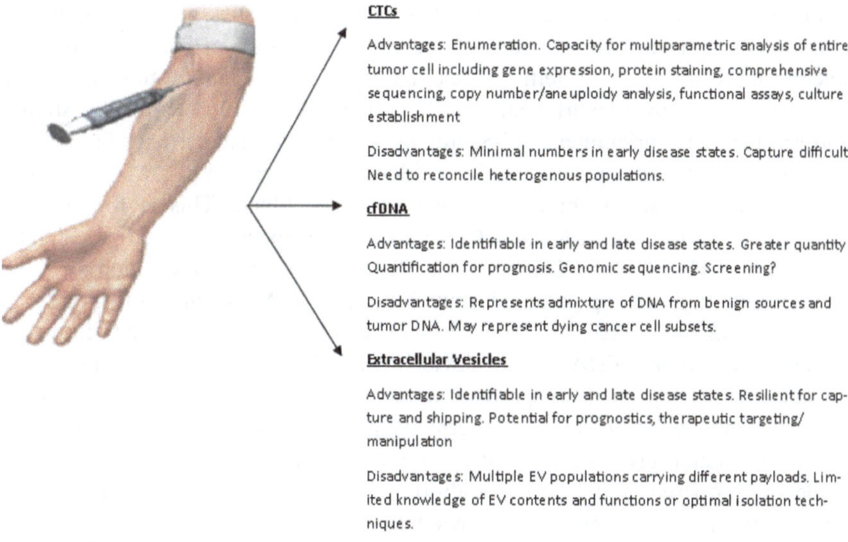

Fig. 1 **Liquid biopsy**. Minimal risk, easily repeatable, low cost, feasible in all patients

RNA and DNA (cfRNA, cfDNA), as well as extracellular vesicles harboring unique cancer-specific materials have each been evaluated in prostate cancer and continue to be developed. Here we examine current applications of these analytes to the evaluation and management of prostate cancer (Fig. 1).

2 Circulating Tumor Cells

2.1 Identification and Enrichment

CTCs are disseminated from a primary or metastatic tumor sites and circulate in the vasculature with potential for distant seeding [7, 8]. These have been identified in the context of virtually all solid malignancies, typically in the advanced state, and conversely are absent in healthy patients [9]. Though clearly essential to the development of metastatic disease which accounts for the majority of cancer-related mortality, the specific mechanisms which drive and enable the proliferation of CTCs remain poorly understood [8, 10]. Although CTCs have been demonstrated to have metastatic potential, not all CTCs are destined to form metastases and additional contributing factors are needed [11]. Nevertheless, the biological and potential clinical value of CTCs is established. CTC capture is technically challenging given their scarcity: usually between 0 and 100, relative to the billions of red and white blood cells within a blood sample [12]. Indeed, though initially recognized almost 200 years ago, only recently has consistent enrichment, identification, and even capture been made possible through technologic advances enabling better understanding of the physical characteristics and phenotypes of CTCs in comparison with other circulating cells [13]. In the evaluation of prostate cancer, the CellSearch system (developed by Janssen Diagnostics, LLC and recently acquired by Menarini-Silicon Biosystems) is the most clinically studied platform for CTC enrichment. CellSearch uses ferrofluid nanoparticles linked with antibodies directed toward epithelial cell adhesion molecule (EpCAM) to separate EpCAM+ cells from the buffy coat of centrifuged blood. This is followed by staining for cytokeratin (CK) and CD45 (leukocyte-specific antigen) to identify CTCs (EpCAM+, CK+, CD45−) [14]. Despite growing appreciation of CTC heterogeneity highlighting potential limitations of EpCAM-dependent identification [15, 16], CellSearch remains the most established platform in the setting of prostate cancer and is the only FDA cleared device for the detection of CTCs in metastatic prostate cancer [17]. It is also approved in the settings of metastatic breast [18] and metastatic colorectal [19] cancers. Alternative platforms isolate cells independent of marker status and rely instead on physical qualities such as size, deformability, or bioelectric properties [20–22]. In an effort to circumvent issues with CTC enrichment platforms have leveraged high-resolution scanning and automated detection algorithms to identify CTCs within whole blood smears or following RBC separation [23, 24]. These systems may prove to better represent total CTC population without regard for physical characteristics or surface antigen expression but limit manipulation and recovery of live cells. It is essential to recognize that all clinical studies must be interpreted with respect to the method of CTC enrichment and identification utilized as this directly impacts the population of cells collected with potentially significant implications. For instance, systems dependent on EpCAM expression fail to capture cancer cells that have undergone epithelial-mesenchymal transition (EMT), a population marked by increased aggressiveness and advanced disease [25]. For the most part, these nuances remain to be explored.

2.2 Clinical Applications of CTCs in Prostate Cancer

2.2.1 Enumeration: CTC Numbers as a Biomarker of Disease Activity

CTC enumeration has been extensively evaluated in localized and advanced prostate cancer states. In localized disease, initial hopes that identification of CTCs may predict disease recurrence were not realized. Davis et al. examined men with localized prostate cancer undergoing radical prostatectomy. Less than 5% had greater than 2 CTCs, and no correlation was found between CTC count and tumor volume, pathological stage, or Gleason score [26]. In another study utilizing the CellSearch enrichment platform, CTCs were detected in just one of twenty patients with high-risk localized prostate cancer (no CTCs were identified in healthy controls) [27]. Overall, CTC detection rates have varied between 5 and 52% in various studies of men with localized prostate cancer [28–31]. No study to date has demonstrated a significant correlation between CTC enumeration and Gleason score, tumor stage or PSA in the pre- or early postoperative time frames. Though enumeration in the localized setting has not proven clinically beneficial, further characterization of CTCs, when identified in this setting, may offer relevant clinical applications as discussed later [30].

More extensive evaluations have been performed in the setting of metastatic prostate cancer wherein ostensibly greater numbers of CTCs may be expected due to increased volume of disseminated cancer. Okegawa et al. found 55% of men with metastatic prostate cancer prior to androgen deprivation therapy to have ≥ 5 CTCs/7.5 ml blood. These men responded to androgen deprivation (by PSA) for just 17 months in comparison with men with ≤ 5 CTCs who responded to ADT for 32 months ($P = 0.007$) [32]. Another study examining this same population by CellSearch found a positive correlation of CTC count with LDH and alkaline phosphatase but not with PSA or testosterone levels. Patients who developed castrate resistance had a median CTC count of 17, while those who did not develop castrate resistance had a median CTC count of 1. On multivariate analysis, only baseline CTC counts were predictive of progression to castration resistance ($P < 0.001$) [33]. Recent evidence supporting the early administration of chemotherapy with hormonal therapy has caused a paradigm shift toward more aggressive initial management of metastatic prostate cancer [34, 35]. Given the demonstrated capacity of CTCs to predict time to castration resistance in this disease state, CTCs may prove beneficial for identifying those patients most likely to benefit from early chemotherapy.

In the castration-resistant setting, the prognostic capacity of CTCs has been most well established. In one of the seminal clinical studies of CTCs in prostate cancer, De Bono et al. enumerated CTCs using CellSearch. A total of 276 men with metastatic castrate-resistant disease prior to initiation of new therapy were enrolled with subsequent evaluation of 231. CTC counts were categorized as favorable (<5 CTCs/7.5 ml blood) and unfavorable (>5 CTCs/7.5 ml blood). CTCs were identified in 219/231 (95%) men at baseline demonstrating the prevalence of CTCs in this advanced disease state. Stratified in this manner, unfavorable initial CTC counts were associated with shorter overall survival (median 11.5 vs. 21.7 months) and outperformed PSA algorithms at all time points. In addition, patients with initially unfavorable CTC counts who converted to favorable counts with treatment experienced similar improvements in median survival (6.8–21.3 months) demonstrating the capacity for CTCs to reflect response to therapy in these patients [17]. Subsequently, the prognostic efficacy of CTCs has been explored in the context of various other systemic treatments for advanced prostate cancer including docetaxel, abiraterone, enzalutamide, and various combinations consistently demonstrating an association with overall survival that rivals or surpasses that of PSA monitoring alone [36–38].

CTC enumeration has not been quickly adopted to clinical practice. Though effective in prognostication, no study to date has demonstrated ability to directly inform management and thereby alter patient outcomes. Increasingly, however, the potential to use CTC counts as surrogate endpoints in clinical trials where they may facilitate shorter trial duration and associated costs is being explored. In evaluating results of COU-AA-301, a large phase III trial of abiraterone plus prednisone versus prednisone alone in patients with mCRPC, Scher et al. found CTC count in combination with lactate dehydrogenase (LDH) level predictive of overall survival at two years [38]. These two measures together met all Prentice criteria required for use as a surrogate endpoint for overall survival [39].

2.2.2 Liquid Biopsy in Practice: Identifying Phenotypes Through CTC Characterization

Simple enumeration of CTCs, while correlated with disease burden, response to treatments, and prognostic among men with advanced prostate cancer, does not capitalize on the nature of CTCs as components of relevant, viable tumor tissue. Characterization of these cells therefore has the capacity to illuminate aspects of individual patient molecular profiles and guide treatment choices even in the localized setting where simple enumeration lacked prognostic significance. Pal et al. performed immunohistochemical staining on enriched CTCs for CD133 (a putative stem-cell marker) and E-cadherin (a marker of epithelial-mesenchymal transition) finding an association between expression of these markers of aggression and biochemical recurrence at one year following prostatectomy in the localized setting, a disease state wherein total enumeration of CTCs was not predictive [30]. Goldkorn et al. evaluated telomerase activity in CTCs in a corollary study of SWOG 0421 (docetaxel with atrasentan versus docetaxel alone in CRPC patients). CTC telomerase activity was prognostic of overall survival in this setting. Though many potential targets for CTC characterization exist, clinical studies have focused on the androgen receptor (AR) given its central role in hormonal therapies for advanced prostate cancer. Immunofluorescent staining of AR on CTCs to determine cellular localization (nuclear vs cytoplasmic) has been linked to chemotherapy response and clinical disease progression on abiraterone [40, 41]. Likewise, classification of AR as "on" vs "off" by immunofluorescent staining identified differences in CTC profiles of hormone-naïve patients and those who had progressed to CRPC [42]. More recently, ligand-independent AR splice variants have been found to play a role in resistance to second-generation antiandrogen therapies enzalutamide and abiraterone [43]. Antonarakis et al. used quantitative reverse-transcriptase polymerase chain reaction (PCR) to evaluate AR-V7 expression in CTCs of men with CRPC. Men with AR-V7 expression had significantly lower PSA response rates, progression-free survival (PFS), and overall survival when treated with enzalutamide or abiraterone, suggesting a possible means of predicting response to these therapies through CTC profiling [44–46]. The association is not entirely clear, however, as other groups have demonstrated clinical response to abiraterone or enzalutamide despite AR-V7 positivity in CTCs [47]. Greater depth of characterization by identifying cellular location of AR-V7 protein may enhance predictive capacity as demonstrated by Scher et al. In their study, nuclear localization of AR-V7 protein was the strongest baseline factor influencing overall survival even in comparison with AR-V7 positive cells without localization [48]. Heterogeneity among these cells and tumors including alterations in specific signaling pathways have been shown to contribute to variable responses through RNA sequencing of single CTCs [49]. Whole-genome and exome sequencing of CTCs from men with prostate cancer has been completed demonstrating a strong capacity for CTC evaluation to recapitulate primary tumor mutations, thus furthering potential clinical applications of CTC analysis [50, 51]. Ongoing work to capture pure CTC samples and better characterize clinical implications of specific CTC characteristics in light of known heterogeneity will enable meaningful application of CTC analysis to patient care (Table 1).

Table 1 Select examples of AR-V7 detection in clinical studies

References	Analyte	Patients analyzed (n)	Method	Findings
Antonarakis et al. [44, 45, 97]	CTCs	62 and 37	RT-PCR to evaluate AR-V7 transcripts in CTCs among men receiving second-generation hormonal therapy or taxane chemotherapy [45, 97]	AR-V7 expression associated with lower PSA response, PFS, and OS among men receiving enzalutamide or abiraterone. Men found AR-V7+ better response to chemotherapy in comparison with antiandrogens
Scher et al. [46, 48]	CTCs	161	Immunofluorescent staining of CTCs for AR-V7 protein [46] with additional evaluation for nuclear-specific signal localization [48]	CTCs expressing AR-V7 found in 34 (18%) samples using nuclear-specific criteria, 56 (29%) without nuclear criteria. AR-V7 associated with resistance to hormonal therapy, decreased PFS, shorter OS among those with nuclear localization of AR-V7+ indicating role for chemotherapy selection
Liu et al. [76]	RNA and CTCs	46	Comparison of PAXgene preserved RNA versus leukocyte depletion and CTC analysis	AR-V7 detected in 68% of samples. Increased expression associated with receipt of second-line hormonal therapies
De Laere [73]	CTCs	30	Low-pass whole-genome sequencing of ctDNA and targeted sequencing of AR gene. Splice variant analysis from CTC RNA	AR alterations identified in 25/30 patients and associated with PFS. AR-V7 negativity more prevalent among poor responders
Del Re et al. [92]	Exosomes	36	Exosomes isolated and RNA extracted for analysis	39% of patients AR-V7+. AR-V7 associated with longer PFS (20 vs. 3 months, $p < 0.001$) and OS (8 months vs. not reached, $p < 0.001$)

3 Plasma Cell-Free Genomic Materials

3.1 Identification

Fragments of DNA circulating freely in the bloodstream are termed cell-free DNA. In the presence of malignancies, the fraction of cell-free DNA (cfDNA) derived from cancerous cells (primary tumor, metastatic sites, or CTCs) is alternatively identified as circulating tumor DNA (ctDNA). cfDNA may be released through a variety of natural and pathologic processes including apoptosis, necrosis, or even physiologic release from viable cells [52–54]. Healthy individuals have cfDNA levels of 1–10 ng/ml [55, 56], whereas cfDNA levels, though greatly variable, are consistently elevated among cancer patients [57, 58]. The role of benign processes in impacting cfDNA levels is significant as intense exercise alone can increase cfDNA levels as can trauma, infections, and inflammatory conditions [59]. cfDNA has been identified in almost all bodily fluids including urine [53]. These DNA fragments can be quantified and analyzed to offer insights regarding prognosis, response to therapy, and tumor mutational status. Identification of the source of DNA fragments is difficult given varied possible sources. Therefore, isolating small fractions of ctDNA within total cfDNA demands highly sensitive approaches targeting specific gene alterations, chromosomal abnormalities, epigenetic alterations or other characteristics to identify the cancerous source [60]. Digital droplet PCR (ddPCR) and associated methods have proven sensitive and can perform well in absolute quantification of ctDNA detecting point mutations at low allele frequencies [54, 58–61]. More recently, next-generation sequencing (NGS) of circulating DNA fragments has allowed comprehensive genomic profiling [62]. The short half-life of cfDNA (<2.5 h) allows accurate characterization of real-time tumor profiles [58, 63]. Extensive clinical evaluations are ongoing to better understand cfDNA and relevance to cancer care. Evaluation of circulating RNA has been performed as well but requires special approaches to collection due to generally quick physiologic degradation of cfRNA. Early studies evaluating cfDNA and ctDNA in the setting of prostate cancer have demonstrated potential for promising clinical applications.

3.2 Clinical Applications of cfDNA in Prostate Cancer

Quantification of cfDNA, especially in the context of temporal changes, offers a means of evaluating tumor burden and response to therapy. A retrospective study analyzed the prognostic significance of cfDNA concentration among men with CRPC prior to initiating chemotherapy and found elevated cfDNA concentration to be associated with poor PSA response and to act as an independent predictor of overall survival on multivariate analysis [64]. Likewise, analysis of cfDNA levels in men with CRPC during chemotherapy in conjunction with serial imaging for treatment response monitoring demonstrated a significant positive relationship between cfDNA levels and tumoral activity as determined by PET/CT [65]. Just as

CTC enumeration reflects disease burden and prognosis, ctDNA quantification can reveal disease burden with potentially even greater sensitivity. By applying an immunospot assay for CTC detection and a PCR-based analysis with a panel of 14 polymorphic markers for detection of allelic imbalances on cfDNA, researchers found a significant relationship between the presence of CTCs and ctDNA levels with meaningful correlation to both tumor stage and Gleason score [66].

The specific relationship of cfDNA and ctDNA concentrations to prognosis remains to be fully defined given evolving techniques for detection. However, in-depth evaluation of these analytes has provided meaningful insights into individual cancer biology with potential therapeutic implications. Examination of cfDNA can demonstrate copy number variations or mutational status of relevant genes for treatment selection. Heitzer et al. completed whole-genome sequencing of cfDNA from patients with advanced prostate cancer and identified multiple copy number alterations and gene rearrangements with potential clinical significance. Most importantly, sequencing of cfDNA demonstrated a capacity to recapitulate the "genomic landscape" of prostate cancer in a more comprehensive fashion than even evaluation of the primary tumor which showed variable copy number changes on multiregional sequencing consistent with multifocal disease [67].

As with CTCs, evaluation of the AR among prostate cancer patients is essential due to its critical role in current treatments and known clinical relevance of various mutations [68]. One study examining CRPC patients undergoing treatment with abiraterone found a significant association between gains of AR copy number or CYP17A1 gene and survival outcomes when evaluating cfDNA prior to treatment [69]. Another group using array comparative genomic hybridization for copy number analysis found AR amplification to be much more common among patients with disease progression on enzalutamide in comparison with those on abiraterone or other treatments. In addition, AR gene aberrations in pretreatment cfDNA were predictive of adverse outcomes including lower rate of PSA decline and shorter time to progression [70]. Likewise, Romanel et al. performed targeted NGS on cfDNA of patients with CRPC receiving treatment with abiraterone and identified plasma DNA AR copy number gains and point mutations that predicted resistance to abiraterone, overall survival, and progression-free survival [71]. Further, emergence of new AR point mutations was identified in 13% of patients progressing on abiraterone without AR copy number change [71]. Therefore, evaluation of AR status prior to treatments can be useful in predicting response to therapy.

cfDNA analysis, due to safety and easy accessibility, lends itself to temporal evaluations not generally feasible when restricted to traditional tissue biopsies. Comparative genomic hybridization for copy number evaluation and sequencing of the AR gene among men treated with enzalutamide revealed clonal selection over the course of treatment. At time of progression, AR mutations or copy number changes were identified in all patients [72]. As in earlier studies, AR amplifications and mutations correlated with worse progression-free survival. De Leare et al. completed comprehensive profiling of the AR from ctDNA of men with CRPC evaluating for any AR perturbation. They identified abnormalities in 25/30 patients and found an association between presence of any AR variant and progression-free survival (PFS). They also analyzed splice variant expression from CTC RNA. Of a minority of poor responding patients who were AR-V7 negative, most were found to have other AR abnormalities [73].

As noted, analysis of whole blood RNA is limited by quick degradation but has been performed with assistance of preservative tubes (e.g., PaxGene, Qiagen; RNA Streck, Streck Inc.). Microarray RNA profiles allowed creation of gene expression signatures which demonstrated prognostic utility in CRPC patients from blood collected in PaxGene tubes [74, 75]. Another study using PaxGene tubes examined select gene expression in men with CRPC by RT-PCR. Transcript detection predicted overall survival and when combined with CTC enumeration had a high concordance probability estimate suggesting potential additive value in liquid biopsy analytes. Liu et al. determined capacity to evaluate AR-V7 expression from PaxGene® preserved blood samples with a correlation to second-line hormonal therapies as demonstrated previously in CTCs [76]. Each of these studies required special attention to the prevention of RNA degradation. Micro RNAs (miRNAs) are small noncoding RNA segments with roles in gene regulation. Known to be altered in virtually all cancers and marked by great stability, miRNAs are now being explored as biomarkers in prostate cancer [77]. Lin et al. identified fourteen miRNAs associated with serum PSA or overall survival among patients with CRPC receiving docetaxel. Detection of high levels of the miR-200 family predicted non-response to docetaxel [78]. Despite these promising early results, further validation in clinical studies is needed prior to clinical applications.

Excitement regarding potential applications of cfDNA analysis must be tempered in light of significant remaining challenges. For instance, in one study modification of sequencing approach enabled identification of multiple new AR mutations with functional characterizations from cfDNA not originally identified highlighting the importance of analytic approach on subsequent findings [79]. In addition, prevalence of false-positive mutations using NGS for low-abundance mutations highlights the need for optimization and standardization of these tests prior to application for clinical decision-making [80]. However, like CTC analysis, cfDNA offers exciting avenues of continued exploration including early disease detection, screening, and disease monitoring. Recent FDA approval of a targeted mutation test from cfDNA (cobas® EGFR Mutation Test v2, Roche Molecular Systems, Inc.) to determine eligibility for specific lung cancer therapy exemplifies the potential applications of cfDNA and the steady drive toward clinical utility which will certainly reach prostate cancer in the near future [81].

4 Extracellular Vesicles (EVs)

4.1 Overview and Preclinical Studies in Prostate Cancer

Increasing clinical interest has been directed to the identification and evaluation of EVs in many disease states including prostate cancer. EVs range in size from 50 nm to 10 μm and are produced by virtually all cells [82]. Appreciation of the unique characteristics and functional roles of various EV populations has grown with mounting evidence demonstrating cell specific vesicular contents as well as roles in intercellular signaling [82–84]. Contrary to early descriptions of EVs as cellular waste, they are now recognized to represent a heterogenous population unique in size, content, and mechanism of cellular release with variable biologic functions. Exosomes, perhaps the most studied EV subtype to date, measure 50–100 nm in diameter and originate from fusion of multivesicular bodies with the plasma membrane [85]. Alternatively, ectosomes and large oncosomes (1–10 μm) originate as direct buds off the plasma membrane which is relevant to isolation and analysis techniques. Each of these vesicles harbors cargo specific to their cells of origin including DNA, RNA, proteins and lipids [86]. While exosomes may originate from both benign and malignant cells, large oncosomes are thought to originate preferentially from malignant cells [87]. Each may supply unique biomarkers due to their highly selective cargos.

Techniques for EV isolation must be tailored to the specific vesicle of interest and continue to be refined. Traditional methods have relied on differential ultracentrifugation, and this remains the gold standard means of isolating EVs. Ultrafiltration- and immunoaffinity-based approaches may prove beneficial due to less technical demands and capacity for improved throughput and scalability. Given recent findings regarding heterogeneity of EVs, appropriate identification and confirmation of particles of interest is essential [88]. Just as for CTC and cfDNA analysis, therefore, clinical results should be interpreted with an eye to method of isolation and purification.

In preclinical settings EVs have been found to exhibit promising potential applications as prostate cancer biomarkers. Examination of EVs from prostate cancer cell lines allows for study of the vesicles in a comparatively pure media as opposed to the diverse milieu of human blood. One group examining EVs from prostate cancer cell lines found high expression levels of surface markers of aggressiveness that were not found in less aggressive lines suggesting capacity to identify specific tumor-derived EVs as well as to function as biomarkers of disease aggression [87, 89]. Other groups have noted alterations in exosome abundance within cell lines following acquisition of resistance to chemotherapy indicating a role for exosome monitoring for detection of drug resistance in addition to potential functional involvement in that process [90]. As EVs are identified and purified with greater consistency, recognition of their differential content and make-ups will enable continued meaningful interpretation and translational applications.

4.2 Clinical Applications of Extracellular Vesicles in Prostate Cancer

Limited trials analyzing EVs in clinical studies have been completed, especially from plasma. Huang et al. performed RNA sequencing of exosomal RNA in men with CRPC and identified two exosomal miRNAs associated with overall survival that they subsequently validated in a larger cohort of patients. miR-1290 and miR-375 were each associated with poor overall survival ($p < 0.004$) demonstrating potential application for exosome analysis [91]. Detection of AR-V7 has been accomplished in exosomal RNA. Del Re et al. extracted RNA from plasma-derived exosomes of CRPC patients and assessed for the presence of AR-V7 by digital PCR. Thirty-nine percent of patients were found AR-V7+ with significantly shorter overall survival among that subset [92]. Validation and comparative studies are required, yet the significant potential of extracellular vesicles as a meaningful liquid biopsy analyte is clear. Many studies have focused on the utility of urinary exosomes or other urinary markers to facilitate improved prostate cancer diagnosis, staging, and prognostication with variable results as well [93–96]. In one study, a prognostic score was developed by comparing urinary exosome gene expression assay by reverse-transcriptase PCR with biopsy outcomes in men with elevated PSAs. The three-gene assay including ERG, SPDEF, and PCA3 was validated in a larger cohort and improved discrimination among Gleason scores and benign disease demonstrating a viable method for determining need of biopsy in that setting [96]. Continued evolution in the differential detection and analysis of EVs will enable further characterization of their roles in prostate cancer signaling, implications for prognosis, prediction of therapeutic response, and clinical application.

5 Summary

The absence of sensitive and accurate biomarkers in the prostate cancer arena has limited clinicians to depend on PSA for disease monitoring and biopsy from primary or metastatic sites for genomic characterization with clear shortcomings. Liquid biopsies are noninvasive, easily repeatable and harbor significant cancer and patient-specific data that, when captured, may provide a near comprehensive representation of individual patients' disease state throughout therapy. Many barriers and challenges remain prior to common clinical use. Optimization of identification, recovery, and analytic approaches is ongoing, and scaling of these approaches and integration to clinical use while maintaining accuracy and precision are challenging. Prospective clinical studies will enable interpretation of detected abnormalities in context of traditional biopsy findings, and various therapeutic settings but optimal applications remain unclear at this time. As seen in AR-V7 evaluation, information gleaned through examination of various available blood analytes may overlap or offer additive value. Therefore, reconciliation through evaluation in the context of translational studies with attention to costs and technical issues is essential when assessing for broad clinical use. Great progress has been made toward establishing applications for liquid biopsy in the clinical care of prostate cancer. Though still limited at this time, liquid biopsies will play a significant role in the care of prostate cancer patients in the near future with direct applications from the level of screening to delivery of precision care in the advanced metastatic state.

References

1. Siegel RL, Miller KD, Jemal A (2016) Cancer statistics, 2016. CA Cancer J Clin 66(1):7–30
2. Aizer AA, Chen M-H, Hattangadi J, D'Amico AV (2014) Initial management of prostate-specific antigen-detected, low-risk prostate cancer and the risk of death from prostate cancer. BJU Int 113(1):43–50
3. Simpkin AJ, Tilling K, Martin RM, Lane JA, Hamdy FC, Holmberg L et al (2015) Systematic review and meta-analysis of factors determining change to radical treatment in active surveillance for localized prostate cancer. Eur Urol 67(6):993–1005
4. Crawford ED, Bennett CL, Andriole GL, Garnick MB, Petrylak DP (2013) The utility of prostate-specific antigen in the management of advanced prostate cancer. BJU Int 112(5): 548–560
5. Kantoff PW, Higano CS, Shore ND, Berger ER, Small EJ, Penson DF et al (2010) Sipuleucel-T immunotherapy for castration-resistant prostate cancer. N Engl J Med 363(5): 411–422
6. Nome R, Hernes E, Bogsrud TV, Bjøro T, Fosså SD (2015) Changes in prostate-specific antigen, markers of bone metabolism and bone scans after treatment with radium-223. Scand J Urol. 49(3):211–217
7. Paget S (1989) The distribution of secondary growths in cancer of the breast. 1889. Cancer Metastasis Rev 8(2):98–101
8. Steeg PS (2006) Tumor metastasis: mechanistic insights and clinical challenges. Nat Med 12(8):895–904
9. Allard WJ, Matera J, Miller MC, Repollet M, Connelly MC, Rao C et al (2004) Tumor cells circulate in the peripheral blood of all major carcinomas but not in healthy subjects or patients with nonmalignant diseases. Clin Cancer Res Off J Am Assoc Cancer Res. 10(20):6897–6904
10. Gupta GP, Massagué J (2006) Cancer metastasis: building a framework. Cell 127(4):679–695
11. Shen MM (2015) Cancer: the complex seeds of metastasis. Nature 520(7547):298–299
12. Alix-Panabières C, Pantel K (2014) Technologies for detection of circulating tumor cells: facts and vision. Lab Chip 14(1):57–62
13. Ashworth T (1869) A case of cancer in which cells similar to those in the tumors were seen in the blood after death. Aust Med J 14:146–147
14. Ignatiadis M, Lee M, Jeffrey SS (2015) Circulating tumor cells and circulating tumor DNA: challenges and opportunities on the path to clinical utility. Clin Cancer Res Off J Am Assoc Cancer Res 21(21):4786–4800
15. Thiery JP (2002) Epithelial-mesenchymal transitions in tumour progression. Nat Rev Cancer 2(6):442–454
16. Mikolajczyk SD, Millar LS, Tsinberg P, Coutts SM, Zomorrodi M, Pham T et al (2011) Detection of EpCAM-negative and cytokeratin-negative circulating tumor cells in peripheral blood. J Oncol 2011:252361
17. de Bono JS, Scher HI, Montgomery RB, Parker C, Miller MC, Tissing H et al (2008) Circulating tumor cells predict survival benefit from treatment in metastatic castration-resistant prostate cancer. Clin Cancer Res Off J Am Assoc Cancer Res. 14(19): 6302–6309
18. Hayes DF, Cristofanilli M, Budd GT, Ellis MJ, Stopeck A, Miller MC et al (2006) Circulating tumor cells at each follow-up time point during therapy of metastatic breast cancer patients predict progression-free and overall survival. Clin Cancer Res Off J Am Assoc Cancer Res 12(14 Pt 1):4218–4224
19. Cohen SJ, Punt CJA, Iannotti N, Saidman BH, Sabbath KD, Gabrail NY et al (2008) Relationship of circulating tumor cells to tumor response, progression-free survival, and overall survival in patients with metastatic colorectal cancer. J Clin Oncol Off J Am Soc Clin Oncol 26(19):3213–3221
20. Karabacak NM, Spuhler PS, Fachin F, Lim EJ, Pai V, Ozkumur E et al (2014) Microfluidic, marker-free isolation of circulating tumor cells from blood samples. Nat Protoc 9(3):694–710

21. Gupta V, Jafferji I, Garza M, Melnikova VO, Hasegawa DK, Pethig R et al (2012) ApoStream^{TM}, a new dielectrophoretic device for antibody independent isolation and recovery of viable cancer cells from blood. Biomicrofluidics 6(2):24133
22. Ferreira MM, Ramani VC, Jeffrey SS (2016) Circulating tumor cell technologies. Mol Oncol 10(3):374–394
23. Epic Sciences [Internet]. Retrieved from http://www.epicsciences.com/what-we-do/technology-overview
24. Campton DE, Ramirez AB, Nordberg JJ, Drovetto N, Clein AC, Varshavskaya P et al (2015) High-recovery visual identification and single-cell retrieval of circulating tumor cells for genomic analysis using a dual-technology platform integrated with automated immunofluorescence staining. BMC Cancer 6(15):360
25. Ring A, Mineyev N, Zhu W, Park E, Lomas C, Punj V et al (2015) EpCAM based capture detects and recovers circulating tumor cells from all subtypes of breast cancer except claudin-low. Oncotarget 6(42):44623–44634
26. Davis JW, Nakanishi H, Kumar VS, Bhadkamkar VA, McCormack R, Fritsche HA et al (2008) Circulating tumor cells in peripheral blood samples from patients with increased serum prostate specific antigen: initial results in early prostate cancer. J Urol 179(6):2187–2191; discussion 2191
27. Thalgott M, Rack B, Maurer T, Souvatzoglou M, Eiber M, Kreß V et al (2013) Detection of circulating tumor cells in different stages of prostate cancer. J Cancer Res Clin Oncol 139 (5):755–763
28. Stott SL, Lee RJ, Nagrath S, Yu M, Miyamoto DT, Ulkus L et al (2010) Isolation and characterization of circulating tumor cells from patients with localized and metastatic prostate cancer. Sci Transl Med 2(25):25ra23
29. Kolostova K, Broul M, Schraml J, Cegan M, Matkowski R, Fiutowski M et al (2014) Circulating tumor cells in localized prostate cancer: isolation, cultivation in vitro and relationship to T-stage and Gleason score. Anticancer Res 34(7):3641–3646
30. Pal SK, He M, Wilson T, Liu X, Zhang K, Carmichael C et al (2015) Detection and phenotyping of circulating tumor cells in high-risk localized prostate cancer. Clin Genitourin Cancer 13(2):130–136
31. Meyer CP, Pantel K, Tennstedt P, Stroelin P, Schlomm T, Heinzer H et al (2016) Limited prognostic value of preoperative circulating tumor cells for early biochemical recurrence in patients with localized prostate cancer. Urol Oncol 34(5):235.e11–e16
32. Okegawa T, Nutahara K, Higashihara E (2008) Immunomagnetic quantification of circulating tumor cells as a prognostic factor of androgen deprivation responsiveness in patients with hormone naive metastatic prostate cancer. J Urol 180(4):1342–1347
33. Goodman OB, Symanowski JT, Loudyi A, Fink LM, Ward DC, Vogelzang NJ (2011) Circulating tumor cells as a predictive biomarker in patients with hormone-sensitive prostate cancer. Clin Genitourin Cancer 9(1):31–38
34. Sweeney CJ, Chen Y-H, Carducci M, Liu G, Jarrard DF, Eisenberger M et al (2015) Chemohormonal therapy in metastatic hormone-sensitive prostate cancer. N Engl J Med 373 (8):737–746
35. James ND, Sydes MR, Clarke NW, Mason MD, Dearnaley DP, Spears MR et al (2016) Addition of docetaxel, zoledronic acid, or both to first-line long-term hormone therapy in prostate cancer (STAMPEDE): survival results from an adaptive, multiarm, multistage, platform randomised controlled trial. Lancet Lond Engl 387(10024):1163–1177
36. Danila DC, Anand A, Sung CC, Heller G, Leversha MA, Cao L et al (2011) TMPRSS2-ERG status in circulating tumor cells as a predictive biomarker of sensitivity in castration-resistant prostate cancer patients treated with abiraterone acetate. Eur Urol 60(5):897–904
37. Goldkorn A, Ely B, Quinn DI, Tangen CM, Fink LM, Xu T et al (2014) Circulating tumor cell counts are prognostic of overall survival in SWOG S0421: a phase III trial of docetaxel with or without atrasentan for metastatic castration-resistant prostate cancer. J Clin Oncol Off J Am Soc Clin Oncol 32(11):1136–1142

38. Scher HI, Heller G, Molina A, Attard G, Danila DC, Jia X et al (2015) Circulating tumor cell biomarker panel as an individual-level surrogate for survival in metastatic castration-resistant prostate cancer. J Clin Oncol Off J Am Soc Clin Oncol 33(12):1348–1355
39. Berger VW (2004) Does the Prentice criterion validate surrogate endpoints? Stat Med 23(10): 1571–1578
40. Darshan MS, Loftus MS, Thadani-Mulero M, Levy BP, Escuin D, Zhou XK et al (2011) Taxane-induced blockade to nuclear accumulation of the androgen receptor predicts clinical responses in metastatic prostate cancer. Cancer Res 71(18):6019–6029
41. Crespo M, van Dalum G, Ferraldeschi R, Zafeiriou Z, Sideris S, Lorente D et al (2015) Androgen receptor expression in circulating tumour cells from castration-resistant prostate cancer patients treated with novel endocrine agents. Br J Cancer 112(7):1166–1174
42. Miyamoto DT, Lee RJ, Stott SL, Ting DT, Wittner BS, Ulman M et al (2012) Androgen receptor signaling in circulating tumor cells as a marker of hormonally responsive prostate cancer. Cancer Discov 2(11):995–1003
43. Qu Y, Dai B, Ye D, Kong Y, Chang K, Jia Z et al (2015) Constitutively active AR-V7 plays an essential role in the development and progression of castration-resistant prostate cancer. Sci Rep 7(5):7654
44. Antonarakis ES, Lu C, Wang H, Luber B, Nakazawa M, Roeser JC et al (2014) AR-V7 and resistance to enzalutamide and abiraterone in prostate cancer. N Engl J Med 371(11): 1028–1038
45. Antonarakis ES, Lu C, Luber B, Wang H, Chen Y, Zhu Y et al (2017) Clinical significance of androgen receptor splice variant-7 mRNA detection in circulating tumor cells of men with metastatic castration-resistant prostate cancer treated with first- and second-line abiraterone and enzalutamide. J Clin Oncol Off J Am Soc Clin Oncol JCO2016701961
46. Scher HI, Lu D, Schreiber NA, Louw J, Graf RP, Vargas HA et al (2016) Association of AR-V7 on Circulating tumor cells as a treatment-specific biomarker with outcomes and survival in castration-resistant prostate cancer. JAMA Oncol
47. Bernemann C, Schnoeller TJ, Luedeke M, Steinestel K, Boegemann M, Schrader AJ et al (2017) Expression of AR-V7 in circulating tumour cells does not preclude response to next generation androgen deprivation therapy in patients with castration resistant prostate cancer. Eur Urol 71(1):1–3
48. Scher HI, Graf RP, Schreiber NA, McLaughlin B, Lu D, Louw J et al (2017) Nuclear-specific AR-V7 protein localization is necessary to guide treatment selection in metastatic castration-resistant prostate cancer. Eur Urol 71(6):874–882
49. Miyamoto DT, Zheng Y, Wittner BS, Lee RJ, Zhu H, Broderick KT et al (2015) RNA-Seq of single prostate CTCs implicates noncanonical Wnt signaling in antiandrogen resistance. Science 349(6254):1351–1356
50. Lohr JG, Adalsteinsson VA, Cibulskis K, Choudhury AD, Rosenberg M, Cruz-Gordillo P et al (2014) Whole-exome sequencing of circulating tumor cells provides a window into metastatic prostate cancer. Nat Biotechnol 32(5):479–484
51. Jiang R, Lu Y-T, Ho H, Li B, Chen J-F, Lin M et al (2015) A comparison of isolated circulating tumor cells and tissue biopsies using whole-genome sequencing in prostate cancer. Oncotarget 6(42):44781–44793
52. Kidess E, Jeffrey SS (2013) Circulating tumor cells versus tumor-derived cell-free DNA: rivals or partners in cancer care in the era of single-cell analysis? Genome Med 5(8):70
53. Alix-Panabières C, Pantel K (2016) Clinical applications of circulating tumor cells and circulating tumor DNA as liquid biopsy. Cancer Discov 6(5):479–491
54. Elshimali YI, Khaddour H, Sarkissyan M, Wu Y, Vadgama JV (2013) The clinical utilization of circulating cell free DNA (CCFDNA) in blood of cancer patients. Int J Mol Sci 14(9): 18925–18958
55. Mouliere F, Rosenfeld N (2015) Circulating tumor-derived DNA is shorter than somatic DNA in plasma. Proc Natl Acad Sci U S A 112(11):3178–3179

56. Wan JCM, Massie C, Garcia-Corbacho J, Mouliere F, Brenton JD, Caldas C et al (2017) Liquid biopsies come of age: towards implementation of circulating tumour DNA. Nat Rev Cancer 17(4):223–238
57. Dawson S-J, Tsui DWY, Murtaza M, Biggs H, Rueda OM, Chin S-F et al (2013) Analysis of circulating tumor DNA to monitor metastatic breast cancer. N Engl J Med 368(13):1199–1209
58. Diehl F, Schmidt K, Choti MA, Romans K, Goodman S, Li M et al (2008) Circulating mutant DNA to assess tumor dynamics. Nat Med 14(9):985–990
59. Tug S, Helmig S, Deichmann ER, Schmeier-Jürchott A, Wagner E, Zimmermann T et al (2015) Exercise-induced increases in cell free DNA in human plasma originate predominantly from cells of the haematopoietic lineage. Exerc Immunol Rev 21:164–173
60. Swarup V, Rajeswari MR (2007) Circulating (cell-free) nucleic acids—a promising, non-invasive tool for early detection of several human diseases. FEBS Lett 581(5):795–799
61. Heitzer E, Ulz P, Geigl JB (2015) Circulating tumor DNA as a liquid biopsy for cancer. Clin Chem 61(1):112–123
62. Ignatiadis M, Dawson S-J (2014) Circulating tumor cells and circulating tumor DNA for precision medicine: dream or reality? Ann Oncol Off J Eur Soc Med Oncol 25(12):2304–2313
63. Yao W, Mei C, Nan X, Hui L (2016) Evaluation and comparison of in vitro degradation kinetics of DNA in serum, urine and saliva: a qualitative study. Gene 590(1):142–148
64. Kienel A, Porres D, Heidenreich A, Pfister D (2015) cfDNA as a prognostic marker of response to taxane based chemotherapy in patients with prostate cancer. J Urol 194(4): 966–971
65. Kwee S, Song M-A, Cheng I, Loo L, Tiirikainen M (2012) Measurement of circulating cell-free DNA in relation to 18F-fluorocholine PET/CT imaging in chemotherapy-treated advanced prostate cancer. Clin Transl Sci 5(1):65–70
66. Schwarzenbach H, Hoon DSB, Pantel K (2011) Cell-free nucleic acids as biomarkers in cancer patients. Nat Rev Cancer 11(6):426–437
67. Heitzer E, Ulz P, Belic J, Gutschi S, Quehenberger F, Fischereder K et al (2013) Tumor-associated copy number changes in the circulation of patients with prostate cancer identified through whole-genome sequencing. Genome Med 5(4):30
68. Schmidt LJ, Tindall DJ (2013) Androgen receptor: past, present and future. Curr Drug Targets 14(4):401–407
69. Salvi S, Casadio V, Conteduca V, Burgio SL, Menna C, Bianchi E et al (2015) Circulating cell-free AR and CYP17A1 copy number variations may associate with outcome of metastatic castration-resistant prostate cancer patients treated with abiraterone. Br J Cancer 112(10): 1717–1724
70. Azad AA, Volik SV, Wyatt AW, Haegert A, Le Bihan S, Bell RH et al (2015) Androgen receptor gene aberrations in circulating cell-free DNA: biomarkers of therapeutic resistance in castration-resistant prostate cancer. Clin Cancer Res Off J Am Assoc Cancer Res 21(10): 2315–2324
71. Romanel A, Gasi Tandefelt D, Conteduca V, Jayaram A, Casiraghi N, Wetterskog D et al (2015) Plasma AR and abiraterone-resistant prostate cancer. Sci Transl Med. 7(312):312re10
72. Wyatt AW, Azad AA, Volik SV, Annala M, Beja K, McConeghy B et al (2016) Genomic alterations in cell-free DNA and enzalutamide resistance in castration-resistant prostate cancer. JAMA Oncol 2(12):1598–1606
73. De Laere B, van Dam P-J, Whitington T, Mayrhofer M, Diaz EH, Van den Eynden G et al (2017) Comprehensive profiling of the androgen receptor in liquid biopsies from castration-resistant prostate cancer reveals novel intra-AR structural variation and splice variant expression patterns. Eur Urol
74. Olmos D, Brewer D, Clark J, Danila DC, Parker C, Attard G et al (2012) Prognostic value of blood mRNA expression signatures in castration-resistant prostate cancer: a prospective, two-stage study. Lancet Oncol 13(11):1114–1124

75. Ross RW, Galsky MD, Scher HI, Magidson J, Wassmann K, Lee G-SM et al (2012) A whole-blood RNA transcript-based prognostic model in men with castration-resistant prostate cancer: a prospective study. Lancet Oncol 13(11):1105–1113
76. Liu X, Ledet E, Li D, Dotiwala A, Steinberger A, Feibus A et al (2016) A whole blood assay for AR-V7 and AR(v567es) in patients with prostate cancer. J Urol 196(6):1758–1763
77. Cortez MA, Bueso-Ramos C, Ferdin J, Lopez-Berestein G, Sood AK, Calin GA (2011) MicroRNAs in body fluids—the mix of hormones and biomarkers. Nat Rev Clin Oncol 8(8): 467–477
78. Lin H-M, Castillo L, Mahon KL, Chiam K, Lee BY, Nguyen Q et al (2014) Circulating microRNAs are associated with docetaxel chemotherapy outcome in castration-resistant prostate cancer. Br J Cancer 110(10):2462–2471
79. Lallous N, Volik SV, Awrey S, Leblanc E, Tse R, Murillo J et al (2016) Functional analysis of androgen receptor mutations that confer anti-androgen resistance identified in circulating cell-free DNA from prostate cancer patients. Genome Biol 17:10
80. Goldstein A, Valda Toro P, Lee J, Silberstein JL, Nakazawa M, Waters I et al (2017) Detection fidelity of AR mutations in plasma derived cell-free DNA. Oncotarget
81. Malapelle U, Sirera R, Jantus-Lewintre E, Reclusa P, Calabuig-Fariñas S, Blasco A et al (2017) Profile of the Roche cobas® EGFR mutation test v2 for non-small cell lung cancer. Expert Rev Mol Diagn 17(3):209–215
82. Minciacchi VR, Freeman MR, Di Vizio D (2015) Extracellular vesicles in cancer: exosomes, microvesicles and the emerging role of large oncosomes. Semin Cell Dev Biol 40:41–51
83. Balaj L, Lessard R, Dai L, Cho Y-J, Pomeroy SL, Breakefield XO et al (2011) Tumour microvesicles contain retrotransposon elements and amplified oncogene sequences. Nat Commun 1(2):180
84. Costa-Silva B, Aiello NM, Ocean AJ, Singh S, Zhang H, Thakur BK et al (2015) Pancreatic cancer exosomes initiate pre-metastatic niche formation in the liver. Nat Cell Biol 17(6): 816–826
85. O'Driscoll L (2015) Expanding on exosomes and ectosomes in cancer. N Engl J Med 372(24):2359–2362
86. Ciardiello C, Cavallini L, Spinelli C, Yang J, Reis-Sobreiro M, de Candia P et al (2016) Focus on extracellular vesicles: new frontiers of cell-to-cell communication in cancer. Int J Mol Sci 17(2):175
87. Minciacchi VR, Zijlstra A, Rubin MA, Di Vizio D (2017) Extracellular vesicles for liquid biopsy in prostate cancer: where are we and where are we headed? Prostate Cancer Prostatic Dis
88. Lötvall J, Hill AF, Hochberg F, Buzás EI, Di Vizio D, Gardiner C et al (2014) Minimal experimental requirements for definition of extracellular vesicles and their functions: a position statement from the International Society for Extracellular Vesicles. J Extracell Vesicles 3:26913
89. Yang L, Dutta SM, Troyer DA, Lin JB, Lance RA, Nyalwidhe JO et al (2015) Dysregulated expression of cell surface glycoprotein CDCP1 in prostate cancer. Oncotarget 6(41):43743–43758
90. Kharaziha P, Chioureas D, Rutishauser D, Baltatzis G, Lennartsson L, Fonseca P et al (2015) Molecular profiling of prostate cancer derived exosomes may reveal a predictive signature for response to docetaxel. Oncotarget 6(25):21740–21754
91. Huang X, Yuan T, Liang M, Du M, Xia S, Dittmar R et al (2015) Exosomal miR-1290 and miR-375 as prognostic markers in castration-resistant prostate cancer. Eur Urol 67(1):33–41
92. Del Re M, Biasco E, Crucitta S, Derosa L, Rofi E, Orlandini C et al (2016) The detection of androgen receptor splice variant 7 in plasma-derived exosomal RNA strongly predicts resistance to hormonal therapy in metastatic prostate cancer patients. Eur Urol
93. Dijkstra S, Birker IL, Smit FP, Leyten GHJM, de Reijke TM, van Oort IM et al (2014) Prostate cancer biomarker profiles in urinary sediments and exosomes. J Urol 191(4): 1132–1138

94. Korzeniewski N, Tosev G, Pahernik S, Hadaschik B, Hohenfellner M, Duensing S (2015) Identification of cell-free microRNAs in the urine of patients with prostate cancer. Urol Oncol 33(1):16.e17–e22
95. Corcoran C, Rani S, O'Driscoll L (2014) miR-34a is an intracellular and exosomal predictive biomarker for response to docetaxel with clinical relevance to prostate cancer progression. Prostate 74(13):1320–1334
96. McKiernan J, Donovan MJ, O'Neill V, Bentink S, Noerholm M, Belzer S et al (2016) A novel urine exosome gene expression assay to predict high-grade prostate cancer at initial biopsy. JAMA Oncol 2(7):882–889
97. Antonarakis ES, Lu C, Luber B, Wang H, Chen Y, Nakazawa M et al (2015) Androgen receptor splice variant 7 and efficacy of taxane chemotherapy in patients with metastatic castration-resistant prostate cancer. JAMA Oncol 1(5):582–591

Management of Small Renal Masses

Avinash Chenam and Clayton Lau

Contents

A. Chenam · C. Lau (✉)
Department of Surgery, Division of Urology and Urologic Oncology, City of Hope National Medical Center, 1500 E. Duarte Rd, MOB L002H, Duarte, CA 91010, USA
e-mail: cllau@coh.org

A. Chenam
e-mail: achenam@coh.org

S. Daneshmand and K. G. Chan (eds.), *Genitourinary Cancers*, Cancer Treatment and Research 175, https://doi.org/10.1007/978-3-319-93339-9_5

Abstract

With the ubiquitous use of cross-sectional abdominal imaging in recent years, the incidence of small renal masses (SRMs) has increased, and the evaluation and management of SRMs have become important clinical issues. Diagnosing a mass in the early stages theoretically allows for high rates of cure but simultaneously risks overtreatment. In the past 20 years, surgical treatment of SRMs has transitioned from radical nephrectomy for all renal tumors, regardless of size, to elective partial nephrectomy whenever technically feasible. Additionally, newer approaches, including renal mass biopsy, active surveillance for select patients, and renal mass ablation, have been increasingly used. In this chapter, we review the current evidence-based papers covering aspects of the diagnosis and management of SRMs.

Keywords

Renal cell carcinoma · Small renal masses · Partial nephrectomy Active surveillance

1 Introduction

In 2015, 61,000 patients were diagnosed with kidney cancer and an estimated 14,000 patients died as a result of the disease in the USA [1]. Renal cell carcinoma (RCC) is the most common type of kidney tumor, accounting for 90% of all malignant kidney masses. In addition, it is the third most common genitourinary malignancy and the most lethal [1, 2]. Over the past three decades, the incidence of RCC in Western populations has increased [2]. Data from the Surveillance, Epidemiology and End Result (SEER) registry shows the incidence of RCC in 1975 was 7.09 (per 100,000 people), while in 2012, that incidence rose to 15.91 (per 100,000 people) [3].

Some have suggested the increased incidence of RCC and other kidney tumors may be attributed to the rise in hypertension and obesity in the US population [4, 5]. In a recent meta-analysis using prospective observation data, the estimated risk of developing RCC increased 24% for men and 34% for women, for every 5 kg/m^2 increase in body mass index (BMI) [6]. However, the increased incidence of RCC is mainly attributed to the increase use of cross-sectional abdominal imaging for unrelated symptoms [2, 7, 8]. Recent studies have shown the use of computed tomography (CT) scans has increased 300% over the last decade in some clinical settings [9]. This has led to more than 50% of RCC cases now being diagnosed incidentally [10, 11]. The increase in incidence of incidentally detected renal masses is seen in all clinical stages; [12]; however, the largest increase is seen with small renal masses, SRMs, defined as masses <4 cm in diameter, which enhance on triphasic computed tomography characteristic of RCC [13].

Given the prevalence and an earlier detection of these masses, evaluation and management of SRMs have become important clinical issues in recent years. Although certain renal tumor histologies have distinct imaging characteristics, current radiologic imaging cannot reliably discriminate benign from indolent or potentially malignant tumors. Reports estimate that, on final pathologic review after excision, 20–30% of the SRMs are benign and thus overtreatment is a legitimate concern [14–16]. In addition to the diagnostic dilemma, the natural history of these lesions is variable, and many tumors demonstrate an indolent course, as the surgical treatment of these small and low-grade tumors has surprisingly not reduced the mortality rate [17]. In the past 20 years, surgical treatment of SRMs has transitioned from radical nephrectomy for all renal tumors, regardless of size, to elective partial nephrectomy whenever technically feasible. Additionally, newer approaches, including renal mass biopsy (RMB), active surveillance for select patients, and renal mass ablation, have been increasingly used. Several groups (American Urological Association [AUA], European Association of Urology [EAU], and National Comprehensive Cancer Network [NCCN]) have released evaluation and management recommendations including these strategies (Fig. 1). Although several patient factors such as age, medical comorbidities, and patient preferences affect the decision-making process, optimal management of SRMs should balance the need to

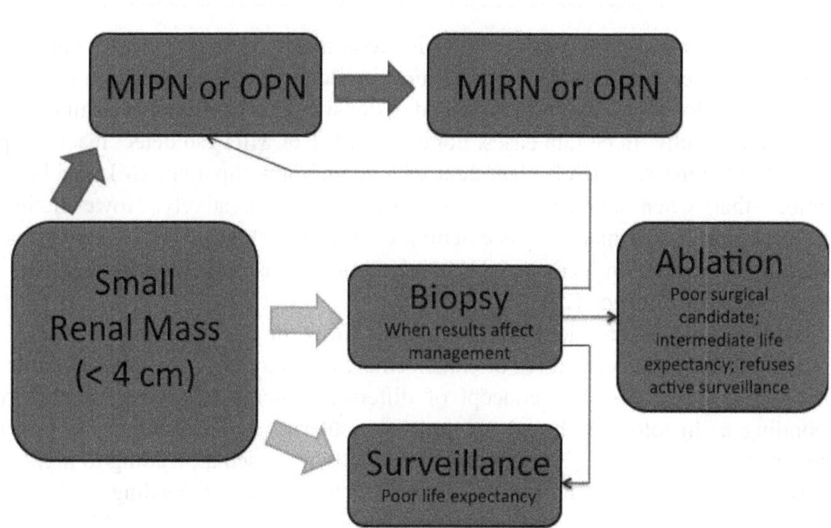

Fig. 1 Small renal mass treatment algorithm. *MIPN* Minimally invasive partial nephrectomy, *OPN* open partial nephrectomy, *MIRN* minimally invasive radical nephrectomy, *ORN* open radical nephrectomy

treat/remove a potential cancer, with the salutary objective of preserving as much renal function as possible [2]. In this chapter, we review the current evidence-based papers covering aspects of the diagnosis and management of SRMs.

2 Diagnosis of Renal Tumors

Historically, patients with RCC presented with a classic triad consisting of hematuria, an abdominal mass, and weight loss, demonstrating later stages of disease and having life expectancies varying between 10 and 15 months [11, 18]. However, with advanced imaging technology, we are now able to identify these SRMs well before they become symptomatic and as a result less than 10% of RCC cases present with the classic triad [11]. Recent estimates suggest that CT scans detect incidental renal lesions measuring at least 1 cm or larger in 14% of asymptomatic adults who undergo imaging for other indications [19]. Alongside the increased incidence of incidental SRMs, there has been a stage and grade migration toward less advanced and less aggressive tumors at presentation. As 25% of SRMs are benign cortical tumors and another 25% are RCC variants that are indolent in nature with limited metastatic potential, there is a need to better characterize these lesions in order to make the most appropriate management decisions and reduce unnecessary harm to patients [20, 21].

2.1 Recent Advances in Imaging Evaluation

Currently, a triphasic CT scan or MRI is recommended for initial assessment and follow-up of renal masses. Both modalities provide valuable information regarding tumor size, location, the presence and extensiveness of tumor thrombus, and lymphadenopathy. In certain cases, noncontrast CT or MRI can detect macroscopic fat within the mass, which is consistent with an angiomyolipoma (AML)—a benign tumor—that, when small, can often be managed conservatively. However, intravenous contrast administration is essential to confirm enhancement of a renal mass, which is defined as an increase in Hounsfield unit measurement of greater than 20 on post-contrast images [22].

Multiphasic CT has demonstrated some utility in distinguishing subtypes of RCC in renal masses via degree of enhancement and may offer a noninvasive means of analysis of SRMs. The concept of differing patterns of enhancement corresponding to histology is based on tumor vascularity. Several authors have concluded that clear cell RCC and oncocytoma are hypervascular, leading to rapid and early enhancement; papillary RCC is mostly hypovascular, leading to low and delayed levels of enhancement; and that chromophobe RCC and AML enhance moderately, correlating with intermediate levels of vascularity [23–25].

CT and MRI are excellent in their depiction of anatomical structures. In the past decade, positron emission tomography (PET) has emerged as a unique imaging modality that provides insight into the biological behavior of tumors rather than their morphological appearance. Using antibody cG250 which reacts against carbonic anhydrase-IX and is over expressed in clear cell carcinomas, Divgi and colleagues reported PET/CT had a higher sensitivity (86.2%) and specificity (85.9%) for identifying clear cell RCC than CT alone (75.5% sensitivity and 46.8% specificity) [26]. Another nuclear medicine test, ^{99m}Tc-sestamibi single-photon emission computed tomography (SPECT)/CT, was recently used for the differentiation of renal histologies in 50 patients with SRMs, and blinded radiologists successfully identified 5 of 6 oncocytomas and 2 of 2 hybrid oncocytic/chromophobe tumors [27].

Even though advances have been made in various imaging modalities, larger prospective studies are needed and as of today reliably differentiating benign and low-risk SRMs from those that will harm a patient's health continues to be imprecise.

2.2 Renal Mass Biopsy

SRMs represent a heterogeneous group of tumors that spans the full spectrum of metastatic and growth potential and include benign, indolent, and more aggressive tumors [28]. As a definitive diagnosis of a malignant SRM on the basis of imaging alone is not possible, renal mass biopsies (RMBs) have been proposed as a safe and useful tool for the pretreatment identification of benign tumors. Ideally, all patients with an SRM, where results may alter management, should be considered for RMB with the goal of avoiding the potential morbidity associated with overtreatment. This is especially true if the patient is a borderline surgical candidate because of medical comorbidities or if the clinician is concerned about the presence of an unusual diagnosis, such as renal lymphoma or a rare metastasis. Further, a patient who is uncertain whether to undergo definitive treatment of a SRM may elect a biopsy, and histopathologic characterization along with prognostic information such as grade can significantly impact management.

Historically, the use of percutaneous sampling of renal tumors was limited due to concerns about its safety, track seeding, diagnostic yield, and accuracy, and for the perceived little impact of RMBs on clinical management [29]. Due to these concerns, RMB has had limited utilization with only 20.7% of SRMs undergoing biopsy from 1992 to 2007 [30, 31]. Recently, however, the role of RMB has been revisited. A meta-analysis of over 5000 patients showed a high overall diagnostic rate for the procedure (92%) with a sensitivity and specificity of 99.7 and 93.2%, respectively, and core needle biopsies were also found to have superior diagnostic rates compared with fine-needle aspiration. In cases where surgical pathology and RMB material were both available, the median concordance rate between tumor histotype and final surgical specimen was 90.7% [32]. In addition to the aforementioned systematic review, Richard et al. also reported on their 13-year experience of 529 patients and showed that RMB had a 93% concordance with final surgical pathology [33]. The same series showed that, conservatively, 10% of patients could have avoided treatment of tumors with confirmed benign pathology.

In terms of safety, the median overall complication rate for RMB in the aforementioned systematic review was reported at 8.1%. The most common complications were Clavien I perirenal hematomas, self-limited hematuria, and lumbar pain. Only three Clavien grade ≥ 2 complications were reported [30]. Richard and colleagues also reported a low associated morbidity (8.5%) with all of them being self-limited with the exception of one [31]. SRMs originating in the collecting system or those with a clinical suspicion for urothelial cancer should not undergo biopsy. Nonetheless, the theoretical risk of tumor cell seeding on the biopsy track has found to be extremely rare, with only a handful of case reports in the literature [30, 34].

Although helpful, there are challenges with RMB. Non-diagnostic biopsies occur in 10–20% of cases, and consideration for repeat biopsy or upfront treatment should be discussed with the patient [20]. However, several series have shown a ~80% diagnostic rate for all re-biopsies of non-diagnostic specimens [31, 35]. Further, recent studies have shown that due to intratumor heterogeneity, RMB may underestimate the grade that the mass truly presents [36–38]. Ball et al. showed that 93% of high-grade specimens (Fuhrman score 3–4) also had low-grade components (Fuhrman score 1–2) [34]. Even though, multicore biopsies may be considered to capture the heterogeneous tissue characteristics of the SRMs, RMB fails to accurately identify high-grade tumors, given the intermixing of high- and low-grade elements in the majority of tumors, resulting in approximately 62% accuracy [2].

Despite the concerns, RMB has gained momentum and has been incorporated into SRM management guidelines. At present, the AUA identifies RMB as an option for SRM management and the EAU recommends RMB in patients in whom AS is pursued (grade C evidence) [2, 39]. As previously mentioned, the incidence of SRMs has increased notably in the past few decades, mainly related to the increased incidence of SRMs identified following abdominal imaging for unrelated reasons [13]. Subsequently, the rates of surgical intervention have also paralleled this increased incidence of SRMs [15, 18, 37]. Wendler and colleagues have estimated an 82% increase in the surgical removal of benign renal masses from 3098 in the year 2000 to 5624 in the year 2009 [15].

In summary, we believe RMB has an increasing role as a decision aide in treatment planning for SRMs. RMB can accurately distinguish malignant from benign lesions as well as provide histology of malignant SRMs prior to developing a treatment plan. The results of RMB reduce unnecessary surgery for benign lesions and guide the selection of patients for active surveillance. The concept of RMB is vital in order to prevent unnecessary treatment and their inherent complication.

3 Active Surveillance

A large proportion of clinically localized renal tumors are diagnosed in older patients or in patients with several comorbidities. In these patients, there is growing understanding and recognition that the competing risk from medical comorbidities may outweigh the potential benefits of surgical intervention [40, 41]. Using SEER-Medicare linked data, Shuch et al. found an increase rate of renal events, cardiovascular events, and secondary cancers in patients who underwent a partial nephrectomy for an SRM [42]. They suggest that intervention with partial nephrectomy may lead to worse non-cancer outcomes. With this consideration of overdiagnosing clinically insignificant disease coupled with additional morbidity due to potentially unnecessary treatments, active surveillance (AS) has been increasingly recommended as an apparently equivalent option in the management of SRMs in the last decade [41, 43–47]. AS is defined as the initial monitoring of tumor size by serial abdominal imaging with delayed intervention reserved for those SRMs that show progression during follow-up [48]. Even though, level I evidence supporting AS of clinically localized renal tumors is absent, institutional studies and pooled analysis have provided robust contemporary data that an initial short-term observation period to determine tumor growth kinetics may be safe for small enhancing tumors in select candidates [49–55].

3.1 Tumor Characteristics and Growth Kinetics

The natural history of prebiopsy SRMs has been documented in several ways. Autopsy series by Mindrup and colleagues report incidentally discovered RCC in 2–3% of cases suggesting indolent growth [56]. Further, Bosniak described the slow growth of many RCCs over a 2- to 8-year period using serial images taken prior to nephrectomy [57]. Additinally, Von Hippel Lindau patients with clear cell RCC are routinely followed until tumors are >3 cm, as growth is usually slow without reported metastases in these clear cell RCC <3 cm [58, 59]. The majority of SRMs, even those histologically proven to be clear cell RCC, demonstrate indolent growth patterns and are unlikely to become symptomatic or metastatic [17, 44, 46, 49, 50, 57, 58, 60, 61].

SRM size appears to be of some prognostic significance as it has correlated with risk of malignancy. In a series of 2770 renal tumors, Frank et al. reported 46.3% of renal masses smaller than 1 cm were benign. Larger tumors carried a higher risk of being malignant, and every 1 cm increase in tumor size was associated with a 17% increase in malignancy risk [62]. Further, tumor size has also shown to predict the risk of metastasis. Bell described the relationship of size to the presence of metastases at autopsy and noted that small tumors were less likely to be associated with metastases [63]. In a review of 287 SRMs, Remzi and colleagues reported the overall risk of distant metastasis in newly diagnosed tumors <3 cm as 2.4% compared with 8.4% for tumors 3.1–4 cm in size [64].

Currently, growth rate, which is assessed by serial axial diameters or tumor volume, is the most commonly used metric for tumor progression. Institutional series have shown that the majority of SRMs demonstrate a slow growth pattern (0.1–0.40 cm per year), that is independent of tumor size at presentation or tumor type [49, 57, 60, 65]. Chawla et al. reported on 234 SRMs with median size of 2.48 cm at presentation and showed an average growth rate of 0.28 cm/year at mean follow-up of 34 months [65]. Jewett and colleagues followed 209 SRMs (mean tumor diameter at diagnosis was 2.2 cm) in a cohort of elderly or infirm patients, and in patients with over 12 months of follow-up, the average growth rate was 0.13 cm/year at a median follow-up of 28 months [60]. Additionally, Kunkle and colleagues followed 106 enhancing renal masses, and they reported the frequency of malignant lesions did not differ significantly between those with growth and those with no growth [66].

3.2 Patient Selection and Surveillance Follow-Up

In a young healthy patient with a long life expectancy, definitive initial treatment (surgery or ablation) remains the standard of care. On the other hand, AS should be considered in elderly patients or in those patients with comorbidities, with limited life expectancy, or high perioperative risk of surgical and medical complications [40, 42, 59, 66]. In addition, patients with baseline chronic kidney disease (CKD) or with a solitary kidney may be offered a period of observation with definitive treatment reserved for patients demonstrating rapid growth [59].

There is a lack of data supporting specific objective criteria for selecting patients managed with AS. Hollingsworth et al. showed that in patients with SRMs, 5% died of RCC compared with 25% who died from unrelated causes and comorbid disease [67]. They also showed that SRM patients older than 70 years of age benefit the least from surgical intervention. To aid with this clinical decision, recent nomograms incorporating age, sex, race, and tumor size have been developed and validated to estimate 5-year outcomes, death from RCC, death from other cancer, and non-cancer death [68, 69]. However, this evaluation should be cautious as life expectancy is difficult to predict in most cases and metastases can develop even in patients with T1a renal tumors in up to 8% of the cases [70].

In regard to surveillance follow-up, there is no clear consensus about the best imaging technique and the optimal follow-up schedule that should be adopted in AS protocols. The AUA recommends follow-up by cross-sectional imaging (CT or MRI) within 6 months after the start of AS followed by CT, MRI, or US at least annually thereafter [39]. The appropriate imaging modality and follow-up protocol should be patient specific, balancing oncologic safety with the risk associated with serial imaging.

Table 1 Active surveillance series for the management of small renal masses

Study	Patients/renal tumors	Mean age (yr)	Mean tumo size (cm)	Mean growth rate (cm/yr)	Mean follow-up (mo)	Progression to metastases n (%)	Disease-specific mortality n (%)
Crispen et al. [44]	154/173	69	2.5	0.29	31	2 (1.3)	0
Abouassaly et al. [46]	110/110	81	2.5	0.24	24	0	0
Volpe et al. [49]	29/32	71	2.5	0.10	38.9	0	0
Abou Youssif et al. [50]	35/44	78.1	2.2	0.21	47.6	2 (5.7)	0
Mason et al. [51]	82/84	74	2.6	0.25	36.0	1 (1.2)	0
Brunocilla et al. [52]	62/64	75	2.0	0.40	91.5	2 (3.2)	2 (3.2)
Haramis et al. [55]	44/51	71.7	2.7	0.15	77.1	0	0
Jewett et al. [60]	178/209	73	2.1	0.13	28	2 (1.1)	2 (1.1)
Rosales et al. [61]	212/223	71	2.8	0.34	35	4 (1.9)	1 (0.5)
Chawla et al. [65]	286	–	2.60	0.28	34	1 (1.6)	–

3.3 Outcomes

With low risk of progression to metastasis and uncommon disease-specific mortality, AS for the management of SRMs is a viable option that appears safe despite limited long-term follow-up data. Table 1 lists the clinical and oncological outcomes of reported SRM series undergoing AS. In a systematic review, Smaldone and colleagues investigated the metastatic progression of SRMs under AS and noted 18 out of 880 patients (2.0%) developed metastases after a mean follow-up of 40 months [43]. Compared with those who had no metastases, patients with metastatic progression had larger tumor size (4.1 + 2.1 cm vs. 2.3 + 1.3 cm; $p < 0.001$) and a faster linear growth rate (0.8 + 0.7 cm/year vs. 0.3 + 0.4 cm/year; $p < 0.001$). Kunkle et al. reported on a meta-analysis evaluating 6471 renal lesions, and there were no statistical differences in the incidence of metastatic progression regardless of whether lesions were managed by surveillance or treated (surgery or ablation) [71].

In regard to delayed intervention after a period of AS, studies have shown delaying intervention does not limit or compromise the feasibility for partial nephrectomy or the ability to undergo a minimally invasive approach, nor did it result in an increased risk of disease progression [72–74]. In an analysis using the DISSRM (Delayed Intervention and Surveillance for Small Renal Masses, a multi-institutional registry) Registry, patients were counseled between primary intervention (nephrectomy or ablation) and AS and then given the option to choose [75]. In the AS cohort, the median tumor growth rate was 0.11 cm/year. At a median follow-up of 2.1 years, cancer-specific survival was 99 and 100% in the primary intervention and AS groups, respectively. Overall, 40% of patients elected for AS once they knew that it was an option, demonstrating that patients could elect for this alternative if they were given more counseling prior to intervention.

3.4 Summary

Although conservative management of suspected RCC is growing in popularity, it should be emphasized that, at this time, the risk of local progression and metastasis with AS is not accurately predictable [13, 39]. While AS represents a reasonable alternative to primary curative intervention, it still necessitates careful patient selection, careful management, patient compliance, and ongoing follow-up.

4 Surgical Excision

4.1 Utilization Trends

Historically, Robson et al. introduced radical nephrectomy (RN) for localized RCC, and since, it has long been the standard treatment for over 50 years [76, 77].

However, as the status of RN has been called into question due to higher risk of CKD and possible overtreatment of SRMs with a significant proportion of benign tumors ($\leq 20\%$), there has been a shift of surgical technique with an increasing utilization of elective nephron sparing surgery (NSS) for the treatment of SRMs. For the first time in 2009, the percentage of partial nephrectomies (PN) exceeded the percentage of RNs performed on patients with renal masses less than 4 cm [77].

The rationale for wider use of NSS is based on data that suggests equal cancer control with RN while preserving renal function [78–81]. A long-term comparison of patients treated with partial nephrectomy versus total/radical nephrectomy for tumors [less than or equal to] 5 cm reported equivalent cancer-specific survival and local recurrence rates at 9 years of follow-up [82]. Lane and colleagues analyzed renal function outcomes for over 2400 patients undergoing PN or RN, and patients in the RN cohort were far more likely ($p < 0.001$) to have an estimated glomerular filtration rate less than 45 ml/min/1.73 m^2 (35%) than any of the partial nephrectomy groups (limited ischemia 11%, unknown ischemia 15%, extended ischemia 19%). Overall, cardiac-specific survival and cancer-specific survival were better with PN of any duration than with RN ($p < 0.001$) [83]. Another study of ~6000 patients compared patients who had been treated with PN to those who had undergone RN. The 3-year and 5-year overall survival probabilities were 83 and 72% in patients treated with RN and 90 and 81%, respectively, in those who received a PN [77]. One of the possible mechanisms by which surgery may increase non-cancer-related deaths is the development of CKD. Studies suggest that RN increases the risk of CKD, which is a significant risk factor for CV events and death [82, 84, 85].

However, a prospective European Organization for Research and Treatment of Cancer (EORTC) randomized trial comparing PN with RN in 541 patients with small (<5 cm) renal masses unexpectedly found higher overall survival in the RN group (81 vs. 76%, respectively; $P < 0.05$) at a mean follow-up of 9.3 years [86]. Additionally, cardiovascular deaths were more common in patients who underwent partial nephrectomy, despite lower burdens of CKD. A recent renal functional follow-up study to the same EORTC trial did demonstrate superior renal function outcomes with PN [87]. The EORTC trial has been criticized for several shortcomings, including marginally statistically significant results and inclusion criteria that were not limited to renal cancers [86]. However, as the only significant randomized trial in this field, it seems that PN does not have a deleterious impact on overall survival compared with RN, and the medical benefits of preserving renal function are potentially important [20]. Thus on the basis of this and other large single- and multicenter nonrandomized studies, current recommendations by the AUA and the EAU continue to state that PN is the standard of care for the surgical treatment of SRMs [2, 39].

4.2 Preservation of Renal Function

The three most important determinants of postoperative renal function are preoperative renal function, volume of renal parenchyma preserved, and vascular damage to nonmalignant parenchyma [88]. The need to preserve renal function was demonstrated in a population-based study of more than 1 million patients, showing elevated incidence of cardiovascular events and mortality with worsening stages of CKD. Preoperative renal function relates to underlying medical renal disease and is unfortunately not modifiable. Ultimately, the two factors that contribute to a decline in renal function after PN are: (1) loss of functional parenchyma associated with excision of the mass and reconstruction (parenchymal volume loss) and (2) incomplete recovery of the preserved nephrons related to ischemic insult.

The volume of remaining parenchyma is largely determined by non-mutable tumor characteristics [89]. For instance, tumor complexity (size/location) is a strong determinant of parenchymal volume loss. Recent studies have suggested that quantity of preserved kidney and quality (preoperative estimated GFR) are the primary determinants of ultimate renal function after PN, with ischemia playing a secondary role as long as it is limited (<25 min) [89–93]. In other words, unless there is an extended warm ischemic interval, most nephrons will eventually recover, leaving parenchymal volume loss as the primary factor responsible for the decline of renal function after PN [93]. In regard to selective clamping, Castaneda and colleagues retrospectively compared renal functional outcomes at 6 months and 1 year postoperatively and found no difference in main renal artery clamping versus selective clamping versus off-clamp methods [94]. Other studies have also showed minimal benefit to zero ischemia [95–97]. A possible explanation for this is due to the lack of clamping, the procedure becomes more difficult, and less parenchymal volume is saved.

4.3 Surgical Approach

Minimally invasive surgical approaches to PN and RN, including laparoscopic and robotic-assisted approaches, are increasingly utilized [98]. In a series analyzing 10-year outcomes of laparoscopic PN (LPN) against open PN (OPN), the choice of operative technique did not impact overall survival [99]. Additionally, in a meta-analysis, the local recurrence-free survival rates for LPN were 98.4% (median tumor size of 2.6 cm, median follow-up of 15 months) versus 97.4% for OPN (median tumor size of 3.1 cm, median follow-up of 46.9 months) [39]. The consistency of the high local RFS rates for surgical excision despite differences in follow-up and tumor size suggests that local recurrence may be minimally influenced by surgical approach as long as complete surgical excision has been performed. However, LPN is a challenging procedure with a long learning curve. In a single surgeon series of 800 procedures performed by one of the leading experts and pioneers of LPN, Gill et al. reported a mean warm ischemia time of about 32 min for the first 500 procedures, and a warm ischemia time shorter than 20 min in about 15% of all procedures. Moreover, the complication rates were as high as 24% in the first 275 cases, falling down to only 15% in the subsequent 289 cases [100].

In the past decade, robotic-assisted laparoscopic partial nephrectomy (RALPN) has increased in popularity and is likely to overtake LPN and OPN as the most common method for PN in regions where the robot is accessible. The key advantages of RALPN appear to be a shorter learning curve and reduced warm ischemic time, while the perioperative and short-term outcomes appear to be at least as good as LPN [101]. The long-term oncological outcomes of RALPN are still awaited, though early markers of surgical success such as positive margin rates are encouraging in experienced hands. In a multicenter series of nearly 350 cases, Ficarra and colleagues demonstrated a warm ischemia time <20 min was achieved in 64% of cases (with median warm ischemia time of only 18 min) and the overall complication rates were as low as 12% (and only 3% of high-grade complications) [102]. In another multi-institutional series of 450 RALPN cases, Spana et al. reported an overall complication rate of 15.8% with only 3.8% being major complications [103].

OPN is still the preferred surgical modality in patients in whom LPN or RALPN approach would be difficult, for example, re-do partial nephrectomies, complex tumors (large or endophytic), and in those with multiple renal tumors (e.g., hereditary renal tumors) [104]. There seems to be a limited role for RN in the management of SRMs [105]. However, in the setting of a normal contralateral kidney, no associated conditions that predispose to CKD, and a complex tumor location, one could consider a RN [106, 107]. In the rare instance that RN is performed for an SRM, a minimally invasive approach is the preferred option given the evidence that supports lower morbidity and equivalent cancer-specific survival [39]. Ultimately, the decision for surgical approach should be made by surgeon's comfort and experience with these goals: (1) excising the SRM with negative surgical margin, (2) maximizing renal parenchymal volume preservation, (3) reconstructing the kidney in a manner that will minimize the risk of postoperative complications, and (4) limiting warm ischemia time to 25 min or less [108].

5 Ablation

Over the past 20 years, minimally invasive ablation therapy has been developed as an alternative to RN and PN for SRMs. As most ablative therapies are performed via a percutaneous or laparoscopic approach, tumor ablative therapy provides a less-invasive treatment option in this group of patients with reasonable oncological control comparable to PN [109]. The two most popular ablative therapy techniques are achieved using application of heat (radiofrequency ablation [RFA]) or cold (cryoablation [CA]).

Typical indications of renal PTA are patients presenting with tumors less than 3 cm in diameter and multiple comorbidity factors (including age), contraindications to surgery, hereditary RCC, bilateral renal tumors, solitary kidney, pre-existing CKD, or high risk of predialysis renal function after PN [110, 111]. Patients should be informed that larger tumors (>3 cm) can require additional ablation sessions [112, 113]. Even in the elderly population of more than 80 years, PTA is safe and effective with estimated cancer-specific survival rates of 100 and

86% at 3 and 5 years, respectively [114]. The AUA and EAU guidelines recommend considering ablative approaches in elderly patients who are at risk of increased surgical morbidity or limited life expectancy [2, 39].

In regard to technical and oncological outcomes, retrospective studies have suggested that partial nephrectomy confers an improved cancer-specific survival compared with ablation [115]. Local recurrence is also more likely following ablation with local recurrence-free survival reported as 8–10% less for RFA and CA compared with PN [39]. However, recent trials have oncological results for PTA comparable to PN. In a cohort of 1424 SRMs (1057 underwent PN, 180 underwent RFA, and 187 underwent CA), the local recurrence-free survival rates at 3 year for PN, RFA, and CA were 98% (95% CI, 97–99), 98% (95% CI, 96–100), and 98% (95% CI, 95–100), respectively [116]. A recent systematic review and meta-analysis of six clinical trials (one randomized and five cohort) reported that recurrence-free survival and cancer-specific survival were similar between patients treated with PN and PTA [117]. The rate of local disease progression was similar (3–4%) in the two groups, but the preservation of the renal function was superior in the ablation group (+14.6 mL/min). The overall complication rate was also significantly lower for PTA (7.4% for ablation versus 11.1% for surgery) as well as the rate of major complications (2.3% for ablation vs. 5% for surgery) [117]. However, it should be noted, however, that there are insufficient data on long-term oncologic outcomes to recommend ablative therapies as a preferred modality [2].

Other emerging techniques include high-intensity focused ultrasound, intestinal laser ablation and microwave therapy. Another recent technology, irreversible electroporation, has been described in small series and may have benefits, given its nonthermal nature [118]. However, these other technologies lack clear evidence currently and can largely be considered to be experimental and evolving [119].

PTA of renal lesions is an alternative to surgical procedures with good short and mid-term outcomes, with an efficacy almost similar to that of PN [116]. It should be proposed to patients with contraindications to general anesthesia and surgery, particularly in the presence of CKD or hereditary renal cancer.

6 Future Considerations

An emerging area that may redefine the evaluation and management of SRMs is personalized and precision-based approaches, such as molecular tumor profiling. Recently, analysis of multidimensional data of over 500 clear cell RCC retrieved from The Cancer Genome Atlas (TCGA) archive has been able to distinguish distinct molecular subclasses of clear cell RCC and to stratify cancer aggressiveness based on genomic profiling [120]. The Cancer Genome Atlas Research Network has identified 19 mutated genes in clear cell RCC, and several genes in papillary RCC correlated to aggressiveness [121, 122]. Additionally, poorer survival in RCC patients has been linked to decreased expression of a new class of small noncoding RNAs called PIWI-interacting RNAs [123]. Clinically, the translation of such research into practice may aid in distinguishing between patients who require treatment for SRMs and patients who do not, obviating the need for expensive treatment, imaging, and surveillance protocols [88].

Currently, there are no readily available or clinically validated screening biomarkers for RCC [124]. Urinary biomarkers including aquaporin 1 and perilipin 2 have shown to be elevated in clear cell and papillary RCC [125, 126]. Morrissey and colleagues have shown these biomarkers to be highly sensitive and specific in distinguishing benign tumors from malignant RCC [125, 127]. Interestingly, the level of biomarker in the urine positively correlated with the size of the clear cell or papillary RCC and decreased significantly after the mass was removed [125]. Currently, the major limitations of these biomarkers is their inability to detect chromophobe RCC and other subtypes, as well as the involved process of the

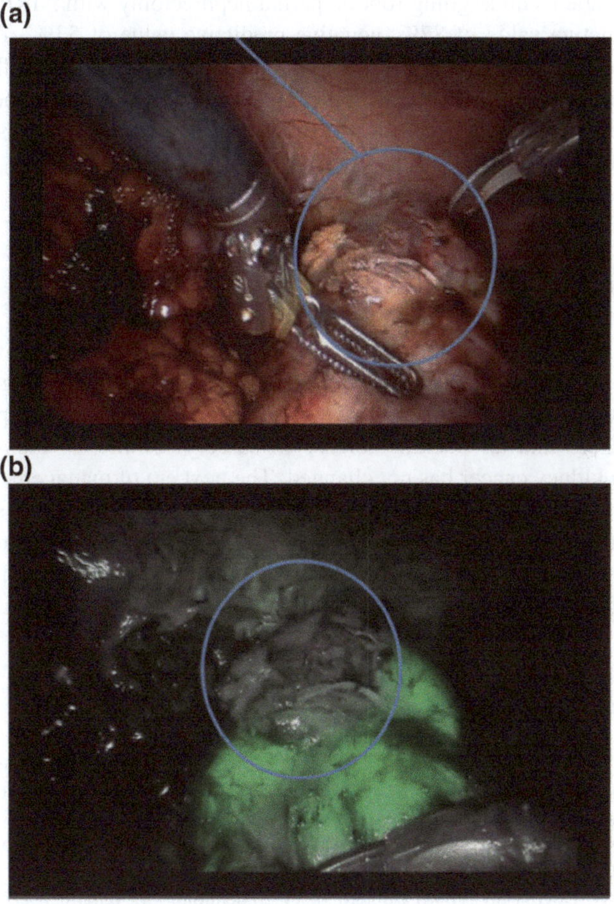

Fig. 2 **a** Exophytic tumor in white light mode. **b** Exophytic tumor in fluorescence mode

Western blot procedure and likely costs associated with it. Otherwise, this test holds great promise for screening patients with SRM to aid in the differential diagnosis.

In regard to advances in surgery, Indocyanine Green (ICG), a water soluble dye, is a popular diagnostic reagent that has been in clinical use for the examination of hepatic function, ophthalmic angiography, cardiac output and circulating blood volume. With the advent of robotic-assisted laparoscopic surgery and near-infrared fluorescence (NIRF) lenses, ICG has found several applications in urologic surgery including enhancing identification of tumor margins during partial nephrectomy. Tobis and colleagues demonstrated the use of intravenous ICG with simultaneous NIRF imaging at the time of partial nephrectomy and demonstrated renal tumors (both benign and malignant) were not only well demarcated by ICG but surprisingly hypo-fluorescent as compared to surrounding normal parenchyma (Fig. 2) [128]. The degree of hypo-fluorescence, however, could not be reliably used to differentiate malignant versus benign tumors according to Manny et al., who found in 100 consecutive patients undergoing robotic partial nephrectomy with NIRF guidance a positive predictive value of 87%, negative predictive value of 53%, sensitivity of 84%, and specificity of 57% [129]. Although the use of intraoperative fluorescence during partial nephrectomy appears appealing, at this time the true benefit remains unclear as pertains to tumor identification and reducing positive margins, especially in experienced hands where positive surgical margin rates are 1–2%.

7 Conclusion

The diagnosis, evaluation, and management of SRMs have evolved over the past few decades. Incidental identification of SRMs has become increasingly common with widespread adoption of cross-sectional imaging. However, despite technological advances and an overall increase in surgery for SRMs, the survival for patients with kidney cancer has not changed. The next era of management of SRMs likely involves renal biopsy and an increased use of surveillance. At some point, every metastatic cancer must have been an SRM, so as we learn more about the molecular signature of renal cancer and the mutations that drive progression, we might eventually manage SRMs differently [121].

References

1. Siegel R, Miller KD, Jemal A (2015) Cancer statistics. CA Cancer J Clin 65:5–29
2. Ljungberg B, Bensalah K, Canfield S et al (2015) EAU guidelines on renal cell carcinoma: 2014 update. Eur Urol 67:913–924
3. Howlader N, Noone A, Krapcho M, et al (2015) Seer Cancer Stat Rev. http://seer.cancer.gov/csr/1975_2013/
4. Chow WH, Devesa SS (2008) Contemporary epidemiology of renal cell cancer. Cancer J 14:288–301

5. Sanfilippo KM, McTique KM, Fidler CJ et al (2014) Hypertension and obesity and the risk of kidney cancer in 2 large cohorts of US men and women. Hypertension 63:934–941
6. Renehan AG, Tyson M, Egger M, Heller RF, Zwahlen M (2008) Body mass index and incidence of cancer: a systematic review and meta-analysis of prospective observational studies. Lancet 371:569–578
7. Kato M, Suzuki T, Suzuki Y et al (2004) Natural history of small renal cell carcinoma: evaluation of growth rate, histological grade, cell proliferation and apoptosis. J Urol 172:863–866
8. Sun M, Thuret R, Abdollah F et al (2011) Age-adjusted incidence, mortality, and survival rates of stage-specific renal cell carcinoma in North America: a trend analysis. Eur Urol 59:135–141
9. Kocher KE, Meurer WJ, Fazel R et al (2011) National trends in use of computed tomography in the emergency department. Ann Emerg Med 58:452–462
10. Luciani LG, Cestari R, Tallarigo C (2000) Incidental renal cell carcinoma-age and stage characterization and clinical implications study of 1092 patients (1982–1997). Urology 56:58–62
11. Jayson M, Sanders H (1998) Increased incidence of serdenipitously discovered renal cell carcinoma. Urology 51:203–205
12. Hock LM, Lynch J, Balaji KC (2002). Increasing incidence of all stages of kidney cancer in the last 2 decades in the United States: an analysis of surveillance, epidemiology and end results program data. J Urol 167:57–60
13. Gill IS, Aron M, Gervais DA et al (2010) Clinical practice. Small renal mass. N Engl J Med 362:624–634
14. Johnson DC, Vukina J, Smith AB et al (2015) Preoperatively misclassified, surgically removed benign renal masses: a systematic review of surgical series and United States population level burden estimate. J Urol 193:30–35
15. Wendler JJ, Porsch M, Nitschke S et al (2015) A prospective phase 2a pilot study investigating focal percutaneous irreversible electroporation (IRE) ablation by NanoKnife in patients with localized renal cell carcinoma (RCC) with delayed interval tumor resection (IRENE trial). Contemp Clin Trials 43:10–19
16. Kutikov A, Fossett LK, Ramchandhani P et al (2006) Incidence of benign pathologic findings at partial nephrectomy for solitary renal mass presumed to be renal cell carcinoma on preoperative imaging. Urology 68:737–740
17. Hollingsworth JM, Miller DC, Daignault S et al (2006) Rising incidence of small renal masses: a need to reassess treatment effect. J Natl Cancer Inst 98:1331–1334
18. Rendon RA, Stanietzky N, Panzarella T et al (2000) The natural history of small renal masses. J Urol 164:1143–1147
19. O'Connor SD, Pickhardt PJ, Kim DH et al (2011) Incidental finding of renal masses at unenhanced CT: prevalence and analysis of features for guiding management. AJR Am J Roentgenol 197:139–145
20. Finelli A, Ismaila N, Bro B et al (2017) Management of small renal masses: American society of clinical oncology clinical practice guideline. J Clin Oncol 35:668–680
21. Marconi L, Dabestani S, Lam TB et al (2011) Systematic review and meta-analysis of diagnostic accuracy of percutaneous renal tumor biopsy. Eur Urol 59:135–141
22. Israel GM, Bosniak MA (2005) How do I do it: evaluating renal masses. Radiology 236:441–450
23. Zhang J, Lefkowitz RA, Ishill NM et al (2007) Solid renal cortical tumors: differentiation with CT. Radiology 244:494–504
24. Jinzaki M, Tanimoto A, Mukai M et al (2000) Double-phase helical CT of small renal parenchymal neoplasms: correlation with pathologic findings and tumor angiogenesis. J Comput Assist Tomogr 24:835–842

25. Pierorazio PM, Hyams ES, Tsai S et al (2013) Multiphasic enhancement patterns of small renal masses (<4 cm) on preoperative computed tomography: utility for distinguishing subtypes of renal cell carcinoma, angiomylipoma, and oncocytoma. Urology 81:1265–1272
26. Divgi CR, Uzzo RG, Gatsonis C et al (2013) Positron emission tomography/computed tomography identification of clear cell renal carcinoma: results from the REDECT trial. J Clin Oncol 31:187
27. Gorin MA, Rowe SP, Baras AS et al (2016) Prospective evaluation of (99 m) Tc-sestamibi SPECT/CT for the diagnosis of renal oncocytomas and hybrid oncocytic/chromophobe tumors. Eur Urol 69:413–416
28. Burruni R, Lhermitte B, Cerantola Y et al (2016) The role of renal biopsy in small renal masses. Can Urol Assoc J 10:E28–E33
29. Herts BR, Baker ME (1995) The current role of percutaneous biopsy in the evaluation of renal masses. Semin Urol Oncol 13:254–261
30. Breau RH, Crispen PL, Jenkins SM, Blute ML, Leibovich BC (2011) Treatment of patients with small renal masses: a survey of the American urological association. J Urol 185:407–413
31. Leppert JT, Hanley J, Wagner TH et al (2014) Utilization of renal mass biopsy in patients with renal cell carcinoma. Urology 185:407–413
32. Marconi L, Dabestani S, Lam TB (2016) Systematic review and meta-analysis of diagnostic accuracy of percutaneous renal tumor biopsy. Eur Urol 69:660–673
33. Richard PO. Jewett MA, Bhatt JR et al (2015) Renal tumor biopsy for small renal masses: a single-center 13-year experience. Eur Urol 68:1007–1013
34. Mullins JK, Rodriguez R (2013) Renal cell carcinoma seeding of a percutaneous biopsy tract. Can Urol Assoc J 7:E176–E179
35. Leveridge MJ, Finelli A, Kachura JR et al (2011) Outcomes of small renal mass needle core biopsy, nondiagnostic percutaneous biopsy, and the role of repeat biopsy. Eur Urol 60:578–584
36. Ball MW, Bezerra SM, Gorin MA et al (2015) Grade heterogeneity in small renal masses: potential implications for renal mass biopsy. J Urol 193:36–40
37. Tomaszewski JJ, Uzzo RG, Smaldone MC (2014) Heterogeneity and renal mass biopsy: a review of its role and reliability. Cancer Biol Med 11:162–172
38. Conti A, Santoni M, Sotte V et al (2015) Small renal masses in the era of personalized medicine: tumor heterogeneity, growth kinetics, and risk of metastasis. Urol Oncol: Semin Original Inv 33:303–309
39. Campbell SC, Novick AC, Belldegrun A et al (2009) Guideline for management of the clinical T1 renal mass. J Urol 182:1271–1279
40. Kutikov A, Egleston BL, Wong YN et al (2010) Evaluating overall survival and competing risks of death in patients with localized renal cell carcinoma using a comprehensive nomogram. J Clin Oncol 28:311
41. Volpe A, Cadeddu JA, Cestari A et al (2011) Contemporary management of small renal masses. Eur Urol 60:501
42. Shuch B, Hanley JM, Lai JC et al (2014) Adverse health outcomes associated with surgical management of the small renal mass. J Urol 191:301–308
43. Smaldone MC, Kutikov A, Egleston BL et al (2012) Small renal masses progressing to metastases under active surveillance: a systematic review and pooled analysis. Cancer 118:997
44. Crispen PL, Viterbo R, Boorjian SA et al (2009) Natural history, growth kinetics, and outcomes of untreated clinically localized renal tumors under active surveillance. Cancer 115:2844
45. Crispen PL, Uzzo RG (2007) The natural history of untreated renal masses. BJU Int 99:1203
46. Abouassaly R, Lane BR, Novick AC (2008) Active surveillance of renal masses in elderly patients. J Urol 180:505

47. Wehle MJ, Thiel DD, Petrou SP et al (2004) Conservative management of incidental contrast enhancing renal masses as safe alternative to invasive therapy. Urology 64:49
48. Volpe A, Jewett MA (2007) The role of surveillance for small renal masses. Nat Clin Pract Urol 4:2–3
49. Volpe A, Panzarella T, Rendon RA, Haider MA, Kondylis FI, Jewett MA (2004) The natural history of incidentally detected small renal masses. Cancer 100:738–745
50. Abou Youssif T, Kassouf W, Steinberg J, Aprikian AG, Laplante MP, Tanguay S (2007) Active surveillance for selected patients with renal masses; updated results with long-term follow up. Cancer 110:1010–1014
51. Mason RJ, Abdolell M, Trottier G et al (2011) Growth kinetics of renal masses analysis of a prospective cohort of patients undergoing active surveillance. Eur Urol 59:863–867
52. Brunocilla E, Borghesi M, Schiavana R et al (2014) Small renal masses initially managed using active surveillance: results from a retrospective study with long-term follow up. Clin Genitourin Cancer 12:178–181
53. Gontero P, Joniau S, Oderda M et al (2013) Active Surveillance for small renal tumors: have clinical concerns been addressed so far? Int J Urol 20:357–361
54. Mehrazin R, Smaldone MC, Kutikov A et al (2014) Growth kinetics and short-term outcomes of cT1b and cT2 renal masses under active surveillance. J Urol 192:659–664
55. Haramis G, Mues AC, Rosales JC et al (2011) Natural history of renal cortical neoplasms during active surveillance with follow-up longer than 5 years. Urology 77:787–791
56. Mindrup SR, Pierre JS, Dahmoush L, Konety BR (2005) The prevalence of renal cell carcinoma diagnosed at autopsy. BJU Int 95:31–33
57. Bosniak MA (1995) Observation of small incidentally detected renal masses. Semin Urol Oncol 13:267–272
58. Duffey BG, Choyke PL, Glenn G et al (2004) The relationship between renal tumor size and metastases in patients with von Hippel-Lindau disease. J Urol 172:63–65
59. Ahmad AE, Finelli A, Jewett M (2016) Surveillance of small renal masses. Urology 98:8–13
60. Jewett MA, Mattar K, Basiuk J et al (2011) Active surveillance of small renal masses: progression patterns of early stage kidney cancer. Eur Urol 60:39–44
61. Rosales JC, Haramis G, Moreno J et al (2010) Active surveillance for renal cortical neoplasms. J Urol 183:1698–1702
62. Frank I, Blute ML, Cheville JC, Lohse CM, Weaver AL, Zincke H (2003) Solid renal tumors: an analysis of pathological features related to tumor size. J Urol 170:2217–2220
63. Bell ER (1938) A classification of renal tumors with observation of the frequency of the various types. J Urol 39:238–243
64. Remzi M, Ozsoy M, Klingler HC et al (2006) Are small renal tumors harmless? Analysis of histopathologic features according to tumors 4 cm or less in diameter. J Urol 176:896–899
65. Chawla SN, Crispen PL, Hanlon AL, Greenberg RE, Chen DY, Uzzo RG (2006) The natural history of observed enhancing renal masses: meta-analysis and review of the world literature. J Urol 175:425–431
66. Kunkle DA, Crispen PL, Li T et al (2007) Tumor size predicts synchronous metastatic renal cell carcinoma: implications for surveillance of small renal masses. J Urol 177:1692
67. Hollingsworth JM, Miller DC, Daignault S, Hollenbeck BK (2007) Five-year survival after surgical treatment for kidney cancer: a population-based competing risk analysis. Cancer 109:1763–1768
68. Kutikov A, Egleston BL, Canter D, Smaldone MC, Wong YN, Uzzo RG (2012) Competing risks of death in patients with localized renal cell carcinoma: a comorbidity based model. J Urol 188:2077–2083
69. Lughezzani G, Sun M, Budaus L, Thuret R, Perrotte P, Karakiewicz PI (2010) Population-based external validation of a competing-risks nomogram for patients with localized renal cell carcinoma. J Clin Oncol 28:e299–e300
70. Klatte T, Patard J-J, de Martino M (2008) Tumor size does not predict risk of metastatic disease or prognosis of small renal cell carcinomas. J Urol 179(5):1719–1726

71. Kunkle DA, Egleston BL, Uzzo RG (2008) Excise, ablate or observe: the small renal mass dilemma- a meta-analysis and review. J Urol 179:1227–1233
72. Rais-Bahrami S, Guzzo TJ, Jarrett TW, Kavoussi LR, Allaf ME (2009) Incidentally discovered renal masses: oncological and perioperative outcomes in patients with delayed surgical intervention. BJU Int 103:1355–1358
73. Crispen PL, Viterbo R, Fox EB, Greenberg RE, Chen DY, Uzzo RG (2008) Delayed intervention of sporadic renal masses undergoing active surveillance. Cancer 112:1051–1057
74. Ambani SN, Morgan TM, Montgomery JS et al (2016) Predictors of delayed intervention for patients on active surveillance for small renal masses: does renal mass biopsy influence our decision. Urology 98:88–96
75. Pierorazio PM, Johnson MH, Ball MW et al (2015) Five-year analysis of a multi-institutional prospective clinical trial of delayed intervention and surveillance for small renal masses: the DISSRM registry. Eur Urol 68:408–415
76. Robson CJ, Churchill BM, Anderson W (1969) The results of radical nephrectomy for renal cell carcinoma. J Urol 101:297–301
77. Huang WC, Atoria CL, Bjurlin M et al (2015) Management of small kidney cancers in the new millennium: contemporary trends and outcomes in a population-based cohort. JAMA Surgery 150:664–672
78. Van Poppel H, Joniau S (2007) Is surveillance an option for the treatment of small renal masses? Eur Urol 52:1323–1330
79. Thompson RH, Boorjian SA, Lohse CM et al (2008) Radical nephrectomy for pT1a renal masses may be associated with decreased overall survival compared with partial nephrectomy. J Urol 179:468–471
80. Poulakis V, Witzsch U, de Vries R et al (2003) Quality of life after surgery for localized renal cell carcinoma: comparison between radical nephrectomy and nephron-sparing surgery. Urology 62:814–820
81. Weight CJ, Lieser G, Larson BT et al (2010) Partial nephrectomy is associated with improved overall survival compared to radical nephrectomy in patients with unanticipated benign renal tumors. Eur Urol 58:293–298
82. Huang WC, Elkin EB, Levey AS et al (2009) Partial nephrectomy versus radical nephrectomy in patients with small renal tumors—Is there a difference in mortality and cardiovascular outcomes? J Urol 181:55–61
83. Lane BR, Fergany AF, Weight CJ, Campbell SC (2010) Renal functional outcomes after partial nephrectomy with extended ischemia intervals are better than after radical nephrectomy. J Urol 184:1286–1290
84. Lau WK, Blute ML, Weaver AL, Torres VE, Zincke H (2000) Matched comparison of radical nephrectomy versus nephron-sparing surgery in patients with unilateral renal cell carcinoma and a normal contralateral kidney. Mayo Clin Proc 75:1236–1242
85. McKiernan J, Simmons R, Katz J, Russo P (2002) Natural history of chronic renal insufficiency after partial and radical nephrectomy. Urology 59:816–820
86. Van Poppel H, Da Pozzo L, Albrecht W et al (2011) A prospective, randomised EORTC intergroup phase 3 study comparing the oncologic outcome of elective nephron-sparing surgery and radical nephrectomy for low-stage renal cell carcinoma. Eur Urol 59:543–552
87. Scosyrev E, Messing EM, Sylvester R et al (2014) Renal function after nephron-sparing surgery versus radical nephrectomy: results from EORTC randomized trial 30904. Eur Urol 65:372–377
88. Leone AR, Diorio GJ, Spiess PE, Gilbert SM (2016) Contemporary issues surrounding small renal masses: evaluation, diagnostic biopsy, nephron sparing, and novel treatment modalities. Oncology 30:507–514
89. Thompson RH, Lane BR, Lohse CM et al (2012) Renal function after partial nephrectomy: effect of warm ischemia relative to quantity and quality of preserved kidney. Urology 79:356–360

90. Aron M, Gill IS, Campbell SC (2012) A nonischemic approach to partial nephrectomy is optimal. J Urol 187:387–390
91. Simmons MN, Fergany AF, Campbell SC (2011) Effect of parenchymal volume preservation on kidney function after partial nephrectomy. J Urol 186:405–410
92. Yossepowitch O, Eggener SE, Serio A et al (2006) Temporary renal ischemia during nephron sparing surgery is associated with short- term but not long-term impairment in renal function. J Urol 176:1339–1343
93. Mir MC, Campbell RA, Sharma N et al (2013) Parenchymal volume preservation and ischemia during partial nephrectomy: functional and volumetric analysis. Urology 82:263–268
94. Castaneda CV, Danzig MR, Finkelstein JB et al (2015) The natural history of renal functional decline in patients undergoing surveillance in the DISSRM registry. Urol Oncol 33:166.e17–e20
95. Ng CK, Gill IS, Patil MB et al (2012) Anatomic renal artery branch microdissection to facilitate zero-ischemia partial nephrectomy. Eur Urol 61:67–74
96. Weight CJ, Thompson RH (2012) The role of ischemia, or the lack thereof, during partial nephrectomy. Eur Urol 61:75–76
97. Simmons MN, Hillier SP, Lee BH, Fergany AF, Kaouk J, Campbell SC (2012) Functional recovery after partial nephrectomy: effects of volume loss and ischemic injury. J Urol 187:1667–1673
98. Liss MA, Wang S, Palazzi K et al (2014) Evaluation of national trends in the utilization of partial nephrectomy in relation to the publication of the American Urologic Association guidelines for the management of clinical T1 renal masses. BMC Urol 14:101
99. Lane BR, Campbell SC, Gill IS (2013) 10-year oncologic outcomes after laparoscopic and open partial nephrectomy. J Urol 190:44–49
100. Gill IS, Kamoi K, Aron M, Desai MM (2010) 800 laparoscopic partial nephrectomies: a single surgeon series. J Urol 183:34–41
101. Novara G, La Falce S, Kungulli A, Gandaglia V, Ficarra V, Mottrie A (2016) Robot-assisted partial nephrectomy. Int J Surg 36:554–559
102. Ficarra V, Bhayani S, Porter J et al (2012) Predictors of warm ischemia time and perioperative complications in a multicenter, international series of robot-assisted partial nephrectomy. Eur Urol Suppl 11:E35–U358
103. Spana G, Haber GP, Dulabon LM et al (2011) Complications after robotic partial nephrectomy at centers of excellence: multi-institutional analysis of 450 cases. J Urol 186:417–421
104. Kasivisvanathan V, Raison N, Challacombe B (2016) The diagnosis and management of small renal masses. Int J Surg 36:493–494
105. Thompson RH (2014) Partial versus radical nephrectomy: the debate regarding renal function ends while the survival controversy continues. Eur Urol 65:378–379
106. Lane BR, Demirjian S, Derweesh IH et al (2015) Survival and functional stability in chronic kidney disease due to surgical removal of nephrons: importance of the new baseline glomerular filtration rate. Eur Urol 68:996–1003
107. Lane BR, Golan S, Eggener S et al (2013) Differential use of partial nephrectomy for intermediate and high complexity tumors may explain variability in reported utilization rates. J Urol 189:2047–2053
108. Zargar H, Allaf ME, Bhayani S et al (2015) Trifecta and optimal perioperative outcomes of robotic and laparoscopic partial nephrectomy in surgical treatment of small renal masses: a multi-institutional study. BJU Int 116:407–414
109. Zargar H, Atwell TD, Cadeddu JA et al (2016) Cryoablation for small renal masses: selection criteria, complications, and functional and oncologic results. Eur Urol 69:116–128
110. Gunn AJ, Gervais DA (2014) Percutaneous ablation of the small renal mass- techniques and outcomes. Semin Interv Radiol 31:33–41
111. Higgins LJ, Hong K (2015) Renal ablation techniques: state of the art. AJR Am J Roentgenol 205:735–741

112. Gervais DA, McGovern FJ, Arellano RS et al (2005) Radiofrequency ablation of renal cell carcinoma: Part 1, indications, results, and role in patient management over a 6-year period and ablation of 100 tumors. AJR Am J Roentgenol 185:64–71
113. Breen DJ, Rutherford EE, Stedman B et al (2007) Management of renal tumors by image-guided radiofrequency ablation: experience in 105 tumors. Cardiovasc Interv Radiol 30:936–942
114. Miller AJ, Kurup AN, Schmit GD et al (2015) Percutaneous clinical T1a renal mass ablation in the octogenarian and nonagenarian: oncologic outcomes and morbidity. J Endourol 29:671–676
115. Whitson JM, Harris CR, Meng MV (2012) Population-based comparative effectiveness of nephron-sparing surgery versus ablation for small renal masses. BJU Int 110:1438–1443
116. Thompson RH, Atwell T, Schmit G et al (2015) Comparison of partial nephrectomy and percutaneous ablation for cT1 renal masses. Eur Urol 67(2):252–259
117. Katsanos K, Mailli L, Krokidis M et al (2014) Systematic review and meta-analysis of thermal ablation versus surgical nephrectomy for small renal tumors. Cardiovasc Interv Radiol 37:427–437
118. Narayanan G, Doshi MH (2016) Irreversible electroporation (IRE) in renal tumors. Curr Urol Rep 17:15
119. Khan F, Sriprasad S, Keeley FX (2012) Cryosurgical ablation for small renal masses, current status and future prospects. Brit J Med Surg Urol 5:S28–S34
120. Christinat Y, Krek W (2015) Integrated genomic analysis identifies subclasses and prognosis signatures of kidney cancer. Oncotarget 6:10521–10531
121. The Cancer Genome Atlas Research Network (2013) Comprehensive molecular characterization of clear cell renal cell carcinoma. Nature 499:43–49
122. The Cancer Genome Atlas Research Network (2016) Comprehensive molecular characterization of papillary renal-cell carcinoma. NEJM 374:135–145
123. Iliev R, Stanik M, Fedorko M et al (2016) Decreased expression levels of PIWIL1, PIWIL2, and PIWIL4 are associated with worse survival in renal cell carcinoma patients. Onco Targets Ther 9:217–222
124. Russo P, Huang W (2008) The medical and oncological rationale for partial nephrectomy for the treatment of T1 renal cortical tumors. Urol Clin N Am 35:635–643
125. Morrissey JJ, Mobley J, Figenshau RS, Vetter J, Bhayani S, Kharasch ED (2015) Urine aquaporin 1 and perilipin 2 differentiate renal carcinomas from other imaged renal masses and bladder and prostate cancer. Mayo Clin Proc 90:35–42
126. Tondel C, Vikse BE, Bostad L, Svarstad E (2012) Safety and complications of percutaneous kidney biopsies in 715 children and 8573 adults in Norway 1988–2010. Clin J Am Soc Nephrol 7:1591–1597
127. Morrissey JJ, Mellnick VM, Luo J et al (2015) Evaluation of urine aquaporin-1 and perilipin-2 concentrations as biomarkers to screen for renal cell carcinoma: a prospective cohort study. JAMA Oncol 1:204–212
128. Tobis S, Knopf JK, Silvers CR et al (2012) Near infrared fluorescence imaging after intravenous indocyanine green: initial clinical experience with open partial nephrectomy for renal cortical tumors. Urology 79:958–964
129. Manny TB, Krane LS, Hemal AK (2013) Indocyanine green cannot predict malignancy in partial nephrectomy: histopathologic correlation with fluorescence pattern in 100 patients. J Endourol Endourol Soc 27:918–921

Advances in the Treatment of Metastatic Renal Cell Carcinoma

Paulo Bergerot, Kathy Burns, Dhruv Prajapati, Rachel Fox, Meghan Salgia and Sumanta K. Pal

Contents

Abstract

The treatment landscape for metastatic renal cell carcinoma has constantly been in flux. In 2005, with the advent of vascular endothelial growth factor (VEGF) tyrosine kinase inhibitor (TKI) therapy, the standard of care shifted to agents such as sunitinib and pazopanib. However, more recently there have been datasets, suggesting that next-generation TKIs such as cabozantinib may play an important role in therapy. Furthermore, immunotherapy has had resurgence with the FDA approval of nivolumab with ipilimumab. In the current chapter, we attempt to contextualize available frontline therapies for metastatic renal cell carcinoma with a focus on the CABOSUN and CheckMate 214 clinical trials.

P. Bergerot · K. Burns · D. Prajapati · R. Fox · M. Salgia · S. K. Pal (✉)
Department of Medical Oncology and Therapeutics Research, City of Hope Comprehensive Cancer Center, 1500 East Duarte Road, Duarte, CA 91010, USA
e-mail: spal@coh.org

S. Daneshmand and K. G. Chan (eds.), *Genitourinary Cancers*, Cancer Treatment and Research 175, https://doi.org/10.1007/978-3-319-93339-9_6

Keywords
CheckMate 214 · CABOSUN · Metastatic

1 Introduction

The management of metastatic renal cell carcinoma (mRCC) underwent a dramatic paradigm shift in the mid-2000s. Around this time, targeted therapies that abrogate signaling through the vascular endothelial growth factor (VEGF) receptor (specifically, sunitinib and sorafenib) were approved [1, 2]. In the years following, a slew of other targeted therapies were approved that also either targeted the VEGF receptor (pazopanib and axitinib) [3–5] VEGF ligand (bevacizumab) [6] or downstream moieties such as the mammalian targeted of rapamycin (mTOR; temsirolimus and everolimus) [7, 8].

These approvals were accompanied by a steady decrease in utilization of conventional immunotherapeutic agents such as interleukin-2 (IL-2) and interferon alpha (IFN alpha). While agents such as high-dose IL-2 offered durable remissions in a small subset of patients (estimated at around 5–7%), there was little gain for the vast majority of patients [9]. In contrast, targeted therapies offered a greater proportion of patients an opportunity for clinical benefit (response or stabilization of disease) [10–12].

Over the past 2 years, there has been yet another renaissance in the management of mRCC. The newest systemic therapies represent the next generation of both immunotherapy and targeted agents. In the former category are checkpoint inhibitors, agents which inhibit specific pathways that contribute to T cell anergy. In the latter category are multikinase inhibitors that target not just VEGF receptor but multiple receptor tyrosine kinases that guide RCC pathogenesis. Multiple existing manuscripts and chapters outline the clinical data for previous generations of immunotherapeutic and targeted therapies [12–14]. Similarly, there are copious publications related to the mechanism of action of the aforementioned novel agents [15, 16]. In the current chapter, we will review the most recent clinical data which shapes the paradigm for first-line systemic treatment.

2 CheckMate 214

In the USA, sunitinib and pazopanib represent the most frequently utilized agents in the first-line setting for patients with mRCC [17]. This is likely to change with results from recent trials including CABOSUN and CheckMate 214. The CheckMate 214 [18] trial randomized 1082 patients with mRCC and clear cell features to receive either sunitinib or nivolumab with ipilimumab. Sunitinib was rendered at the standard dose of 50 mg oral daily, 4 weeks on and 2 weeks off. Nivolumab and ipilimumab were rendered at 3 and 1 mg/kg, respectively, and given intravenously every 3 weeks for a total of 12 weeks. Thereafter, nivolumab was continued at the same dose on a 2-weekly cycle until the time of disease progression or unacceptable toxicity.

The study used the International mRCC Database Consortium (IMDC) [19] criteria to risk-stratify patients. These criteria include (1) time from diagnosis to initiation of systemic therapy, (2) performance status, (3) hemoglobin level, (4) calcium level, (5) neutrophil level, and (6) platelet count. The study was designed with 3 primary endpoints (objective response rate [ORR], progression-free survival [PFS], and overall survival [OS]), each explored within the subset of patients with intermediate- and poor-risk disease by these criteria. From a statistical perspective, the study utilized an overall alpha of 0.05, split across the 3 co-primary endpoints (0.001 for ORR, 0.009 for PFS, and 0.04 for OS).

Ultimately, 847 patients with intermediate- and poor-risk disease were included for assessment of the primary endpoints. Characteristics of patients on the control and experimental arms were similar, with 79 and 21% of patients possessing intermediate- and poor-risk disease, respectively, on each arm. Programmed death-ligand 1 (PD-L1) expression on tumor cells was quantified using a threshold of 1%. Roughly one-quarter of patients on both arms had elevated PD-L1 expression ($\geq 1\%$).

In the intermediate- and poor-risk subset, there was an improvement in RR with nivolumab/ipilimumab versus sunitinib (42 vs. 27%; $P < 0.0001$). Among responders, 9% of patients receiving nivolumab/ipilimumab garnered a complete response (CR), as compared to just 1% of patients receiving sunitinib. Duration of response (DOR) was also more prolonged in patients receiving nivolumab/ipilimumab—the median DOR was not reached in this subset, versus 18.2 months in patients receiving sunitinib. With the stringent *P*-value used to evaluate PFS, a significant difference was not identified, although there was a trend toward benefit with nivolumab/ipilimumab (11.6 vs. 8.4 months). Finally, OS was significantly improved in patients receiving nivolumab/ipilimumab, with the median value not reached in this cohort versus 26.0 months with sunitinib ($P < 0.0001$).

Several differences were noted with respect to dose intensity and drug discontinuation. In the overall study population, a larger proportion of patients receiving nivolumab/ipilimumab discontinued therapy on account of toxicity (24 vs. 12%). Given that patients on the experimental arm received a median of 4 doses of ipilimumab, the regimen was likely discontinued in a latent fashion after receipt of the combination. Furthermore, although grade 3–5 treatment-related adverse events were more frequent in patients receiving sunitinib as compared to nivolumab/ipilimumab (63 vs. 46%), there were a higher number of treatment-related deaths on the nivolumab/ipilimumab arm (7 vs. 4). Multiple immune-related grade 3–4 adverse events were also noted with nivolumab/ipilimumab, with the most frequent being hepatitis, diarrhea/colitis, rash, adrenal insufficiency, and hyopophysitis. Approximately 60% of patients receiving this regimen required corticosteroids for management of adverse events, and more intensive agents (e.g., mycophenolate and infliximab) were rendered in approximately 4% of patients.

Beyond the analysis of the primary endpoint and toxicity data, several subset analyses are informative in deciphering appropriate populations for receipt of nivolumab/ipilimumab [20]. Firstly, an analysis of patients with good-risk disease (excluded from the analysis of primary endpoint) suggests a marked benefit in PFS with sunitinib versus nivolumab/ipilimumab (25.1 vs. 15.3 months; $P < 0.0001$). Similarly, RR was improved with sunitinib in this subset (52 vs. 29%; $P = 0.0002$). A second important analysis segregated patients based on PD-L1 status. Recalling that roughly one-fourth of patients were PD-L1 positive, the largest benefit in OS was observed in this subset with nivolumab/ipilimumab relative to sunitinib (median OS not reached vs. 19.6 months; HR 0.45, $P < 0.001$). A survival benefit was noted in patients who were PD-L1 negative with nivolumab/ipilimumab versus sunitinib, but this difference was more subtle (median OS not reached for either group; HR 0.73, $P = 0.0249$). Notably, there was no difference in PFS between nivolumab/ipilimumab and sunitinib in this subset.

3 CABOSUN

Another trial that has had a dramatic impact on the first-line treatment paradigm for mRCC is CABOSUN [21–23]. This randomized, phase II trial compared sunitinib and cabozantinib in mRCC patients with no prior therapy and was restricted to patients with intermediate- and poor-risk disease by IMDC criteria. Patients with known brain metastases were permitted in this study, provided there was documented stability for 3 months. Permissible ECOG performance status ranged from 0 to 2. Patients received standard starting doses of sunitinib and cabozantinib at 50 and 60 mg oral daily, respectively. As in CheckMate 214, sunitinib was dosed at the conventional 4-week on, 2-week off schedule.

The primary endpoint of the study was PFS with secondary endpoints of OS, objective RR and safety. With a planned enrollment of 140 patients, the study had 85% power to detect a HR of 0.67 with a one-sided type I error of 0.12. The authors anticipated that this would translate to a PFS of 8 months with sunitinib versus 12 months with cabozantinib. Ultimately, 157 patients were enrolled. Most patients were ECOG 0-1, although 12.7% of patients enrolled were classified as ECOG 2. Intermediate-risk disease patients constituted 80.9% of the overall sample. The study possessed a relatively high frequency of patients with bone metastases, amounting to 36.3% of patients enrolled. Approximately one-fourth of patients enrolled had not had nephrectomy.

The initial assessment of PFS was based solely on investigator review. The study met its primary endpoint, with an improvement in PFS from 5.6 months with sunitinib to 8.6 months with cabozantinib ($P = 0.012$). Cabozantinib was associated with a significant improvement in RR relative to sunitinib, as well (46 vs. 18%). A trend toward improvement in median OS was observed with cabozantinib (31.3 months vs. 21.8 months), but this difference was not statistically significant. With respect to toxicity, the frequency of grade 3 and 4 adverse events was similar between sunitinib (68%) and cabozantinib (67%). The nature of side effects was typical for VEGF-directed therapies, with the most common toxicities across both groups including hypertension, fatigue, and diarrhea. Treatment-related grade 5 events were recorded with both cabozantinib and sunitinib. Among patients receiving cabozantinib, 3 treatment-related deaths were recorded secondary to acute kidney injury, sepsis, and jejunal perforation. For patients receiving sunitinib, 3 treatment-related deaths were attributed to sepsis, respiratory failure, and vascular disorders, respectively.

The encouraging phase II data from cabozantinib led many to question whether the agent would be granted FDA approval. To appease one of the principal critiques of the trial, which centered on investigator review of imaging data, the ALLIANCE cooperative group worked to collect and perform independent review of scans obtained on CABOSUN [22]. This recently reported review suggested a similar PFS benefit with cabozantinib (8.6 vs. 5.3 months), now with a two-sided *P*-value of 0.0008. This rigorous validation was also applied to assessment of RR. Although fewer responses were observed on both treatment arms, it is noteworthy that the RR associated with cabozantinib was double that observed with sunitinib (20 vs. 9%), akin to the original analysis. These data ultimately led to FDA approval of cabozantinib for previously untreated mRCC on December 19, 2017.

4 Other First-Line Studies

The results of the CABOSUN and CheckMate 214 trials provide fuel for vigorous debate regarding first-line standards for mRCC. While these two studies are independently practice-changing, it should be noted that there are multiple other regimens that are being aggressively explored in this setting. Table 1 summarizes the current and ongoing landscape of trials [24]. As can be seen, the preponderance focuses on the combination of VEGF blockade with PD-1/PD-L1 blockade or other immunotherapeutic strategies. The only of these studies to report so far is the phase III ADAPT trial, which evaluated sunitinib with or without the autologous dendritic cell vaccine AGS-003 in patients receiving cytoreductive nephrectomy. While a phase II assessment of sunitinib with AGS-003 had shown encouraging clinical outcomes, the phase III study failed to show any difference in OS (the primary endpoint).

Table 1 Current and ongoing landscape of trials

Study	Phase	Masking	Status	First posted date	Last update posted date	Experimental arm 1	Experimental arm 2	Comparator	Objective
NCT01582672 ADAPT	III	Open label	Active, not recruiting	April 2012	June 2017	AGS-003 + standard treatment	NA	Standard treatment	OS benefit between rocapuldencel-T in combination with standard treatment versus standard treatment alone
NCT00678119	II	Open label	Completed	May 2008	July 2013	AGS-003 + Sunitinib	NA	Single arm study	Investigate AGS-003, when used in combination with sunitinib in subjects with previously untreated advanced stage RCC.
NCT01984242 IMmotion150	II	Open label	Completed	Nov 2013	Dec 2017	Atezolizumab + Bevacizumab	Atezolizumab	Sunitinib	Evaluate the efficacy, safety, and tolerability of atezolizumab monotherapy or in combination with bevacizumab versus sunitinib in inoperable, locally advanced, or metastatic RCC who have not received prior systemic therapy.
NCT02420821 IMmotion151	III	Open label	Recruiting	Apr 2015	Jan 2018	Atezolizumab + Bevacizumab	NA	Sunitinib	Evaluate the efficacy and safety of atezolizumab plus bevacizumab versus sunitinib in participants with inoperable, locally advanced, or metastatic RCC who have not received prior systemic therapy.
NCT02133742	I	Open label	Active, not recruiting	May 2014	Dec 2017	Axitinib + Pembrolizumab	NA	Single arm study	Evaluate safety, pharmacokinetics and pharmacodynamics of axitinib in combination with pembrolizumab in patients with advanced RCC.

(continued)

Table 1 (continued)

Study	Phase	Masking	Status	First posted date	Last update posted date	Experimental arm 1	Experimental arm 2	Comparator	Objective
NCT02684006 JAVELIN Renal 101	III	Open label	Recruiting	Feb 2016	Jan 2018	Avelumab + Axitinib	NA	Sunitinib	Evaluate anti-tumor activity and safety of avelumab in combination with axitinib versus sunitinib monotherapy, administered as first-line treatment, in patients with advanced RCC.
NCT02811861	III	Open label	Recruiting	June 2016	Dec 2017	Lenvatinib 18 mg + Everolimus 5 mg	Lenvatinib 20 mg + Pembrolizumab 200 mg	Sunitinib 50 mg	Compare the efficacy and safety of lenvatinib in combination with everolimus (Arm A) or pembrolizumab (Arm B) versus sunitinib (Arm C) as first-line treatment in patients with advanced RCC.

The premise for combining VEGF-directed therapies with PD-1/PD-L1 antibodies is predicated on the immunomodulatory effects of both classes of drugs. To date, the only randomized data comes from IMmotion150, a randomized, phase II study comparing sunitinib to atezolizumab and to the combination of bevacizumab with atezolizumab. The study was powered to assess investigator-assessed PFS in the intention-to-treat and PD-L1-positive study populations. In the PD-L1-positive population, the study met the primary endpoint with an improvement from 6.8 months with sunitinib to 11.1 months with bevacizumab/atezolizumab. These data bode well for the phase III IMmotion151 trial, which directly compares sunitinib and bevacizumab/atezolizumab (the study does not evaluate atezolizumab monotherapy). Given that bevacizumab is relatively infrequently used in the metastatic setting, it will be curious to see whether (in the face of positive data) the agent will be employed in combinations. Several studies are underway which use different VEGF-tyrosine kinase inhibitors (TKIs) at their base. A phase III study comparing sunitinib to axitinib with avelumab is bolstered by very encouraging phase Ib data, suggesting 58.2% response rate in previously untreated patients [25]. Similarly, compelling data is available for the combinations of axitinib with pembrolizumab [26] and lenvatinib with pembrolizumab [27], each being compared to sunitinib in separate phase III assessments.

5 Future Management Paradigms for mRCC

As the data in this chapter demonstrate, the paradigm for first-line therapy of mRCC has evolved once again. Agents such as sunitinib and pazopanib may potentially find a niche among good-risk patients, given that data from CheckMate 214 suggests that a TKI-based approach may supersede checkpoint inhibition in this setting. However, one might make the argument that a more potent TKI, such as cabozantinib, could be employed in this setting—there is little reason to think cabozantinib would not offer superiority to sunitinib in the good-risk population.

In intermediate- and poor-risk patients, many argue that nivolumab/ipilimumab represents an obvious choice. Certainly, the complete responses observed with this therapy are compelling. However, several considerations must be kept in mind. First, the rate of severe immunologic toxicities is non-negligible, and the large proportion of patients requiring steroids (60%) suggest that this is a pervasive phenomenon. Second, the studies that have been done to date all utilize a comparator arm of sunitinib. While cross-trial comparisons are challenging, it is difficult to fathom whether a significant difference in RR and OS would have been identified had nivolumab/ipilimumab been compared to cabozantinib. Finally, cost may ultimately become a major determinant. Dual checkpoint inhibition takes a substantial financial toll, and it is unclear whether all healthcare systems are equipped to bear this burden. For these reasons, a healthy debate should precede the decision to employ cabozantinib or nivolumab/ipilimumab in the front-line setting.

Although somewhat cliché, the future of mRCC may ultimately be predicated on use of biomarkers. Data from the previously cited IMmotion150 trial offers a unique circumstance in which to compare biomarkers in a TKI-treated cohort and in a cohort exposed to dual VEGF and checkpoint inhibition. Rich genomic profiling studies accompanying this effort suggest that there may be an immune profile predictive of response to checkpoint inhibition and a separate angiogenic profile predictive of response to VEGF-TKIs [15, 28, 29]. While further validation or prospective evaluation of these biomarkers is warranted, it hints to the possibility of a biomarker-based approach in the future. A recently reported collaboration between Dana Farber, Johns Hopkins, and Memorial Sloan Kettering investigators pooled together response to patients receiving nivolumab for mRCC and identified alterations in *PBRM1* as potential predictors of response [15]. These biomarkers may therefore serve to identify ideal candidates for checkpoint inhibition. With the multitude of ongoing studies and the sea of therapies likely to emerge, a biologically driven approach to treatment would be most useful.

Acknowledgements None.
Conflict of Interest SKP declares consulting agreements with Genentech, Roche, Exelixis, BMS, Ipsen, Novartis, Astellas, Eisai and Pfizer.

References

1. Escudier B, Eisen T, Stadler WM et al (2007) Sorafenib in advanced clear-cell renal-cell carcinoma. New Engl J Med 356:125–134
2. Motzer RJ, Hutson TE, Tomczak P et al (2007) Sunitinib versus interferon alfa in metastatic renal-cell carcinoma. New Engl J Med 356:115–124
3. Motzer RJ, Hutson TE, Cella D et al (2013) Pazopanib versus sunitinib in metastatic renal-cell carcinoma. New Engl J Med 369:722–731
4. Sternberg CN, Davis ID, Mardiak J et al (2010) Pazopanib in locally advanced or metastatic renal cell carcinoma: results of a randomized phase III trial. J Clin Oncol: Official J Am Soc Clin Oncol 28:1061–1068
5. Rini BI, Escudier B, Tomczak P, et al (2011) Comparative effectiveness of axitinib versus sorafenib in advanced renal cell carcinoma (AXIS): a randomised phase 3 trial. Lancet (London, England) 378:1931–1939
6. Escudier B, Pluzanska A, Koralewski P, et al (2007) Bevacizumab plus interferon alfa-2a for treatment of metastatic renal cell carcinoma: a randomised, double-blind phase III trial. Lancet (London, England) 370:2103–2111
7. Hudes G, Carducci M, Tomczak P et al (2007) Temsirolimus, interferon alfa, or both for advanced renal-cell carcinoma. New Engl J Med 356:2271–2281
8. Motzer RJ, Escudier B, Oudard S, et al (2008) Efficacy of everolimus in advanced renal cell carcinoma: a double-blind, randomised, placebo-controlled phase III trial. Lancet (London, England) 372:449–456
9. Atzpodien J, Kirchner H, Jonas U et al (2004) Interleukin-2- and interferon alfa-2a-based immunochemotherapy in advanced renal cell carcinoma: a Prospectively Randomized Trial of the German Cooperative Renal Carcinoma Chemoimmunotherapy Group (DGCIN). J Clin Oncol: Official J Am Soc Clin Oncol 22:1188–1194

10. Pal SK, Bergerot P, Figlin RA (2015) Renal cell carcinoma: An update for the practicing urologist. Asian J Urol 2:19–25
11. Choueiri TK, Motzer RJ (2017) Systemic therapy for metastatic renal-cell carcinoma. New Engl J Med 376:354–366
12. Singh P, Agarwal N, Pal SK (2015) Sequencing systemic therapies for metastatic kidney cancer. Curr Treat Options Oncol 16:316
13. McDermott DF (2011) Immunotherapy and targeted therapy combinations in renal cancer. Current Clin Pharmacool 6:207–213
14. Albouy B, Gross Goupil M, Escudier B, Massard C (2010) Renal cell carcinoma management and therapies in 2010. Bull Cancer 97:17–28
15. Ho TH, Choueiri TK, Wang K et al (2016) Correlation between molecular subclassifications of clear cell renal cell carcinoma and targeted therapy response. Eur Urol Focus 2:204–209
16. Cancer Genome Atlas Research Network (2013) Comprehensive molecular characterization of clear cell renal cell carcinoma. Nature 499:43–49
17. Pal SK, Signorovitch JE, Li N et al (2017) Patterns of care among patients receiving sequential targeted therapies for advanced renal cell carcinoma: A retrospective chart review in the USA. Int J Urol: Official J Jpn Urol Assoc 24:272–278
18. Hammers HJ, Plimack ER, Sternberg C, et al (2015) CheckMate 214: A phase III, randomized, open-label study of nivolumab combined with ipilimumab versus sunitinib monotherapy in patients with previously untreated metastatic renal cell carcinoma. J Clin Oncol 33:TPS4578–TPS
19. Heng DY, Xie W, Regan MM et al (2009) Prognostic factors for overall survival in patients with metastatic renal cell carcinoma treated with vascular endothelial growth factor-targeted agents: results from a large, multicenter study. J Clin Oncol: Official J Am Soc Clin Oncol 27:5794–5799
20. Motzer RJ, Tannir NM, McDermott DF, Frontera OA, Melichar B, Plimack ER, Barthelemy P, George S, Neiman V, Porta C, Choueiri TK, Powles T, Donskov F, Salman P, Kollmannsberger CK, Rini B, Mekan S, McHenry MB, Wind-Rotolo M, Hammers HJ, Escudier B (2017) Nivolumab + Ipilimumab (N + I) versus Sunitinib (S) for treatment-naïve advanced or metastatic renal cell carcinoma (aRCC): results from CheckMate 214, including overall survival by subgroups. SITC 2017 ANNUAL MEETING ABSTRACTS BOOK. Maryland: Society for Immunotherapy of Cancer p 103
21. Choueiri TK, Escudier B, Powles T et al (2015) Cabozantinib versus everolimus in advanced renal-cell carcinoma. New Engl J Med 373:1814–1823
22. Choueiri TK, Halabi S, Sanford BL et al (2017) Cabozantinib versus sunitinib as initial targeted therapy for patients with metastatic renal cell carcinoma of poor or intermediate risk: the alliance A031203 CABOSUN trial. J Clin Oncol 35:591–597
23. Choueiri TK, Escudier B, Powles T et al (2016) Cabozantinib versus everolimus in advanced renal cell carcinoma (METEOR): final results from a randomised, open-label, phase 3 trial. Lancet Oncol 17:917–927
24. NIH U.S. National library of medicine https://clinicaltrials.gov/ Accessed January 10, 2018
25. Choueiri TK, Rini BI, Larkin JMG, et al (2017) Avelumab plus axitinib versus sunitinib as first-line treatment of advanced renal cell carcinoma: Phase 3 study (JAVELIN Renal 101). J Clin Oncol 35:TPS4594–TPS
26. Atkins MB, Gupta S, Choueiri TK et al (2015) Phase Ib dose-finding study of axitinib plus pembrolizumab in treatment-naïve patients with advanced renal cell carcinoma. J Immuno Ther Cancer 3:353
27. Lee CVM, Rasco D, Taylor M, Dutcus C, Shumaker R., Schmidt EV, Stepan D., Li D, Motzer RJ (2017) Anti-Cancer Agents & Biologic Therapy Renal Cell Cancer Cancer Immunology and Immunotherapy Genitourinary Cancers. ESMO 2017 Congress. Madrid, Spain: Annals of Oncology v295–v329. 10.1093

28. Hahn AW, Gill DM, Maughan B et al (2017) Correlation of genomic alterations assessed by next-generation sequencing (NGS) of tumor tissue DNA and circulating tumor DNA (ctDNA) in metastatic renal cell carcinoma (mRCC): potential clinical implications. Oncotarget 8:33614–33620
29. Becerra MF, Reznik E, Redzematovic A, et al (2017) Comparative genomic profiling of matched primary and metastatic tumors in renal cell carcinoma. Eur Urol Focus

Optical and Cross-Sectional Imaging Technologies for Bladder Cancer

Bernhard Kiss, Gautier Marcq and Joseph C. Liao

Contents

B. Kiss · G. Marcq · J. C. Liao
Department of Urology, Stanford University School of Medicine, Stanford, CA 94305, USA

B. Kiss · G. Marcq · J. C. Liao
Veterans Affairs Palo Alto Health Care System, Palo Alto, CA 94304, USA

J. C. Liao (✉)
300 Pasteur Dr., Room S-287, Stanford, CA 94305-5118, USA
e-mail: jliao@stanford.edu

S. Daneshmand and K. G. Chan (eds.), *Genitourinary Cancers*, Cancer Treatment and Research 175, https://doi.org/10.1007/978-3-319-93339-9_7

Abstract

Optical and cross-sectional imaging plays critical roles in bladder cancer diagnostics. White light cystoscopy remains the cornerstone for the management of non-muscle-invasive bladder cancer. In the last decade, significant technological improvements have been introduced for optical imaging to address the known shortcomings of white light cystoscopy. Enhanced cystoscopy modalities such as blue light cystoscopy and narrowband imaging survey a large area of the urothelium and provide contrast enhancement to detect additional lesions and decrease cancer recurrence. However, higher false-positive rates accompany the gain of sensitivity. Optical biopsy technologies, including confocal laser endomicroscopy and optical coherence tomography, provide cellular resolutions combined with subsurface imaging, thereby enabling optical-based cancer characterization, and may lead to real-time cancer grading and staging. Coupling of fluorescently labeled binding agents with optical imaging devices may translate into high molecular specificity, thus enabling visualization and characterization of biological processes at the molecular level. For cross-sectional imaging, upper urinary tract evaluation and assessment potential extravesical tumor extension and metastases are currently the primary roles, particularly for management of muscle-invasive bladder cancer. Multi-parametric MRI, including dynamic gadolinium-enhanced and diffusion-weighted sequences, has been investigated for primary bladder tumor detection. Ultrasmall superparamagnetic particles of iron oxide (USPIO) are a new class of contrast agents that increased the accuracy of lymph node imaging. Combination of multi-parametric MRI with positron emission tomography is on the horizon to improve accuracy rates for primary tumor diagnostics as well as lymph node evaluation. As these high-resolution optical and cross-sectional technologies emerge and develop, judicious assessment and validation await for their clinical integration toward improving the overall management of bladder cancer.

Keywords

Bladder cancer · Optical imaging · Cross-sectional imaging
Molecular imaging · Enhanced cystoscopy · Optical biopsy

1 Introduction

Imaging plays an integral role in all aspects of bladder cancer management. As the standard optical imaging modality, white light cystoscopy (WLC) is utilized for office-based identification of bladder tumors and enables transurethral resection (TUR) for local staging. Cross-sectional imaging, primarily computed tomography

(CT), complements WLC to assess the upper urinary tract and potential extravesical tumor extension and metastases.

Over the past two decades, new optical and cross-sectional imaging technologies have emerged to complement and augment current standards, particularly in improving cancer diagnostic accuracy. New technologies provide enhanced spatial and temporal resolutions and hold the potential to highlight the dynamic cellular and molecular differences between cancerous and non-cancerous tissues. This chapter aims to review the current state of the art of new and developing optical and cross-sectional imaging technologies for bladder cancer.

2 Optical Imaging

In 2017, white light cystoscopy (WLC) remains the standard for evaluation of bladder urothelium and management of non-muscle-invasive bladder cancer (NMIBC), both in the office setting with flexible cystoscopy and TUR in the operating room. Despite its central role, WLC has well-recognized limitations [54, 59]. For papillary lesions, WLC is unreliable for the determination of low- and high-grade cancer and cannot assess level of invasion [22]. Differentiation of non-papillary and flat malignant lesions, particularly carcinoma in situ (CIS), from inflammations can be difficult, with detection rates of CIS as low as 58–68% by WLC [30, 43, 83]. Furthermore, smaller or satellite tumors can be missed, which contributes to the up to 40% rate of residual bladder cancer found at the time of second-look TUR [6, 25]. Finally, indistinct borders and inadequate submucosal margins during TUR can lead to incomplete tumor resection and understaging [21, 51]. These limitations of WLC contribute to the increased risk of cancer persistence, recurrence, and in the case of high-grade bladder disease, progression to metastatic disease [11, 47, 49]. Hence, there is significant interest to develop adjunctive imaging techniques to augment conventional WLC for more precise diagnostic and surveillance of bladder cancer.

2.1 Enhanced Cystoscopy Technologies

Adjunctive optical imaging technologies that go beyond WLC may be classified based on their field of view and spatial resolution. Enhanced cystoscopy technologies survey a large area of the urothelium and provide contrast enhancement beyond WLC to distinguish suspicious lesions from benign transformations. Blue light cystoscopy (BLC) and narrowband imaging (NBI) are approved examples of this modality.

2.1.1 Blue Light Cystoscopy (BLC)

Also known as photodynamic diagnosis or fluorescence cystoscopy, BLC provides wide field of view similar to WLC. It requires preoperative intravesical instillation of a photosensitizer that is preferentially metabolized by neoplastic cells. Once taken up by the urothelium, the photosensitizer (i.e., protoporphyrin IX precursor) accumulates, whereby in neoplastic cells the absorption of blue fluorescent light (375–440 nm) induces emission of red light, thus allowing visualization of the neoplastic tissue [14, 64] (Fig. 1). In bladder imaging, two protoporphyrin analogues, 5-aminolevulinic acid (5-ALA), and its ester derivate hexaminolevulinate (HAL) have been extensively investigated clinically. HAL, which is more lipophilic with greater local bioavailability and superior fluorescence intensity, is approved for clinical use.

BLC has been demonstrated to improve detection of papillary lesions and CIS in numerous multi-institutional randomized studies [53, 76]. In a meta-analysis, the detection of CIS was significantly higher by the combination of BLC and WLC compared to WLC alone (87 vs. 75%) [57]. Furthermore, significantly reduced residual tumor rates were found in patients who underwent BLC-assisted TUR (relative risk of 2.77-fold higher for WLC compared to BLC) in meta-analyses [45, 86]. A prospective randomized multi-institutional study (n = 300) failed to demonstrate a significant benefit in tumor recurrence and progression for BLC compared to WLC after 12-month follow-up [84], while another prospective randomized study (n = 551) found an increased time to recurrence of 16.4 months with BLC using HAL compared to 9.4 months with WLC ($p = 0.04$) [38]. In a meta-analysis of the prospective trials, Burger et al. found significantly lower overall recurrence rates at 12 months with BLC compared to WLC in 1345 patients with NMIBC (34.5 vs. 45.4% pooled sensitivity, $p = 0.006$) [12]. Main limitation of BLC is the non-cancer-specific fluorescence from inflammatory lesions, previous biopsies, or pretreatment with bacillus Calmette–Guérin (BCG) [53, 59] leading to

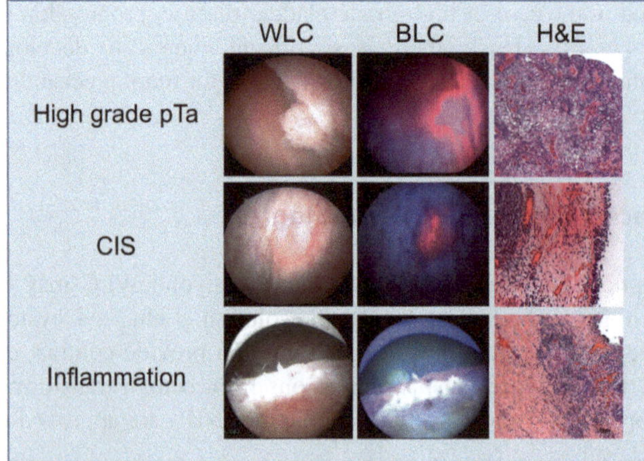

Fig. 1 Blue light cystoscopy facilitates detection of papillary and flat bladder cancer but increases false-positive rate. Endoscopic images of high-grade pTa, carcinoma in situ (CIS) and inflammation under white light cystoscopy (WLC), blue light cystoscopy (BLC), and corresponding hematoxylin and eosin (H&E) histology

false-positive diagnosis in 10–12% on a per-patient basis [88]. HAL-assisted BLC is currently not approved for patients within 90 days of intravesical chemotherapy or BCG instillations. In the 2016 AUA guidelines on NMIBC, HAL-assisted BLC received moderate recommendation [17].

2.1.2 Narrowband Imaging (NBI)

Narrowband imaging (NBI) was developed in 1999 [35] by Olympus (Tokyo, Japan) and first applied to gastrointestinal endoscopy [34]. The technology relies on a light filter that provides narrow (blue, green), instead of broad illumination (blue, green, and red) as in standard white light, thereby highlighting vascularized lesions (Fig. 2) [103]. In contrast to BLC, NBI does not need exogenous fluorescent dyes. A prospective randomized trial in 178 patients with NMIBC showed significantly lower recurrence rates at 3 and 12 months for patients who underwent NBI-assisted TUR than patient who underwent standard TUR [62]. At 3-month follow-up, the recurrence rates were 5.8% in the NBI group compared with 18.5% in the WLC-only group. At 1-year follow-up, the recurrence rates were 18.6% in the NBI group compared with 38.04% in the WLC. The recurrence rate of CIS was significantly lower in the NBI group (2.3 vs. 14.1%, $p < 0.05$).

A meta-analysis [100] has shown that compared to WLC alone, NBI increased NMIBC detection by 9.9%, increased diagnostic sensitivity from 81.6 to 95.8%, reduced tumor persistence rate at 1 month at re-resection (RR = 0.43), and reduced recurrence rate at 12 months (RR = 0.81). A recent multi-institutional, prospective, randomized study of 965 patients with primary diagnosis of NMIBC found a significantly higher recurrence rate in patients with low-risk NMIBC treated by WLC-assisted compared to NBI-assisted TURBT (27.3 vs. 5.6%, $p = 0.002$) at 12 months [69]. However, no overall difference in recurrence rates was found at 12 months (27.1% WLC vs. 25.4% NBI, $p = 0.585$). Increasing sensitivity frequently leads to higher false-positive rates, and NBI was shown to have higher false-positive rates of 21.8–50% per patient compared to WLC [40, 100, 101] even if a recent study found an increased detection of CIS up to 28% without increased false-positive rates with NBI [58]. Table 1 summarizes performance of enhanced cystoscopy technologies compared to WLC alone when analyzing accuracy on the patient level as well as on the biopsy level.

2.2 Optical Biopsy Technologies

Whereas enhanced cystoscopy technologies improve identification and enumeration of suspicious bladder lesions, their overall field of view and spatial resolutions are comparable to standard WLC and hence relatively minimal learning curve. In contrast, optical biopsy technologies provide cellular resolutions combined with subsurface imaging, thereby raising the possibility of real-time, optical-based cancer characterization including grading and staging. For integration into the clinical workflow, the high-resolution imaging data require real-time interpretation, thereby increasing the associated learning curve with the technology adaptation.

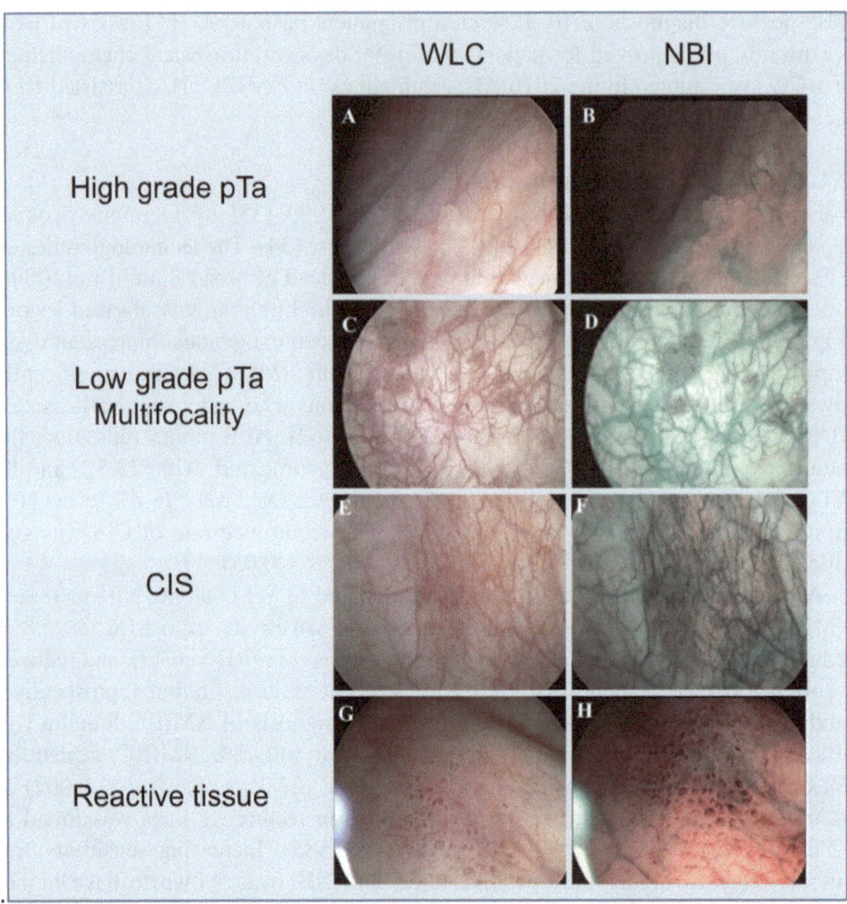

Fig. 2 NBI-enhanced cystoscopy facilitates detection of papillary and flat bladder cancer but increases false-positive rate. **a** Small papillary tumor (pathology pTa) poorly visualized under WLC but improved under NBI (**b**); multi-focal papillary tumors (pathology pTa) under WLC (**c**) and NBI (**d**); **e** WLC image of CIS and NBI (**f**); **g** false-positive lesion near the right orifice identified by WLC; **h** same lesion identified by NBI (reactive tissue in pathology). Figures obtained from [15] with permission

Confocal laser endomicroscopy (CLE) and optical coherence tomography (OCT) are examples of optical biopsy technologies with early stage clinical experience. Importantly, these technologies complement wide field imaging (i.e., WLC, BLC, and NBI) to provide a more comprehensive evaluation of tissue of interest.

2.2.1 Confocal Laser Endomicroscopy (CLE)

Confocal laser endomicroscopy (CLE) is based on the well-established confocal microscopy technique commonly used in laboratory settings [67]. Configuration of

Table 1 Comparison table between blue light cystoscopy, narrowband imaging, and white light cystoscopy

Authors	Year of publication	Type	No of patient	Group	Lesion	Sensitivity (%)	Specificity (%)
Mowatt et al. [68]	2011	Meta-analysis	2949	BLC +WLC	All type patient level	92	57
		27 studies		WLC		71	72
				BLC +WLC	All type biopsy level	93	60
				WLC		65	81
				BLC +WLC	CIS patient level	83	–
				WLC		32	–
				BLC +WLC	CIS biopsy level	86	–
				WLC		50	–
Xiong et al. [100]	2017	Meta-analysis	1518	NBI + WLC	All type patient level	96	74
		25 studies		WLC		82	79
				NBI + WLC	All type biopsy level	95	66
				WLC		72	79
Zheng et al. [102]	2012	Meta-analysis	1022	NBI + WLC	CIS patient level	93	77
		Eight studies		WLC		–	–
				NBI + WLC	CIS biopsy level	–	–
				WLC		–	–

Performance of each technique is given by sensitivity and specificity. BLC = blue light cystoscopy, WLC = white light cystoscopy, CIS = carcinoma in situ, NBI = narrowband imaging. Patient-level analysis shows the accuracy of the technology to diagnose all lesions in the bladder. Biopsy-level analysis shows the accuracy of the technology to diagnose one lesion in the bladder the technology into probe-based devices compatible with standard endoscopic instruments has enabled clinical translation and in vivo imaging of cellular and subcellular structures (2001). The CLE system (Cellvizio®, Mauna Kea Technologies, France) in clinical use has been coupled with endoscopy of the gastrointestinal, respiratory, and urinary tracts. The technology is based on a fiber-optic imaging probe coupled to a 488-nm laser-scanning unit. The reusable probe has a 1–5μm spatial resolution. Fluorescein is used as the contrast agent and can be applied either topically via intravesical instillation or systemically via intravenous injection [95]. Bladder application of CLE has been described in detail [19]. Pilot studies have shown that CLE can discriminate normal mucosa from benign lesions (scar, inflammatory lesion) and malignant lesion (CIS, low and high grade) after training (Fig. 3) [18, 99]. The inter-observer agreement to diagnose cancer was 90% in urologists experienced in using CLE compared with 80% in urologists not-experienced in CLE after one-hour training session [18]. To assess the learning curve of CLE image interpretation more broadly, crowdsourcing has been applied to assess the diagnostic accuracy to distinguish normal urothelium from cancer. After a shorting training module, of 92% diagnostic accuracy was obtained 1173 ratings from 602 participants [18, 20]. Current limitations of CLE include the lack of multi-institutional studies in order to validate diagnosis criteria and accuracy. Additional future directions include combining CLE with molecular imaging

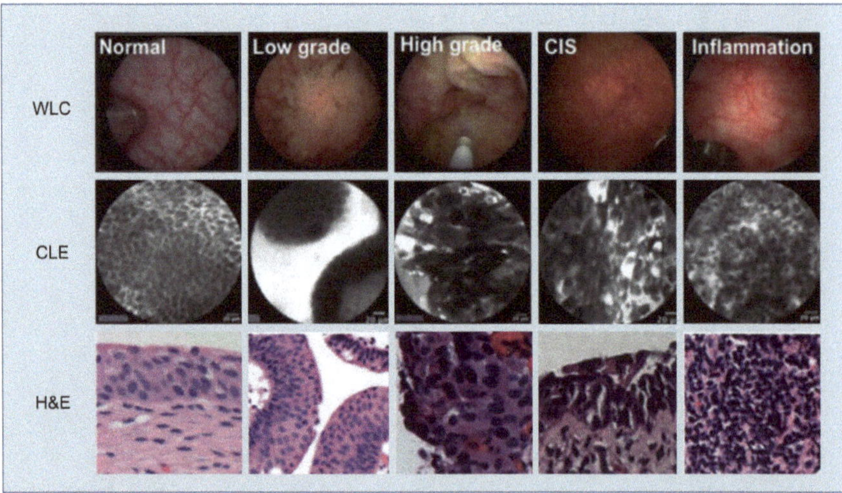

Fig. 3 Optical biopsy of bladder mucosa using probe-based confocal laser endomicroscopy (CLE). CLE of normal, low-/high-grade papillary bladder cancer, CIS, and inflammation shown with corresponding white light cystoscopy (WLC) and hematoxylin and eosin (H&E) staining of the biopsy. Low-grade cancer shows characteristic-organized papillary structure, whereas high-grade cancer and CIS show pleomorphic cells and distorted micro-architecture. Inflammatory mucosa shows lymphocytic infiltrates. Figure from [42] with permission

modalities such as monoclonal antibodies bound to fluorescein-labeled monoclonal antibodies for targeted binding of cancer-specific antigens.

2.2.2 Optical Coherence Tomography (OCT)

OCT provides real-time high-resolution subsurface imaging of tissue using near-infrared light with wavelengths between 890 and 1300 nm. Analogous to B-mode ultrasound, the technique measures the backscatter properties of tissue layers thus providing a cross-sectional imaging with an image resolution of 10–20 μm and a depth of penetration of 2 mm [63]. Originally described for imaging of the retina [56], OCT has been demonstrated in a variety of organ systems including gastrointestinal, respiratory, and urinary tracts. In cancerous lesions, the anatomic layers of the urothelium are lost and therefore enable real-time cancer diagnostic. The reported overall sensitivity for cancer diagnosis is 84–100% and overall specificity 65–89% [32, 39, 44, 63, 75, 85]. Goh et al. reported 32 patients a 100% negative predictive value for the detection of muscle invasion [32], whereas another trial involving 24 patients at high risk for bladder cancer found a positive predictive value for tumor invasion into the lamina propria of 90% [63]. Schmidbauer and colleagues investigated combining enhanced cystoscopy (i.e., BLC) with OCT and found increased specificity in cancer diagnosis compared to BLC alone [82]. Current limitations include availability of clinical systems for bladder applications and relatively slow image acquisition time. Similar to CLE, further larger scale prospective studies are needed for OCT to demonstrate clinical utilities.

2.3 Molecular Imaging

Molecular imaging modalities enable visualization and characterization of biological processes at the molecular level, which may precede micro- or macroscale anatomic changes [37, 103]. Coupling of fluorescently labeled binding agents such as antibodies, peptides, or small molecules with optical imaging devices may translate into high molecular specificity. Urinary bladder, as an easily accessible hollow organ, is amenable to intravesical applications of therapeutic or imaging agents. The ideal molecular imaging agent has good safety profile, high sensitivity and specificity for cancer detection, suitable pharmacokinetics, and excellent in vivo stability.

Surface antigens are ideal targets for fluorescently labeled antibodies. Epidermal growth factor (EGFR) and prostate stem cell antigen (PSCA) show differential distribution and expression patterns in benign urothelium and bladder cancer [2, 13, 55, 65, 73]. Their relatively low expression rate in bladder cancer, however, makes them suboptimal targets for cancer molecular imaging. A recently described promising target is CD47, a cell surface protein involved in immune functions including neutrophil migration and T-cell co-stimulation, and a negative regulator of phagocytosis. Binding of CD47 on target cells with the native ligand SIRP-α on macrophages inhibits macrophage activation and phagocytosis. Blocking the CD47-SIRP-α interaction with an anti-CD47 antibody promotes phagocytosis of

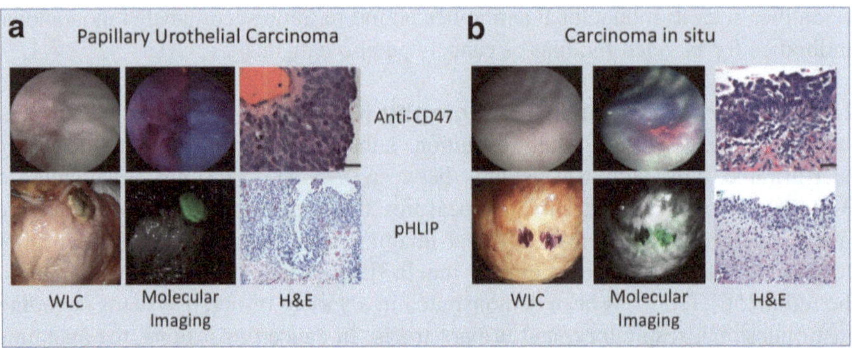

Fig. 4 Molecular imaging of human bladder tumors. Ex vivo molecular imaging of human bladder using anti-CD47-Qdot625 (anti-CD47) imaged with BLC and indocyanine green with pH low insertion peptide (pHLIP) agent imaged with da Vinci Si NIRF imaging system. The respective imaging systems for the two molecular imaging strategies are capable of detecting both **a** papillary tumors and **b** CIS with high sensitivity and specificity. Anti-CD47 images from [72] and pHLIP images obtained from [33] with permission

the CD47 expressing cells and prevents metastasis in mouse xenograft models [16, 98]. CD47 expression is upregulated in bladder cancer, and it is expressed in more than 80% of bladder cancer cells and absent on the luminal cell layer of normal urothelium [16, 72]. In an ex vivo study to validate CD47 as an imaging target, fluorescently labeled anti-CD47 was instilled in 25 fresh radical cystectomy specimens followed by endoscopic fluorescence imaging of the intact bladders (Fig. 4) [72]. CLE and BLC were used as the imaging modalities and fluorescently labeled mouse monoclonal anti-CD47 as the targeting agent. Using the combination with BLC and anti-CD47 conjugated to a quantum dot (Qdot626) with matching spectra, an overall diagnostic sensitivity of 82.9% and a specificity of 90.5% were found for CD47-targeted imaging of bladder cancer.

pH low insertion peptides (pHLIPs) are a class of membrane-binding peptides that preferentially target acidic cells by inserting across cellular membranes at low extracellular pH [3, 97]. Due to increased metabolic activities, a wide variety of cancer cells exhibit acidic pH, thereby providing a versatile strategy for tumor targeting [8]. A recent study used a pHLIP conjugated to indocyanine green (ICG) for ex vivo imaging of bladder tumors from radical cystectomy specimen of 22 patients using a clinical grade near-infrared fluorescence (NIRF) imaging system (Firefly™) (Fig. 4). Sensitivity of targeting cancerous tissue versus normal urothelium was 97%, and specificity was 100% irrespective of urothelial tumor subtype. However, considering necrotic and previously treated tissues as false positives, the specificity was decreased to 80%. In vivo, studies and results particularly low-grade tumors are pending. While molecular imaging may represent the future given the improved cancer specificity, biosafety and regulatory hurdles remain to be overcome for clinical translation.

2.4 Other Early Stage Optical Imaging Technologies

Raman Spectroscopy. Raman spectroscopy (RS) provides optical diagnostics through generation of tissue-specific spectra (i.e., molecular fingerprinting) without the need for exogenous contrast agents. RS is based on the Raman effect, a phenomenon of inelastic scattering of photons that occurs when the incident light is deflected by molecules [74]. These scattered photons are detected to generate spectra specific to the sample (i.e., cancer vs. non-cancer) [28]. For bladder cancer, ex vivo RS studies have demonstrated differentiation of normal urothelial layers, identification of low- and high-grade bladder cancer, and assessment of tumor invasiveness [23, 26]. In a pilot in vivo study of 62 suspicious lesions, an increase in the intensity of specific amino acid peaks and possibly in the DNA-specific peaks demonstrated sensitivity and specificity of 85 and 79%, respectively, for bladder cancer detection [26]. To further increase in sensitivity and specificity, surface-enhanced Raman spectroscopy (SERS), through coupling of molecular targeting nanoparticles, can significantly increase the overall signal-to-noise ratio and enable multiplexed detection of several molecular targets [94].

Ultraviolet Autofluorescence. Differences in tissue autofluorescence, derived from endogenous fluorophores and variations in tissue metabolism and cell types, have been investigated for optical diagnosis of bladder cancer using an ultraviolet (UV) laser [4, 81]. In a pilot in vivo feasibility study of 14 patients with bladder tumors, a UV imaging probe (360 and 450 nm excitation) was inserted in the working channel of a standard rigid cystoscope and placed in close proximity of suspicious bladder lesions. Compared to normal urothelium, decrease in overall fluorescence intensity was observed in bladder cancer, regardless of tumor stage and grade. The fluorescence signal was converted to an intensity ratio of the emitted light at abovementioned wavelengths and color coded, thus facilitating real-time interpretation [81].

Three-Dimensional (3D) bladder reconstruction. While cystoscopy video sequences contain a large volume of data, their documentations are generally suboptimal using non-standardized medical recordkeeping. A more precise strategy to document bladder tumors and suspicious mucosal changes may improve TUR surgical planning, tumor surveillance, trainee education and reduce inter-observer variance. Toward that goal, a variety of hardware and software-based approaches have been investigated. An 'image stitching' algorithm has been described based on an ultrathin preclinical endoscope called scanning fiber endoscope [87]. Using ex vivo pig bladders, full-surface mosaics were generated with a projection error of 1.66 pixels on average and covered 99.6% of the bladder surface area. In another study using TUR videos derived from human subjects, the software algorithm successfully created panoramic images with a resolution of 4096 $\times$ 2048 pixel in 10 out of 12 cases [52]. Notable drawbacks include decreased illustration of the anterior bladder wall as well as low image quality in patients with significant gross hematuria. More recently, a Stanford group described a complete software-based strategy for high-resolution 3D reconstruction of the bladder using standard WLC videos using standard clinical hardware with only a minor modification to the

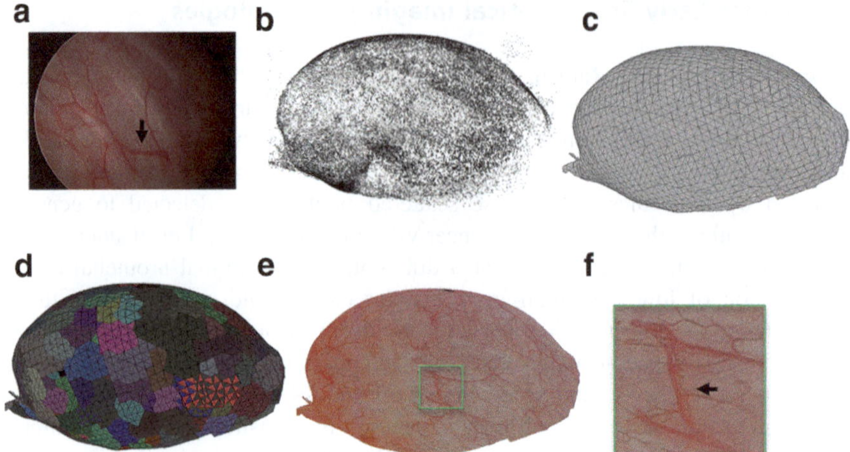

Fig. 5 Software-based 3D bladder reconstruction from WLC videos. Output from individual steps of the reconstruction pipeline from a clinical dataset of human bladder: **a** a representative, original WLC image, **b** point cloud from the structure-from-motion step before outlier removal, **c** mesh from the mesh-generation step, **d** labeled texture (faces with the same color are labeled with the same input image), and **e–f** textured mesh from texture-generation steps. The green box shows a similar region between subfigures **d–f** indicating clear continuity of vessels despite the use of multiple input images to construct this region. The green box is approximately the size of a single WLC image. Black arrows in **a** and **f** indicate similar regions of the bladder. From [61] with permission

standard clinical scan pattern. The images were processed through a customized software algorithm called structure from motion (SfM) to generate a 3D point cloud, followed by mesh and texture generation (Fig. 5). The authors reported that successful reconstruction was achieved for 66.7% of the datasets, whereat the definition of successful was that at least 25% of the camera poses could be computed [60, 61] making this technique broadly applicable to endoscopy and thus may represent a significant advance in cancer surveillance opportunities for big data cancer research.

3 Cross-Sectional Imaging

Current roles for cross-sectional imaging in bladder cancer include evaluation of the upper urinary tract (UUT) and assessment potential extravesical tumor extension and metastases in patients with MIBC. For primary bladder tumor, cross-sectional imaging currently does not have the spatial resolution to replace cystoscopy, particularly for detection of small and flat urothelial lesions. For staging, cross-sectional imaging complements tissue diagnosis obtained via TUR under WLC and other optical imaging technologies. CT, and to a lesser extent magnetic resonance imaging (MRI), is the standard for staging.

CT staging of the primary tumor has been reported both overstage and understage in 23.4 and 24.7% of patients, respectively, and accuracy in predicting pathological tumor stage was 49% [92]. Furthermore, up to 25% of bladder cancer patients who were initially staged with clinical N0 disease preoperatively by cross-sectional imaging were found to have lymph node (LN) metastases in the final pathologic specimen [5]. Research on new cross-sectional imaging technologies, including new imaging agents and multimodal imaging, is progressing and poised for clinical translation in the near future.

3.1 Primary Bladder Cancer Diagnosis Using CT or MRI

CT urography (CTU) represents the cornerstone of urologic imaging for hematuria work-up. Sensitivity and specificity of CTU to correctly diagnose the source of hematuria showed large variations and are reported between 78 and 95% and 83 and 99%, respectively [10, 80, 93]. However, CTU shows inadequate accuracy in diagnosing small and flat lesions (i.e., CIS) [96]. Furthermore, cross-sectional imaging performed right after a TUR further decreases diagnostic accuracy to 60% [41]. Thus, CTU for primary bladder cancer diagnostics is clearly inferior to optical imaging of the bladder.

Newer MRI sequences, including dynamic gadolinium-enhanced MRI (DGE-MRI) and diffusion-weighted MRI, have been investigated for primary bladder tumor. In a prospective study in 122 patients with bladder cancer who were scheduled for a radical cystectomy, Daneshmand et al. investigated the diagnostic accuracy of preoperative DGE-MRI to predict final pathological staging [24]. The authors report an overall accuracy of 74%, sensitivity of 87.5%, and specificity of 47.6% to correctly diagnosing organ-confined disease. The authors concluded that this technology still lacks significant predictive power.

Another group investigated diagnostic accuracy of diffusion-weighted MRI in bladder cancer to differentiate between NMIBC and MIBC (Fig. 6). DW-MRI is an imaging sequence that analyzes tissue diffusion properties, which provides information on the microstructure of the underlying tissue, without the need for exogenous contrast agent. The authors report a diagnostic accuracy between 78.8 and 81.7% within two different radiologists [50]. In a study comparing WLC to CTU or MRI, respectively, and CTU to MRI, the authors conclude that cross-sectional imaging (either by CTU or MRI) is not able to replace WLC and that MRI showed better accuracy rates compared to CTU (sensitivity 76.9 vs. 61.5%, specificity 93.4 vs. 94.9%, respectively) [31].

3.2 Lymph Node Imaging Using MRI or CT

CT and MRI are the standard for preoperative detection of LN metastases in patients with invasive bladder cancer. These conventional imaging techniques rely mainly on morphologic criteria including LN size, shape, and morphological

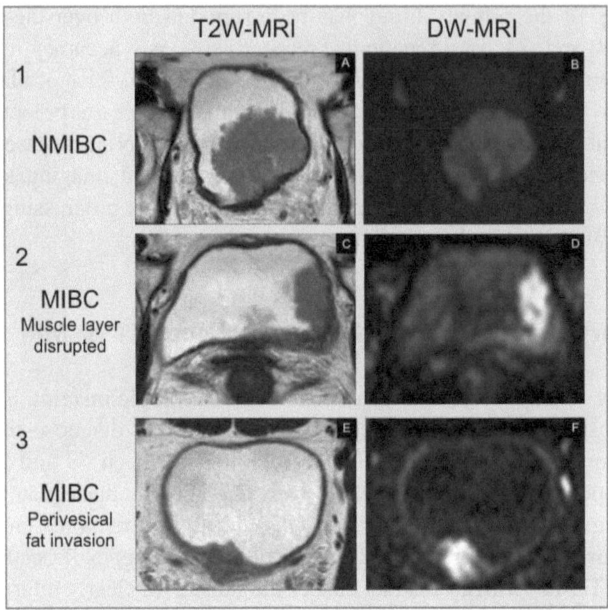

Fig. 6 Cross-sectional imaging of primary bladder tumor using multi-parametric MRI. (1) A large papillary NMIBC (pathology low-grade Ta) on T2 W-MRI (**a**) and DW-MRI sequences (**b**). DW-MRI shows a high-intensity area; (2) MIBC showing focal disruption of the muscle layer under T2 W-MRI (**c**) and a high-intensity area without submucosal components on transverse DW-MRI (**d**); (3) MIBC with perivesical fat invasion in T2 W-MRI (**e**) and DW-MRI (**f**), showing a high-intensity area with an irregular margin on transverse DW-MRI. Modified from [50] with permission. NMIBC = non-muscle-invasive bladder cancer; MIBC = muscle-invasive bladder cancer; T2 W = T2 weighted; DWI = diffusion weighted

features including LN-calcification or necrosis. However, the size of non-metastatic LNs varies widely and may overlap with the size of LN containing metastases. A lack of consensus regarding the normal size limit diagnostic of pelvic LN metastases is another shortcoming [66]. Using the short-axis diameter of the LN, which is generally used as criterion for metastases, the sensitivity and specificity vary between 78 and 97%, respectively, with a 6 mm cutoff [71] to 86 and 78%, respectively, with a 5 mm cutoff [66].

Small metastases often remain undetected, and enlarged LNs due to reactive hyperplasia may be misinterpreted as metastatic LNs [89]. Accordingly, upstaging in pelvic urologic malignancies of clinical N0 to pathological N + is frequently found despite the fact that negative preoperative imaging and diagnostic accuracy are low [7, 29]. Importantly, accuracy of LN imaging may only be drawn if a meticulous PLND has been performed and reported. Otherwise, the true rate of positive and negative LNs, and thus the accuracy of the imaging, remains unknown. A meticulous PLND depends on more than just the number of removed LNs. However, the reported number of removed LNs may represent a surrogate if a complete PLND was aimed and the benchmark imaging technique compared to.

3.3 Diffusion-Weighted MRI (DW-MRI)

In a prospective study to evaluate the diagnostic performance of DW-MRI for LN staging, 120 patients with bladder or prostate cancer and normal-sized LNs on conventional imaging techniques (CT and/or MRI) were evaluated with DW-MRI [91]. The authors found a sensitivity and specificity ranging between the three different radiologists who independently evaluated the images and were blinded for the pathological results from 64 to 79% and 79 to 85%, respectively, on a per-patient basis. This study shows that detection of small LN metastases in normal-sized LNs that would have been missed with conventional imaging modalities is enabled with DW-MRI alone. Currently, DW-MRI cannot replace a meticulous PLND in terms of accuracy because of the possibility of obtaining false-negative results with DW-MRI.

3.4 Ultrasmall Superparamagnetic Particles of Iron Oxide (USPIO) with MRI

USPIOs (e.g., ferumoxtran-10) are iron oxide nanoparticles with a diameter <50 nm which can be used for MR contrast-enhanced imaging [70]. The iron oxide crystalline core of the USPIO produces strong susceptibility leading to a signal decrease in T2-weighted images. USPIOs are transported through the vascular endothelium into the interstitial space after intravenous injection. Subsequently, the particles are taken up by macrophages and transported into LNs. Therefore, lymphotropic USPIO can be used as MRI contrast agent for detection of metastases in normal-sized pelvic LNs. Non-malignant LNs, which contain significant amounts of USPIO within the macrophages, appear hypointense. Malignant LNs, in contrast, have fewer macrophages and show a total or partial lack of USPIO uptake, thus not showing a change in signal intensity after USPIO injection. The lack of USPIO uptake in metastatic LNs, therefore, is indicative of metastatic LNs, highlighting and potentially facilitating the identification of metastases in normal-sized LNs [9].

An initial study using ferumoxtran-10 as USPIO for preoperative staging in BC reports about sensitivity and specificity of 96 and 95% [27]. Although the numbers are very encouraging, no backup PLND was performed in this study and thus the true false-negative rate remains unknown even more because PLND was mostly limited to enlarged (which would have been detected by conventional MRI as well) or suspicious LNs in selected patients.

A Swiss group combined USPIO and diffusion-weighted DW-MRI for the detection of metastases in normal-sized pelvic LNs of patients with BC or PC and clinically staged N0 [9]. Combining those two techniques enables characterization of metastatic LNs according to a high signal intensity on DW-MRI and a lack of signal decrease after USPIO injection. After an extended PLND (median 39 LNs removed per patient), pathologically confirmed LN metastases were found in 20 patients and the long-axis diameter of the LN metastases was ≤ 5 mm in 83 and

≤ 3 mm in 50%. On a per-patient basis, sensitivity and specificity ranged from 65 to 75% and 93 to 96%, respectively, between the three different radiologists who independently evaluated the images and were blinded for the pathological results. Thus, the combination of USPIO and DW-MRI improved the detection rate of LN metastases in normal-sized LNs. Nevertheless, 25–35% of the LN-positive patients were incorrectly staged as LN negative, which remains too high. Furthermore, two MRI examinations are needed and USPIOs are not without side effects and have limited commercial availability [48].

3.5 Positron Emission Tomography (PET)

The diagnostic efficiency of PET does not depend on traditional parameters such as size or shape, but on the increased metabolic rate of specific tissues and their volume. As an intravenous imaging agent, ^{18}F-fluorodeoxyglucose (FDG) highlights anatomic regions of increased metabolic activity. In bladder cancer, FDG-PET is predominantly used for detection of LN metastases. In a small 2010 prospective study, 51 bladder cancer patients received a FDG-PET/CT scan before radical cystectomy and pelvic LN dissection (a mean of 16 LN per patient removed) and the authors described a sensitivity and specificity in the detection of pelvic LN metastases of 46 and 97%, respectively [90]. Thus, the false-negative rate was over 50%, and even in some enlarged metastatic LNs up to 25 mm in size, no abnormal FDG uptake was found. Recently, another trial [1] compared preoperative FDG-PET/CT and conventional CT with pathological results in 54 patients who underwent radical cystectomy and PLND (a mean of 28 LNs removed per patient), and the same low sensitivity for both imaging techniques (41 vs. 41%) in the detection of regional LN metastases was reported. In line with these results is another study comparing preoperative CT scan with FDG-PET/CT in 207 patients with BC who underwent radical cystectomy and PLND (a mean of 17 LNs removed per patient) [36]. Although an increased sensitivity detecting LN metastases from 45% using CT alone to 69% with FDG-PET/CT was found, the additional diagnostic yield of 5% on a per-patient basis was small. Thus, FDG-PET/CT provides no or only minimal additional benefit in the loco-regional LN staging in BC (as the authors of this study claim). Other trials, however, have reported an increased detection rate of metastases using FDG-PET/CT for preoperative LN staging. The sensitivity rates in these trials varied from 50 to 70% [46, 79]. Only one of these trials [79], however, reports a median of 12 resected LNs per patient; the others did not perform (or did not report) a backup PLND. So, the true rate of false-negative LN metastases remains unknown. In summary, for patients with BC, currently available FDG-PET/CT techniques offer no substantial diagnostic benefit for the detection of pelvic LN metastases [48].

Recently, FDG-PET in combination with MRI has been investigated prospectively in a small pilot study of bladder cancer patients [78]. In a series of 22 patients with known bladder cancer, Rosenkrantz et al. report increased accuracy of primary tumor detection from 77 to 86%, increased accuracy of detection of metastatic pelvic lymph nodes from 76 to 95%, and increased accuracy of detection of non-nodal pelvic malignancy from 91 to 100% when combining ^{18}F FDG-PET with MRI compared to MRI alone (Fig. 7). The combination of multi-parametric MRI which offers high-contrast resolution with ^{18}F FDG-PET which offers metabolic information seems to be a promising technology allowing to increase accuracy rates significantly. However, the sample size is small and a pathologic evaluation of the LNs has not been done in all cases. Therefore, final conclusions on the real advantages of this new combination of technologies are much too premature.

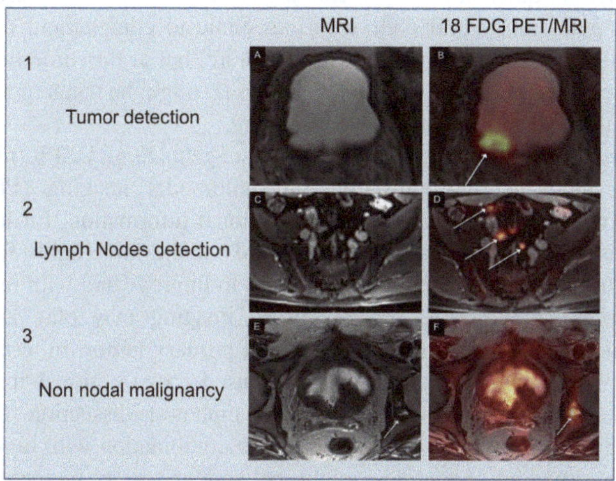

Fig. 7 Cross-sectional imaging the example of ^{18}F-FDG-PET/MRI in pre-TURBT setting. (1) *Tumor detection*: A 68-year-old man with muscle-invasive high-grade bladder cancer on prior biopsy, undergoing simultaneous ^{18}F-FDG-PET/MRI. **a** and **b**, Axial T2-weighted images show regions of mild nonspecific mural thickening (arrow, **b**) that was considered equivocal for the presence of tumor. (2) *Lymph node detection*: A 62-year-old man with prior biopsy showing high-grade non-muscle-invasive bladder cancer, undergoing simultaneous ^{18}F-FDG-PET/MRI. **c** On postcontrast axial T1-weighted image of the pelvis, potential pelvic lymph nodes are difficult to differentiate from surrounding vessels and bowel loops. **d** Fused ^{18}F-FDG-PET/MR image shows marked increased activity within numerous pelvic lymph nodes (arrows), which raised suspicion for nodal metastases. The nodes decreased in size following treatment with systemic chemotherapy. (3) *Non-nodal malignancy*: An 82-year-old man with prior biopsy showing high-grade non-muscle-invasive bladder cancer, undergoing simultaneous ^{18}F-FDG-PET/MRI. **e** Axial T2-weighted image shows a left acetabular lesion (arrow) that was considered possibly degenerative, given its proximity to the hip joint, and equivocal for bone metastasis. **f** Fused PET/MR image shows corresponding marked increased metabolic activity (arrow), raising suspicion that the lesion represents a bone metastasis. Subsequent bone biopsy demonstrated metastatic urothelial carcinoma. From [78] with permission

4 Conclusion

Judicious applications of optical and cross-sectional imaging technologies play a paramount role in the management of patients with bladder cancer. Over the past 20 years, significant advances have taken place in both areas to improve their diagnostic yield for patients with NMIBC and MIBC. Level 1 evidence exists that enhanced cystoscopy such as BLC and NBI improves tumor detection and resection and reduces recurrence. However, in case of repeated intravesical chemotherapy instillations or post-BCG results are not that expedient and further validation in this setting has to be undertaken. To improve preoperative planning and standardize documentation at the same time, computer-assisted diagnostic algorithm (e.g., 3D reconstruction, machine learning) to enhance image processing will be increasingly studied. Numerous other emerging technologies (e.g., CLE, OCT) are promising and hold the potential to find their way into clinic to complement the currently available optical imaging technologies in the future, but at this time they still lack clinical efficacy data. Diagnostic accuracy, however, might be taken to another level in the future through molecular targeted imaging.

In cross-sectional imaging, while new contrast agents (e.g., USPIO) improve the detection of micro-metastatic disease and multimodal imaging (PET-CT and PET-MRI) provides superb anatomic and functional information, for local staging TUR with tissue diagnosis remains the standard for the foreseeable future. However, as resolution of MRI technology continues to improve and with integration of molecular tracers, noninvasive cross-sectional imaging may play an important adjunctive role in the future for the diagnosis of primary tumor. In terms of lymph node staging accuracy, none of the currently used cross-sectional imaging technologies have the potential to substitute pelvic lymph node dissection. Thus, similar to optical imaging, molecular targeting agents in combination with high-resolution cross-sectional imaging modalities might be anticipated to increase diagnostic accuracy.

Acknowledgements We thank Dharati Trivedi for her helpful assistance with editing the figures. Bernhard Kiss was funded by Swiss National Foundation (P300 PB 167793/1) and Bern Cancer League. Gautier Marcq was funded by Lille 2 University mobility grant.

References

1. Aljabery F, Lindblom G, Skoog S, Shabo I, Olsson H, Rosell J, Jahnson S (2015) PET/CT versus conventional CT for detection of lymph node metastases in patients with locally advanced bladder cancer. BMC Urol 15:87. https://doi.org/10.1186/s12894-015-0080-z
2. Amara N, Palapattu GS, Schrage M, Gu Z, Thomas GV, Dorey F, Said J, Reiter RE (2001) Prostate stem cell antigen is overexpressed in human transitional cell carcinoma. Can Res 61 (12):4660–4665
3. Andreev OA, Engelman DM, Reshetnyak YK (2014) Targeting diseased tissues by pHLIP insertion at low cell surface pH. Frontiers in Physiol 5:97. https://doi.org/10.3389/fphys.2014.00097

4. Anidjar M, Cussenot O, Blais J, Bourdon O, Avrillier S, Ettori D, Villette JM, Fiet J, Teillac P, Le Duc A (1996) Argon laser induced autofluorescence may distinguish between normal and tumor human urothelial cells: a microspectrofluorimetric study. J Urol 155 (5):1771–1774
5. Babjuk M, Bohle A, Burger M, Capoun O, Cohen D, Comperat EM, Hernandez V, Kaasinen E, Palou J, Roupret M, van Rhijn BW, Shariat SF, Soukup V, Sylvester RJ, Zigeuner R (2017) EAU guidelines on non-muscle-invasive urothelial carcinoma of the bladder: update 2016. Eur Urol 71(3):447–461. https://doi.org/10.1016/j.eururo.2016.05.041
6. Babjuk M, Soukup V, Petrik R, Jirsa M, Dvoracek J (2005) 5-aminolaevulinic acid-induced fluorescence cystoscopy during transurethral resection reduces the risk of recurrence in stage Ta/T1 bladder cancer. BJU Int 96(6):798–802. https://doi.org/10.1111/j.1464-410X.2004.05715.x
7. Bader P, Burkhard FC, Markwalder R, Studer UE (2002) Is a limited lymph node dissection an adequate staging procedure for prostate cancer?. J Urol 168 (2):514–518; discussion 518
8. Bailey KM, Wojtkowiak JW, Hashim AI, Gillies RJ (2012) Targeting the metabolic microenvironment of tumors. Advances in pharmacology (San Diego, Calif) 65:63–107. https://doi.org/10.1016/b978-0-12-397927-8.00004-x
9. Birkhauser FD, Studer UE, Froehlich JM, Triantafyllou M, Bains LJ, Petralia G, Vermathen P, Fleischmann A, Thoeny HC (2013) Combined ultrasmall superparamagnetic particles of iron oxide-enhanced and diffusion-weighted magnetic resonance imaging facilitates detection of metastases in normal-sized pelvic lymph nodes of patients with bladder and prostate cancer. Eur Urol 64(6):953–960. https://doi.org/10.1016/j.eururo.2013.07.032
10. Blick CG, Nazir SA, Mallett S, Turney BW, Onwu NN, Roberts IS, Crew JP, Cowan NC (2012) Evaluation of diagnostic strategies for bladder cancer using computed tomography (CT) urography, flexible cystoscopy and voided urine cytology: results for 778 patients from a hospital haematuria clinic. BJU Int 110(1):84–94. https://doi.org/10.1111/j.1464-410X.2011.10664.x
11. Brausi M, Collette L, Kurth K, van der Meijden AP, Oosterlinck W, Witjes JA, Newling D, Bouffioux C, Sylvester RJ (2002) Variability in the recurrence rate at first follow-up cystoscopy after TUR in stage Ta T1 transitional cell carcinoma of the bladder: a combined analysis of seven EORTC studies. Eur Urol 41(5):523–531
12. Burger M, Grossman HB, Droller M, Schmidbauer J, Hermann G, Dragoescu O, Ray E, Fradet Y, Karl A, Burgues JP, Witjes JA, Stenzl A, Jichlinski P, Jocham D (2013) Photodynamic diagnosis of non-muscle-invasive bladder cancer with hexaminolevulinate cystoscopy: a meta-analysis of detection and recurrence based on raw data. Eur Urol 64 (5):846–854. https://doi.org/10.1016/j.eururo.2013.03.059
13. Carlsson J (2012) Potential for clinical radionuclide-based imaging and therapy of common cancers expressing EGFR-family receptors. Tumour Biol: J Int Soc Oncodevelopmental Biol Med 33(3):653–659. https://doi.org/10.1007/s13277-011-0307-x
14. Cauberg EC, de Bruin DM, Faber DJ, van Leeuwen TG, de la Rosette JJ, de Reijke TM (2009) A new generation of optical diagnostics for bladder cancer: technology, diagnostic accuracy, and future applications. Eur Urol 56(2):287–296. https://doi.org/10.1016/j.eururo.2009.02.033
15. Cauberg EC, Kloen S, Visser M, de la Rosette JJ, Babjuk M, Soukup V, Pesl M, Duskova J, de Reijke TM (2010) Narrow band imaging cystoscopy improves the detection of non-muscle-invasive bladder cancer. Urology 76(3):658–663. https://doi.org/10.1016/j.urology.2009.11.075
16. Chan KS, Espinosa I, Chao M, Wong D, Ailles L, Diehn M, Gill H, Presti J Jr, Chang HY, van de Rijn M, Shortliffe L, Weissman IL (2009) Identification, molecular characterization, clinical prognosis, and therapeutic targeting of human bladder tumor-initiating cells. Proc Natl Acad Sci USA 106(33):14016–14021. https://doi.org/10.1073/pnas.0906549106

17. Chang SS, Boorjian SA, Chou R, Clark PE, Daneshmand S, Konety BR, Pruthi R, Quale DZ, Ritch CR, Seigne JD, Skinner EC, Smith ND, McKiernan JM (2016) Diagnosis and Treatment of Non-Muscle Invasive Bladder Cancer: AUA/SUO Guideline. J Urol 196 (4):1021–1029. https://doi.org/10.1016/j.juro.2016.06.049
18. Chang TC, Liu JJ, Hsiao ST, Pan Y, Mach KE, Leppert JT, McKenney JK, Rouse RV, Liao JC (2013) Interobserver agreement of confocal laser endomicroscopy for bladder cancer. J Endourol 27(5):598–603. https://doi.org/10.1089/end.2012.0549
19. Chang TC, Liu JJ, Liao JC (2013) Probe-based confocal laser endomicroscopy of the urinary tract: the technique. J Visualized Exp: Jove 71:e4409. https://doi.org/10.3791/4409
20. Chen SP, Kirsch S, Zlatev DV, Chang T, Comstock B, Lendvay TS, Liao JC (2016) Optical Biopsy of Bladder Cancer Using Crowd-Sourced Assessment. JAMA Surgery 151(1):90–93. https://doi.org/10.1001/jamasurg.2015.3121
21. Cheng L, Neumann RM, Weaver AL, Cheville JC, Leibovich BC, Ramnani DM, Scherer BG, Nehra A, Zincke H, Bostwick DG (2000) Grading and staging of bladder carcinoma in transurethral resection specimens. Correlation with 105 matched cystectomy specimens. Am J Clin Pathol 113(2):275–279. https://doi.org/10.1309/94b6-8vfb-mn9j-1nf5
22. Cina SJ, Epstein JI, Endrizzi JM, Harmon WJ, Seay TM, Schoenberg MP (2001) Correlation of cystoscopic impression with histologic diagnosis of biopsy specimens of the bladder. Hum Pathol 32(6):630–637. https://doi.org/10.1053/hupa.2001.24999
23. Crow P, Uff JS, Farmer JA, Wright MP, Stone N (2004) The use of Raman spectroscopy to identify and characterize transitional cell carcinoma in vitro. BJU Int 93(9):1232–1236. https://doi.org/10.1111/j.1464-410X.2004.04852.x
24. Daneshmand S, Ahmadi H, Huynh LN, Dobos N (2012) Preoperative staging of invasive bladder cancer with dynamic gadolinium-enhanced magnetic resonance imaging: results from a prospective study. Urology 80(6):1313–1318. https://doi.org/10.1016/j.urology.2012.07.056
25. Daniltchenko DI, Riedl CR, Sachs MD, Koenig F, Daha KL, Pflueger H, Loening SA, Schnorr D (2005) Long-term benefit of 5-aminolevulinic acid fluorescence assisted transurethral resection of superficial bladder cancer: 5-year results of a prospective randomized study. J Urol 174(6):2129–2133, discussion 2133. https://doi.org/10.1097/01.ju.0000181814.73466.14
26. de Jong BW, Bakker Schut TC, Wolffenbuttel KP, Nijman JM, Kok DJ, Puppels GJ (2002) Identification of bladder wall layers by Raman spectroscopy. J Urol 168(4 Pt 2):1771–1778. https://doi.org/10.1097/01.ju.0000030059.28948.c6
27. Deserno WM, Harisinghani MG, Taupitz M, Jager GJ, Witjes JA, Mulders PF, Hulsbergen van de Kaa CA, Kaufmann D, Barentsz JO (2004) Urinary bladder cancer: preoperative nodal staging with ferumoxtran-10-enhanced MR imaging. Radiology 233(2):449–456. https://doi.org/10.1148/radiol.2332031111
28. Draga RO, Grimbergen MC, Vijverberg PL, van Swol CF, Jonges TG, Kummer JA, Ruud Bosch JL (2010) In vivo bladder cancer diagnosis by high-volume Raman spectroscopy. Anal Chem 82(14):5993–5999. https://doi.org/10.1021/ac100448p
29. Fleischmann A, Thalmann GN, Markwalder R, Studer UE (2005) Extracapsular extension of pelvic lymph node metastases from urothelial carcinoma of the bladder is an independent prognostic factor. J Clin Oncol: Official J Am Soc Clin Oncol 23(10):2358–2365. https://doi.org/10.1200/jco.2005.03.084
30. Fradet Y, Grossman HB, Gomella L, Lerner S, Cookson M, Albala D, Droller MJ (2007) A comparison of hexaminolevulinate fluorescence cystoscopy and white light cystoscopy for the detection of carcinoma in situ in patients with bladder cancer: a phase III, multicenter study. J Urol178(1):68–73; discussion 73. https://doi.org/10.1016/j.juro.2007.03.028
31. Gandrup KL, Logager VB, Bretlau T, Nordling J, Thomsen HS (2015) Diagnosis of bladder tumours in patients with macroscopic haematuria: a prospective comparison of split-bolus computed tomography urography, magnetic resonance urography and flexible cystoscopy. Scand J Urol 49(3):224–229. https://doi.org/10.3109/21681805.2014.981203

32. Goh AC, Tresser NJ, Shen SS, Lerner SP (2008) Optical coherence tomography as an adjunct to white light cystoscopy for intravesical real-time imaging and staging of bladder cancer. Urology 72(1):133–137. https://doi.org/10.1016/j.urology.2008.02.002
33. Golijanin J, Amin A, Moshnikova A, Brito JM, Tran TY, Adochite RC, Andreev GO, Crawford T, Engelman DM, Andreev OA, Reshetnyak YK, Golijanin D (2016) Targeted imaging of urothelium carcinoma in human bladders by an ICG pHLIP peptide ex vivo. Proc Natl Acad Sci USA 113(42):11829–11834. https://doi.org/10.1073/pnas.1610472113
34. Gono K (2015) Narrow band imaging: technology basis and research and development history. In: Clin Endosc, vol 48. vol 6. pp 476–480. https://doi.org/10.5946/ce.2015.48.6.476
35. Gono K, Obi T, Yamaguchi M, Ohyama N, Machida H, Sano Y, Yoshida S, Hamamoto Y, Endo T (2004) Appearance of enhanced tissue features in narrow-band endoscopic imaging. J Biomed Opt 9(3):568–577. https://doi.org/10.1117/1.1695563
36. Goodfellow H, Viney Z, Hughes P, Rankin S, Rottenberg G, Hughes S, Evison F, Dasgupta P, O'Brien T, Khan MS (2014) Role of fluorodeoxyglucose positron emission tomography (FDG PET)-computed tomography (CT) in the staging of bladder cancer. BJU Int 114(3):389–395. https://doi.org/10.1111/bju.12608
37. Greco F, Cadeddu JA, Gill IS, Kaouk JH, Remzi M, Thompson RH, van Leeuwen FW, van der Poel HG, Fornara P, Rassweiler J (2014) Current perspectives in the use of molecular imaging to target surgical treatments for genitourinary cancers. Eur Urol 65(5):947–964. https://doi.org/10.1016/j.eururo.2013.07.033
38. Grossman HB, Stenzl A, Fradet Y, Mynderse LA, Kriegmair M, Witjes JA, Soloway MS, Karl A, Burger M (2012) Long-term decrease in bladder cancer recurrence with hexaminolevulinate enabled fluorescence cystoscopy. J Urol 188(1):58–62. https://doi.org/10.1016/j.juro.2012.03.007
39. Hermes B, Spoler F, Naami A, Bornemann J, Forst M, Grosse J, Jakse G, Knuchel R (2008) Visualization of the basement membrane zone of the bladder by optical coherence tomography: feasibility of noninvasive evaluation of tumor invasion. Urology 72(3):677–681. https://doi.org/10.1016/j.urology.2008.02.062
40. Herr HW, Donat SM (2008) A comparison of white-light cystoscopy and narrow-band imaging cystoscopy to detect bladder tumour recurrences. BJU Int 102(9):1111–1114. https://doi.org/10.1111/j.1464-410X.2008.07846.x
41. Hilton S, Jones LP (2014) Recent advances in imaging cancer of the kidney and urinary tract. Surg Oncol Clin N Am 23(4):863–910. https://doi.org/10.1016/j.soc.2014.06.001
42. Hsu M, Gupta M, Su LM, Liao JC (2014) Intraoperative optical imaging and tissue interrogation during urologic surgery. Curr Opin Urol 24(1):66–74. https://doi.org/10.1097/MOU.0000000000000010
43. Jocham D, Witjes F, Wagner S, Zeylemaker B, van Moorselaar J, Grimm MO, Muschter R, Popken G, Konig F, Knuchel R, Kurth KH (2005) Improved detection and treatment of bladder cancer using hexaminolevulinate imaging: a prospective, phase III multicenter study. J Urol 174(3):862–866; discussion 866. https://doi.org/10.1097/01.ju.0000169257.19841.2a
44. Karl A, Stepp H, Willmann E, Buchner A, Hocaoglu Y, Stief C, Tritschler S (2010) Optical coherence tomography for bladder cancer—ready as a surrogate for optical biopsy? Results of a prospective mono-centre study. Eur J Med Res 15(3):131–134
45. Kausch I, Sommerauer M, Montorsi F, Stenzl A, Jacqmin D, Jichlinski P, Jocham D, Ziegler A, Vonthein R (2010) Photodynamic diagnosis in non-muscle-invasive bladder cancer: a systematic review and cumulative analysis of prospective studies. Eur Urol 57(4):595–606. https://doi.org/10.1016/j.eururo.2009.11.041
46. Kibel AS, Dehdashti F, Katz MD, Klim AP, Grubb RL, Humphrey PA, Siegel C, Cao D, Gao F, Siegel BA (2009) Prospective study of [18F]fluorodeoxyglucose positron emission tomography/computed tomography for staging of muscle-invasive bladder carcinoma. J Clin Oncol: Official J Am Soc Clin Oncol 27(26):4314–4320. https://doi.org/10.1200/jco.2008.20.6722

47. Kirkali Z, Chan T, Manoharan M, Algaba F, Busch C, Cheng L, Kiemeney L, Kriegmair M, Montironi R, Murphy WM, Sesterhenn IA, Tachibana M, Weider J (2005) Bladder cancer: epidemiology, staging and grading, and diagnosis. Urology 66(6 Suppl 1):4–34. https://doi.org/10.1016/j.urology.2005.07.062
48. Kiss B, Thoeny HC, Studer UE (2016) Current status of lymph node imaging in bladder and prostate cancer. Urology 96:1–7. https://doi.org/10.1016/j.urology.2016.02.014
49. Klan R, Loy V, Huland H (1991) Residual tumor discovered in routine second transurethral resection in patients with stage T1 transitional cell carcinoma of the bladder. J Urol 146 (2):316–318
50. Kobayashi S, Koga F, Yoshida S, Masuda H, Ishii C, Tanaka H, Komai Y, Yokoyama M, Saito K, Fujii Y, Kawakami S, Kihara K (2011) Diagnostic performance of diffusion-weighted magnetic resonance imaging in bladder cancer: potential utility of apparent diffusion coefficient values as a biomarker to predict clinical aggressiveness. Eur Radiol 21(10):2178–2186. https://doi.org/10.1007/s00330-011-2174-7
51. Kolozsy Z (1991) Histopathological "self control" in transurethral resection of bladder tumours. Br J Urol 67(2):162–164
52. Kriegmair MC, Bergen T, Ritter M, Mandel P, Michel MS, Wittenberg T, Bolenz C (2017) Digital mapping of the urinary bladder: potential for standardized cystoscopy reports. Urology. https://doi.org/10.1016/j.urology.2017.02.019
53. Lapini A, Minervini A, Masala A, Schips L, Pycha A, Cindolo L, Giannella R, Martini T, Vittori G, Zani D, Bellomo F, Cosciani Cunico S (2012) A comparison of hexaminolevulinate (Hexvix(R)) fluorescence cystoscopy and white-light cystoscopy for detection of bladder cancer: results of the HeRo observational study. Surg Endosc 26(12):3634–3641. https://doi.org/10.1007/s00464-012-2387-0
54. Lee CS, Yoon CY, Witjes JA (2008) The past, present and future of cystoscopy: the fusion of cystoscopy and novel imaging technology. BJU Int 102(9 Pt B):1228–1233. https://doi.org/10.1111/j.1464-410x.2008.07964.x
55. Lepin EJ, Leyton JV, Zhou Y, Olafsen T, Salazar FB, McCabe KE, Hahm S, Marks JD, Reiter RE, Wu AM (2010) An affinity matured minibody for PET imaging of prostate stem cell antigen (PSCA)-expressing tumors. Eur J Nucl Med Mol Imaging 37(8):1529–1538. https://doi.org/10.1007/s00259-010-1433-1
56. Lerner SP, Goh A (2015) Novel endoscopic diagnosis for bladder cancer. Cancer 121 (2):169–178. https://doi.org/10.1002/cncr.28905
57. Lerner SP, Liu H, Wu MF, Thomas YK, Witjes JA (2012) Fluorescence and white light cystoscopy for detection of carcinoma in situ of the urinary bladder. Urol Oncol 30(3):285–289. https://doi.org/10.1016/j.urolonc.2010.09.009
58. Li K, Lin T, Fan X, Duan Y, Huang J (2013) Diagnosis of narrow-band imaging in non-muscle-invasive bladder cancer: a systematic review and meta-analysis. Int J Urol: Official J Jpn Urol Assoc 20(6):602–609. https://doi.org/10.1111/j.1442-2042.2012.03211.x
59. Liu JJ, Droller MJ, Liao JC (2012) New optical imaging technologies for bladder cancer: considerations and perspectives. J Urol 188(2):361–368. https://doi.org/10.1016/j.juro.2012.03.127
60. Lurie KL, Angst R, Seibel EJ, Liao JC, Ellerbee Bowden AK (2016) Registration of free-hand OCT daughter endoscopy to 3D organ reconstruction. Biomed Opt Express 7 (12):4995–5009. https://doi.org/10.1364/boe.7.004995
61. Lurie KL, Angst R, Zlatev DV, Liao JC, Ellerbee Bowden AK (2017) 3D reconstruction of cystoscopy videos for comprehensive bladder records. Biomed Opt Express 8(4):2106–2123. https://doi.org/10.1364/BOE.8.002106
62. Ma T, Wang W, Jiang Z, Shao G, Guo L, Li J, Zhang L, Liu Y (2015) Narrow band imaging-assisted holmium laser resection reduced the recurrence rate of non-muscle invasive bladder cancer: a prospective, randomized controlled study. Zhonghua yi Xue za Zhi 95 (37):3032–3035

63. Manyak MJ, Gladkova ND, Makari JH, Schwartz AM, Zagaynova EV, Zolfaghari L, Zara JM, Iksanov R, Feldchtein FI (2005) Evaluation of superficial bladder transitional-cell carcinoma by optical coherence tomography. J Endourol 19(5):570–574. https://doi.org/10.1089/end.2005.19.570
64. Mark JR, Gelpi-Hammerschmidt F, Trabulsi EJ, Gomella LG (2012) Blue light cystoscopy for detection and treatment of non-muscle invasive bladder cancer. Can J Urol 19(2):6227–6231
65. Mazzucchelli R, Barbisan F, Santinelli A, Lopez-Beltran A, Cheng L, Scarpelli M, Montironi R (2009) Immunohistochemical expression of prostate stem cell antigen in cystoprostatectomies with incidental prostate cancer. Int J Immunopathology Pharmacology 22(3):755–762. https://doi.org/10.1177/039463200902200321
66. McMahon CJ, Rofsky NM, Pedrosa I (2010) Lymphatic metastases from pelvic tumors: anatomic classification, characterization, and staging. Radiology 254(1):31–46. https://doi.org/10.1148/radiol.2541090361
67. Minsky M (1988) Memoir on inventing the confocal scanning microscope. Scanning 10 (4):128–138
68. Mowatt G, NDow J, Vale L, Nabi G, Boachie C, Cook JA, Fraser C, Griffiths TR, Aberdeen Technology Assessment Review G (2011) Photodynamic diagnosis of bladder cancer compared with white light cystoscopy: Systematic review and meta-analysis. Int J Technol Assess Health Care 27(1):3–10. https://doi.org/10.1017/s0266462310001364
69. Naito S, Algaba F, Babjuk M, Bryan RT, Sun YH, Valiquette L, de la Rosette J (2016) The clinical research office of the endourological society (CROES) multicentre randomised trial of narrow band imaging-assisted transurethral resection of bladder tumour (TURBT) versus conventional white light imaging-assisted turbt in primary non-muscle-invasive bladder cancer patients: trial protocol and 1-year results. Eur Urol 70(3):506–515. https://doi.org/10.1016/j.eururo.2016.03.053
70. Neuwelt EA, Hamilton BE, Varallyay CG, Rooney WR, Edelman RD, Jacobs PM, Watnick SG (2009) Ultrasmall superparamagnetic iron oxides (USPIOs): a future alternative magnetic resonance (MR) contrast agent for patients at risk for nephrogenic systemic fibrosis (NSF)? Kidney Int 75(5):465–474. https://doi.org/10.1038/ki.2008.496
71. Oyen RH, Van Poppel HP, Ameye FE, Van de Voorde WA, Baert AL, Baert LV (1994) Lymph node staging of localized prostatic carcinoma with CT and CT-guided fine-needle aspiration biopsy: prospective study of 285 patients. Radiology 190(2):315–322. https://doi.org/10.1148/radiology.190.2.8284375
72. Pan Y, Volkmer JP, Mach KE, Rouse RV, Liu JJ, Sahoo D, Chang TC, Metzner TJ, Kang L, van de Rijn M, Skinner EC, Gambhir SS, Weissman IL, Liao JC (2014) Endoscopic molecular imaging of human bladder cancer using a CD47 antibody. Science translational medicine 6 (260):260ra148. https://doi.org/10.1126/scitranslmed.3009457
73. Pfost B, Seidl C, Autenrieth M, Saur D, Bruchertseifer F, Morgenstern A, Schwaiger M, Senekowitsch-Schmidtke R (2009) Intravesical alpha-radioimmunotherapy with 213Bi-anti-EGFR-mAb defeats human bladder carcinoma in xenografted nude mice. J Nucl Med 50(10):1700–1708. https://doi.org/10.2967/jnumed.109.065961
74. Rao AR, Hanchanale V, Javle P, Karim O, Motiwala H (2007) Spectroscopic view of life and work of the Nobel Laureate Sir C.V. Raman. J Endourol 21(1):8–11. https://doi.org/10.1089/end.2006.9998
75. Ren H, Waltzer WC, Bhalla R, Liu J, Yuan Z, Lee CS, Darras F, Schulsinger D, Adler HL, Kim J, Mishail A, Pan Y (2009) Diagnosis of bladder cancer with microelectromechanical systems-based cystoscopic optical coherence tomography. Urology 74(6):1351–1357. https://doi.org/10.1016/j.urology.2009.04.090
76. Rink M, Babjuk M, Catto JW, Jichlinski P, Shariat SF, Stenzl A, Stepp H, Zaak D, Witjes JA (2013) Hexyl aminolevulinate-guided fluorescence cystoscopy in the diagnosis and follow-up of patients with non-muscle-invasive bladder cancer: a critical review of the current literature. Eur Urol 64(4):624–638. https://doi.org/10.1016/j.eururo.2013.07.007

77. Robinson JP (2001) Chapter 4 Principles of confocal microscopy. Methods Cell Biol 63:89–106. https://doi.org/10.1016/s0091-679x(01)63008-5
78. Rosenkrantz AB, Friedman KP, Ponzo F, Raad RA, Jackson K, Huang WC, Balar AV (2017) Prospective pilot study to evaluate the incremental value of PET information in patients with bladder cancer undergoing 18F-FDG simultaneous PET/MRI. Clin Nucl Med 42(1):e8–e15. https://doi.org/10.1097/RLU.0000000000001432
79. Rouanne M, Girma A, Neuzillet Y, Vilain D, Radulescu C, Letang N, Yonneau L, Herve JM, Botto H, Le Stanc E, Lebret T (2014) Potential impact of 18F-FDG PET/CT on patients selection for neoadjuvant chemotherapy before radical cystectomy. Eur J Surgical Oncology: J Eur Soc Surgical Oncol Br Assoc Surgical Oncol 40(12):1724–1730. https://doi.org/10.1016/j.ejso.2014.08.479
80. Sadow CA, Silverman SG, O'Leary MP, Signorovitch JE (2008) Bladder cancer detection with CT urography in an Academic Medical Center. Radiology 249(1):195–202. https://doi.org/10.1148/radiol.2491071860
81. Schafauer C, Ettori D, Roupret M, Phe V, Tualle JM, Tinet E, Avrillier S, Egrot C, Traxer O, Cussenot O (2013) Detection of bladder urothelial carcinoma using in vivo noncontact, ultraviolet excited autofluorescence measurements converted into simple color coded images: a feasibility study. J Urol 190(1):271–277. https://doi.org/10.1016/j.juro.2013.01.100
82. Schmidbauer J, Remzi M, Klatte T, Waldert M, Mauermann J, Susani M, Marberger M (2009) Fluorescence cystoscopy with high-resolution optical coherence tomography imaging as an adjunct reduces false-positive findings in the diagnosis of urothelial carcinoma of the bladder. Eur Urol 56(6):914–919. https://doi.org/10.1016/j.eururo.2009.07.042
83. Schmidbauer J, Witjes F, Schmeller N, Donat R, Susani M, Marberger M (2004) Improved detection of urothelial carcinoma in situ with hexaminolevulinate fluorescence cystoscopy. J Urol 171(1):135–138. https://doi.org/10.1097/01.ju.0000100480.70769.0e
84. Schumacher MC, Holmang S, Davidsson T, Friedrich B, Pedersen J, Wiklund NP (2010) Transurethral resection of non-muscle-invasive bladder transitional cell cancers with or without 5-aminolevulinic Acid under visible and fluorescent light: results of a prospective, randomised, multicentre study. Eur Urol 57(2):293–299. https://doi.org/10.1016/j.eururo.2009.10.030
85. Sengottayan VK, Vasudeva P, Dalela D (2008) Intravesical real-time imaging and staging of bladder cancer: use of optical coherence tomography. Ind J Urol: IJU: J Urol Soc Ind 24 (4):592–593
86. Shen P, Yang J, Wei W, Li Y, Li D, Zeng H, Wang J (2012) Effects of fluorescent light-guided transurethral resection on non-muscle-invasive bladder cancer: a systematic review and meta-analysis. BJU Int 110(6 Pt B):E209–215. https://doi.org/10.1111/j.1464-410x.2011.10892.x
87. Soper TD, Porter MP, Seibel EJ (2012) Surface mosaics of the bladder reconstructed from endoscopic video for automated surveillance. IEEE Trans Bio-med Eng 59(6):1670–1680. https://doi.org/10.1109/tbme.2012.2191783
88. Stenzl A, Burger M, Fradet Y, Mynderse LA, Soloway MS, Witjes JA, Kriegmair M, Karl A, Shen Y, Grossman HB (2010) Hexaminolevulinate guided fluorescence cystoscopy reduces recurrence in patients with nonmuscle invasive bladder cancer. J Urol 184(5):1907–1913. https://doi.org/10.1016/j.juro.2010.06.148
89. Studer UE, Scherz S, Scheidegger J, Kraft R, Sonntag R, Ackermann D, Zingg EJ (1990) Enlargement of regional lymph nodes in renal cell carcinoma is often not due to metastases. J Urol 144(2 Pt 1):243–245
90. Swinnen G, Maes A, Pottel H, Vanneste A, Billiet I, Lesage K, Werbrouck P (2010) FDG-PET/CT for the preoperative lymph node staging of invasive bladder cancer. Eur Urol 57(4):641–647. https://doi.org/10.1016/j.eururo.2009.05.014
91. Thoeny HC, Froehlich JM, Triantafyllou M, Huesler J, Bains LJ, Vermathen P, Fleischmann A, Studer UE (2014) Metastases in normal-sized pelvic lymph nodes:

detection with diffusion-weighted MR imaging. Radiology 273(1):125–135. https://doi.org/10.1148/radiol.14132921

92. Tritschler S, Mosler C, Straub J, Buchner A, Karl A, Graser A, Stief C, Tilki D (2012) Staging of muscle-invasive bladder cancer: can computerized tomography help us to decide on local treatment? World J Urol 30(6):827–831. https://doi.org/10.1007/s00345-011-0817-6
93. Turney BW, Willatt JM, Nixon D, Crew JP, Cowan NC (2006) Computed tomography urography for diagnosing bladder cancer. BJU Int 98(2):345–348. https://doi.org/10.1111/j.1464-410X.2006.06216.x
94. Vendrell M, Maiti KK, Dhaliwal K, Chang YT (2013) Surface-enhanced Raman scattering in cancer detection and imaging. Trends Biotechnol 31(4):249–257. https://doi.org/10.1016/j.tibtech.2013.01.013
95. Wallace MB, Meining A, Canto MI, Fockens P, Miehlke S, Roesch T, Lightdale CJ, Pohl H, Carr-Locke D, Lohr M, Coron E, Filoche B, Giovannini M, Moreau J, Schmidt C, Kiesslich R (2010) The safety of intravenous fluorescein for confocal laser endomicroscopy in the gastrointestinal tract. Aliment Pharmacol Ther 31(5):548–552. https://doi.org/10.1111/j.1365-2036.2009.04207.x
96. Wang LJ, Wong YC, Ng KF, Chuang CK, Lee SY, Wan YL (2010) Tumor characteristics of urothelial carcinoma on multidetector computerized tomography urography. J Urol 183(6):2154–2160. https://doi.org/10.1016/j.juro.2010.02.028
97. Weerakkody D, Moshnikova A, Thakur MS, Moshnikova V, Daniels J, Engelman DM, Andreev OA, Reshetnyak YK (2013) Family of pH (low) insertion peptides for tumor targeting. Proc Natl Acad Sci USA 110(15):5834–5839. https://doi.org/10.1073/pnas.1303708110
98. Willingham SB, Volkmer JP, Gentles AJ, Sahoo D, Dalerba P, Mitra SS, Wang J, Contreras-Trujillo H, Martin R, Cohen JD, Lovelace P, Scheeren FA, Chao MP, Weiskopf K, Tang C, Volkmer AK, Naik TJ, Storm TA, Mosley AR, Edris B, Schmid SM, Sun CK, Chua MS, Murillo O, Rajendran P, Cha AC, Chin RK, Kim D, Adorno M, Raveh T, Tseng D, Jaiswal S, Enger PO, Steinberg GK, Li G, So SK, Majeti R, Harsh GR, van de Rijn M, Teng NN, Sunwoo JB, Alizadeh AA, Clarke MF, Weissman IL (2012) The CD47-signal regulatory protein alpha (SIRPa) interaction is a therapeutic target for human solid tumors. Proc Natl Acad Sci USA 109(17):6662–6667. https://doi.org/10.1073/pnas.1121623109
99. Wu K, Liu JJ, Adams W, Sonn GA, Mach KE, Pan Y, Beck AH, Jensen KC, Liao JC (2011) Dynamic real-time microscopy of the urinary tract using confocal laser endomicroscopy. Urology 78(1):225–231. https://doi.org/10.1016/j.urology.2011.02.057
100. Xiong Y, Li J, Ma S, Ge J, Zhou L, Li D, Chen Q (2017) A meta-analysis of narrow band imaging for the diagnosis and therapeutic outcome of non-muscle invasive bladder cancer. PLoS ONE 12(2):e0170819. https://doi.org/10.1371/journal.pone.0170819
101. Ye Z, Hu J, Song X, Li F, Zhao X, Chen S, Wang X, He D, Fan J, Ye D, Xing J, Pan T, Wang D (2015) A comparison of NBI and WLI cystoscopy in detecting non-muscle-invasive bladder cancer: A prospective, randomized and multi-center study. Sci Rep 5:10905. https://doi.org/10.1038/srep10905
102. Zheng C, Lv Y, Zhong Q, Wang R, Jiang Q (2012) Narrow band imaging diagnosis of bladder cancer: systematic review and meta-analysis. BJU Int 110(11 Pt B):E680–687. https://doi.org/10.1111/j.1464-410x.2012.11500.x
103. Zlatev DV, Altobelli E, Liao JC (2015) Advances in imaging technologies in the evaluation of high-grade bladder cancer. The Urol Clinics North Am 42(2):147–157, vii. https://doi.org/10.1016/j.ucl.2015.01.001

Molecular Prognostication in Bladder Cancer

Anirban P. Mitra and Siamak Daneshmand

Contents

Abstract

Clinical outcomes for patients with bladder cancer have largely remained unchanged over the last three decades despite improvements in surgical techniques, perioperative therapies, and postoperative management. Current

A. P. Mitra (✉) · S. Daneshmand
Institute of Urology, Keck School of Medicine of the University of Southern California, 1441 Eastlake Avenue, Suite 7416, MC 9178, Los Angeles, CA 90033, USA
e-mail: apmitra@gmail.com

S. Daneshmand and K. G. Chan (eds.), *Genitourinary Cancers*, Cancer Treatment and Research 175, https://doi.org/10.1007/978-3-319-93339-9_8

management still heavily relies on pathologic staging that does not always reflect an individual patient's risk. The genesis and progression of bladder cancer is now increasingly recognized as being a result of alterations in several pathways that affect the cell cycle, apoptosis, cellular signaling, gene regulation, immune modulation, angiogenesis, and tumor cell invasion. Multiplexed assessment of biomarkers associated with alterations in these pathways offers novel insights into tumor behavior while identifying panels that are capable of reproducibly predicting patient outcomes. Future management of bladder cancer will likely incorporate such prognostic molecular models for risk stratification and treatment personalization.

Keywords
Urinary bladder neoplasms · Cellular pathways · Immunohistochemistry Expression profiling · Multimarker analysis · Prognosis · Risk stratification Therapeutic targeting

1 Introduction

There have been several advances in the management of bladder cancer over the last decade. Improvements in detection and visualization modalities now allow for more detailed localization of tumors within the bladder [1, 2], and novel methods of urine-based cancer detection offer the opportunity for precise and noninvasive surveillance [3, 4]. Neoadjuvant chemotherapy has shown some oncologic benefit [5], and improved perioperative management protocols have enhanced patient recovery after surgery without significantly increasing hospital readmissions [6]. Despite such developments, survival outcomes for patients undergoing radical surgery for bladder cancer have, however, remained unchanged over the last 30 years [7]. Cancer of the urinary bladder remains the sixth-most common malignancy in the USA and the eight-most frequent cause of cancer-related deaths [8]. Worldwide, the disease accounts for over 165,000 deaths annually [9].

Several risk factors have been attributed to the genesis and progression of bladder cancer, and some of them have been linked to distinct molecular alterations [10]. While the use of molecular correlates as a guide to treatment has become mainstay in several other cancer types, management of urothelial carcinoma of the bladder (UCB) is still largely based on tumor stage and other histopathological parameters. Extensive research has now shown that molecular alterations in UCB dictate the rate of tumor progression and may therefore help substratify patients into risk groups based on the aggressiveness of their disease [11].

2 Molecular Pathways of Bladder Cancer Development and Progression

UCB can present as a noninvasive phenotype where malignant cells are restricted to the urothelial layer and an invasive phenotype wherein tumor cells breach the basement membrane and may invade the subepithelial connective tissue and underlying muscle [12]. Development and progression of UCB involves alterations is several cellular pathways that normally maintain tissue homeostasis. Noninvasive UCB may present as two distinct forms: Papillary (Ta) tumors are generally exophytic, tend to recur locally, but rarely invade the basement membrane or metastasize. However, the flat carcinoma in situ (CIS) is a lesion with high propensity for invasion and metastasis if left untreated. Patients with only CIS lesions in their urinary tract may also have synchronous and/or develop metachronous tumors [13]. Ta tumors potentially develop due to molecular aberrations that are distinct from CIS and invasive (T1–T4) cancers, although these pathways may not always be mutually exclusive [14, 15]. Low-grade papillary tumors often have a constitutively active receptor tyrosine kinase–Ras pathway, with activating mutations in *HRAS* and fibroblast growth factor receptor 3 (*FGFR3*) genes [16–18]. High-grade Ta tumors may be characterized by homozygous deletion of $p16^{INK4a}$ [19]. CIS and invasive tumors may often show alterations in the *TP53* and retinoblastoma (*RB*) genes and pathways [20]. While loss of heterozygosity of chromosome 9q is more frequently noted in low-grade Ta tumors, some investigators have found chromosome 9 deletions in both dysplastic urothelium and CIS lesions [21, 22]. When the occasional papillary tumor does transform to an invasive phenotype, it is often due to accumulation of additional p53 pathway alterations. p16 alterations have also been identified in invasive tumors [23]. Muscle-invasive (T2–T4) tumors are characterized by alterations in cadherins, matrix metalloproteinases (MMPs), vascular endothelial growth factors (VEGFs), and thrombospondin-1 (TSP-1), which remodel the extracellular matrix and promote tumor angiogenesis and nodal metastasis [14]. Post-cystectomy tumor recurrence rates are higher for patients with muscle-invasive cancers than those with non-muscle-invasive tumors, and prognosis following such recurrence is generally poor [24].

3 Prognostic Impact of Molecular Alterations in Bladder Cancer

Bladder tumorigenesis involves alterations in multiple homeostatic pathways with profound deregulations within a complex molecular circuitry. Distinct molecular alterations have been documented in noninvasive and invasive UCB. Investigations by The Cancer Genome Atlas (TCGA) project and other groups have greatly advanced our understanding of the complex molecular circuitry associated with UCB development; these efforts are further highlighted in a latter chapter [25, 26].

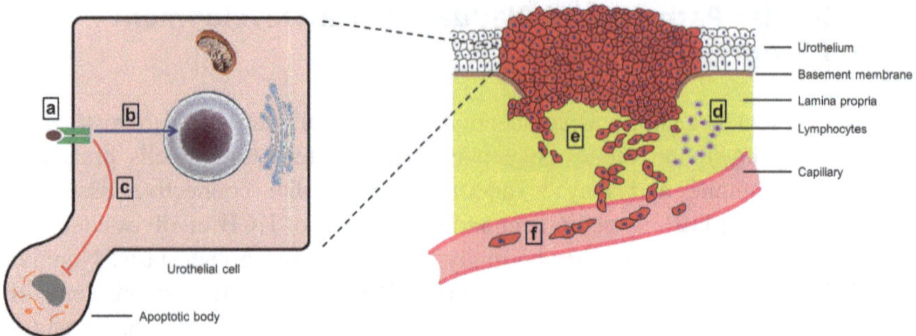

Fig. 1 Model for urothelial tumorigenesis and progression. Aberrations resulting from **a** extrinsic and intrinsic cues through cell receptors and signaling mechanisms get transmitted intracellularly resulting in **b** alterations in cell-cycle regulation and **c** inhibition of apoptosis. Tumor progression may also involve **d** modulation of the body's immune response, **e** facilitation of direct tumor cell invasion, and **f** tumor-mediated angiogenesis

Alterations in cellular signaling and their associated receptors can cause profound aberrations in cell-cycle regulation and inhibition of apoptotic mechanisms. This can lead to uncontrolled urothelial cell proliferation that leads to the genesis of UCB. Additional modulations of the immune system and promotion of angiogenesis can result in tumor cell invasion of the stroma that ultimately contributes toward disease progression (Fig. 1). The net effect of such deregulations on key cellular processes establishes the ultimate fate of the tumor (Table 1). These alterations therefore often serve as predictors of outcome and may also act as therapeutic targets [27–29].

3.1 Alterations in Cell-Cycle Regulation

The most extensively characterized cellular process in UCB involves the pathways that control cell-cycle progression [30]. The cell cycle is primarily controlled by the p53 and Rb pathways, which closely interact with mediators of apoptosis, signal transduction, and gene regulation.

Encoded by *TP53* located on chromosome 17p13.1, the p53 tumor-suppressor protein inhibits cell-cycle progression at the G_1-S transition by transcriptionally activating $p21^{WAF1/CIP1}$ [31]. While UCB generally exhibits loss of a single 17p allele, mutation in the remaining allele can lead to *TP53* inactivation and loss of its tumor-suppressor function [32]. Loss of heterozygosity on chromosome 17 generally occurs in advanced UCB and is associated with an aggressive phenotype. Wild-type p53 has a half-life of <30 min, which prevents its accumulation in the cell nucleus [33]. However, *TP53* mutations result in an altered protein that is resistant to normal ubiquitin-mediated degradation. This causes increased intranuclear p53 accumulation that can be detected by immunohistochemistry.

Table 1 Alterations in markers associated with urothelial carcinoma of the bladder and their prognostic impact

Marker	Function	Association of alteration with disease and prognosis				
		Advanced tumor grade	Advanced tumor stage	Higher nodal metastasis probability	Higher recurrence probability	Lower survival probability
Cell cycle						
p53[a]	Inhibits G_1-S progression				✓	✓
p21[b]	Cyclin-dependent kinase inhibitor				✓	✓
Mdm2[c]	Mediates proteasomal degradation of p53	✓	✓			
p14[b]	Inhibits *MDM2*					✓
p16[b]	Cyclin-dependent kinase inhibitor				✓	✓
Rb[d]	Sequesters E2F; inhibits cell-cycle progression				✓	✓
p27[b]	Cyclin-dependent kinase inhibitor				✓	✓
Apoptosis						
Caspase-3[b]	Promotes apoptosis				✓	✓
Survivin[c]	Inhibits apoptosis				✓	✓
Bcl-2[c]	Inhibits caspase activation					✓
Bax[b]	Releases cytochrome c from mitochondria; promotes apoptosis					✓
Apaf-1[b]	Promotes apoptosis					✓
Cell signaling and gene regulation						
FGFR3[e]	Receptor for fibroblast growth factor; transmits growth signals				✓	
ErbB-1[c]	Epidermal growth factor receptor; transmits growth signals				✓	✓
ErbB-2[c]	Epidermal growth factor receptor; transmits growth signals					✓*

(continued)

Table 1 (continued)

Marker	Function	Association of alteration with disease and prognosis				
		Advanced tumor grade	Advanced tumor stage	Higher nodal metastasis probability	Higher recurrence probability	Lower survival probability
Estrogen receptor-β[c]	Sex hormone receptor; regulates transcription	✓	✓			
AR[b]	Sex hormone receptor; regulates transcription	✓*	✓*			
STAT3[c]	Regulates gene expression; increases Bcl-2 expression				✓	✓
Inflammation and immune modulation						
IL-6, IL-6sR[c]	Lymphocyte proliferation, production of acute-phase proteins		✓	✓	✓	✓
NFKBIA[c]	Regulates gene expression				✓	
CRP[c]	Promotes phagocytosis by macrophages, activates complement system					✓
Angiogenesis						
Microvessel density[c]	Histological marker of angiogenesis			✓	✓*	✓*
VEGF[c]	Promotes angiogenesis through nitric oxide synthase	✓	✓	✓	✓	✓
VEGFR2[c]	VEGF receptor; transmits angiogenic signals		✓	✓		
uPA[c]	Degrades extracellular matrix			✓	✓	✓
bFGF[c]	Growth factor stimulating angiogenesis		✓	✓	✓	
aFGF[c]	Growth factor stimulating angiogenesis		✓			
TSP-1[b]	Inhibits angiogenesis				✓	✓

(continued)

Table 1 (continued)

Marker	Function	Association of alteration with disease and prognosis				
		Advanced tumor grade	Advanced tumor stage	Higher nodal metastasis probability	Higher recurrence probability	Lower survival probability
Invasion						
E-cadherin[b]	Mediates intercellular adhesion				✓	✓
Protocadherin 19[b]	Mediates intercellular adhesion			✓		✓
Thymidine phosphorylase[c]	Promotes VEGF and interleukin-8 secretion; induces MMP				✓	
MMP-2[c]	Degrades extracellular matrix	✓			✓	✓
MMP-9[c]	Degrades extracellular matrix	✓	✓			✓
MMP-7[c]	Degrades extracellular matrix				✓	✓
ICAM1[c]	Binds integrins	✓		✓		
α6β4 integrin[d]	Links collagen VII to cytoskeleton; transduces regulatory signals					✓
CA 19-9[c]	Unknown				✓	✓
CEA[c]	Mediates intercellular adhesion					✓

Abbreviations *aFGF* acidic fibroblast growth factor; *AR* androgen receptor; *bFGF* basic fibroblast growth factor; *CA 19-9* carbohydrate antigen 19-9; *CEA* carcinoembryonic antigen; *CRP* C-reactive protein; *FGFR3* fibroblast growth factor receptor 3; *ICAM1* intercellular adhesion molecule 1; *IL-6* interleukin-6; *IL-6sR* IL-6 soluble receptor; *MMP* matrix metalloproteinase; *NFKBIA* NF-κB inhibitor a; *Rb* retinoblastoma protein; *STAT* signal transducer and activator of transcription; *TSP-1* thrombospondin-1; *uPA* urokinase-type plasminogen activator; *VEGF* vascular endothelial growth factor; *VEGFR2* VEGF receptor 2

[a]Altered

[b]Underexpressed/lost

[c]Overexpressed/increased

[d]Lost/hyperphosphorylated

[e]Overactivated

* Conflicting data

✓ Positive association

Retrospective studies have reported that p53 nuclear accumulation is prognostic in UCB, especially in patients treated with radical cystectomy [34–39]. The rate of altered p53 expression in tumors has been shown to increase progressively from normal urothelium to non-muscle-invasive UCB, to muscle-invasive disease and metastatic lymph nodes [40–42]. An analysis of high-grade muscle-invasive UCB specimens by TCGA Research Network identified *TP53* mutations in nearly half of the samples, which were mutually exclusive in their relationship with amplification and overexpression of *MDM2*; hence, *TP53* function was noted to be inactivated in 76% of samples [25]. However, at this time, the use of p53 as a prognostic marker in UCB is still not clinically established despite over 100 studies evaluating its utility. Indeed, discordance in p53 nuclear accumulation and *TP53* mutations has been documented [43]. A meta-analysis of the role of p53 in UCB that examined data from 117 studies noted that observational discrepancies may be related to the choice of p53 antibody used in immunohistochemical assays, variability in interpretation and stratification criteria, and other technical and specimen handling inconsistencies [44]. A phase III trial designed to evaluate the benefit of stratifying organ-confined invasive UCB patients based on their p53 status for adjuvant cisplatin-containing chemotherapy could not confirm the prognostic value of the protein alteration or any association with chemotherapeutic response [45]. However, this trial had several limitations including high patient refusal rate, lower than expected event rate, and failures to receive assigned therapy that compromised the study's power.

The $p21^{WAF1/CIP1}$ gene encodes for the p21 cyclin-dependent kinase inhibitor (CDKI). This is transcriptionally regulated by p53, and loss of p21 expression is a potential mechanism by which p53 alterations influence tumor progression [20]. Loss of p21 expression has been reported to be an independent predictor of UCB progression, and maintenance of its expression can abrogate the deleterious effects of altered p53 [46]. In patients with muscle-invasive UCB, p21 is an independent predictor of recurrence and cancer-specific mortality [42]. The prognostic value of p21 may be most useful in patients with pT2-3N0 disease, especially in combination with other markers [40].

Mdm2 is involved in an autoregulatory feedback loop with p53, thereby controlling its activity. Increased levels of p53 upregulate *MDM2* by transactivating its promoter, and the translated protein mediates proteasomal degradation of p53. The resultant lowered p53 levels then reduce the levels of Mdm2. *MDM2* amplification has been observed in UCB, and its frequency increases with increasing tumor stage and grade [47]. *MDM2* is transcriptionally inhibited by p14. The protein is encoded by $p14^{ARF}$, one of the two splice variants derived from the *CDKN2A* locus that is situated on chromosome 9p21. $p14^{ARF}$ is induced by the E2F transcription factor, thereby making it the molecular link between the Rb and p53 pathways [48]. $p14^{ARF}$ may be inactivated by homozygous deletion or by varying degrees of methylation of the promoter region [27]. The other splice variant, $p16^{INK4a}$, encodes for p16 that is a CDKI. Reports suggest that homozygous $p16^{INK4a}$ deletions in non-muscle-invasive UCB have higher recurrence rates, but deletions that affect both p16 and p14, which deregulate both Rb and p53 pathways, correlate with the worst outcomes [19]. Hemizygous and homozygous deletions of the *CDKN2A* locus have been found in 40–60% and 10–30% of cases, respectively [49].

Encoded on chromosome 13q14, the Rb protein interacts with regulatory proteins involved in the G_1-S transition of the cell cycle. Dephosphorylated Rb sequesters the transcription factor E2F. Upon phosphorylation of Rb by cyclin-dependent kinases, E2F is released leading to transcription of genes required for DNA synthesis. Inactivating *RB* mutations resulting in loss of protein expression have been noted in UCB [50]. In conjunction with other cell-cycle regulatory proteins, Rb has also been shown to be prognostic in UCB [37, 38]. Rb phosphorylation is facilitated by cyclin/cyclin-dependent kinase complexes. Negative regulation of cyclin-dependent kinases is achieved by CDKIs such as p21, p16, and p27, which act as tumor suppressors. Low p27 levels have been associated with advanced stage bladder adenocarcinomas [51]. p27 alterations have also been linked with shortened disease-free and overall survival in UCB [52]. In patients with pT1 tumors treated with radical cystectomy, p27 alterations in combination with other immunohistochemical markers improved the predictive value of a nomogram based on standard clinicopathological variables [53]. Combined immunohistochemical assessment of p53, p21, Rb, cyclin E1, and p27 has been shown to yield predictive accuracies superior to that of any single molecular marker in patients with UCB treated with radical cystectomy and can improve risk stratification [54, 55].

3.2 Alterations in Apoptotic Pathways

Apoptosis is a complex and highly regulated process that involves a series of coordinated steps throughout normal development and in response to a variety of initiation stimuli resulting in programmed cell death. Apoptosis can be initiated by two pathways. The extrinsic pathway involves activation of cell-surface death receptors, whereas the intrinsic pathway is mediated by mitochondria. Both pathways activate caspases that cleave cellular substrates and lead to the characteristic apoptotic changes. In vitro tumor-specific caspase-8 expression has been shown to induce apoptosis in urothelial carcinoma cell lines [56]. Decreased caspase-3 expression has also been associated with a higher probability of disease recurrence and cancer-specific mortality [57]. Survivin is a member of the inhibitor of apoptosis family, and inhibits the process, at least partly, by blocking downstream caspase activity. Survivin overexpression was present in 64% of cases and was associated with higher probability of disease recurrence and cancer-specific mortality in 226 bladder cancer patients [57]. Further, the proportion of specimens with survivin overexpression increased progressively from non-muscle-invasive to muscle-invasive disease and to metastatic lymph nodes [58]. In a multicenter validation study, addition of survivin improved the accuracy of standard clinicopathologic features for prediction of disease recurrence and cancer-specific survival in a subgroup of patients with pT1-3N0M0 disease [59].

The Bcl-2 family of proteins is involved in the intrinsic apoptotic pathway; it includes antiapoptotic members such as Bcl-2 as well as proapoptotic members such as Bax and Bad. Bcl-2 overexpression has been associated with poor prognosis in UCB patients treated with radiotherapy or synchronous chemoradiotherapy [60, 61]. Bcl-2 may also serve as a marker in patients with advanced UCB undergoing radiotherapy who may benefit from neoadjuvant chemotherapy [62]. However, other findings have suggested that Bcl-2 overexpression confers worse all-cause survival and lower response rates to chemotherapy [63]. Bcl-2 expression has been associated with decreased tumor-free survival in high-grade T1 disease and may serve as a good prognostic indicator in non-muscle-invasive disease in combination with p53 [64, 65]. A prognostic index that included Mdm2, p53, and Bcl-2 has been proposed where aberrations in all three markers corresponded to the worst survival probability in UCB [66]. On the other hand, Bax expression is an independent predictor of a more favorable prognosis in invasive UCB [65, 67, 68]. Bax mediates its proapoptotic role through the activation of Apaf-1 [69]. Decreased Apaf-1 expression has been associated with higher mortality in UCB [70].

3.3 Alterations in Cell Signaling and Gene Regulation Mechanisms

Several cell-surface receptors modulate signals from external cues and transmit them via transduction pathways to the nuclei of urothelial cells. Aberrations in these receptors and/or the transmitted signals can lead to abnormal regulation of genes, thereby causing uncontrolled cellular proliferation and tumor formation.

Of the FGFR family members, activating mutations of *FGFR3* are the most extensively studied alterations in UCB. Nearly 60–70% of low-grade papillary Ta tumors harbor *FGFR3* mutations [71, 72]. *FGFR3* activation results in downstream signaling through the Ras–mitogen-activated protein kinase (MAPK) pathway. *FGFR3* and *Ras* mutations may be mutually exclusive; nearly 82% of grade 1 tumors and Ta tumors have mutations in either a *Ras* gene or *FGFR3*, suggesting that MAPK pathway activation may be an obligate event in most of these cases [73]. *HRAS* expression has also been associated with noninvasive UCB recurrence at initial presentation [74].

Epidermal growth factor receptor (EGFR) family members include ErbB-1 and ErbB-2 (Her2/neu), which are overexpressed in invasive UCB [75–77]. ErbB-1 overexpression has been associated with higher probability of progression and mortality [78, 79]. ErbB-2 overexpression has also been associated with aggressive UCB and poor disease-specific survival [80–83]. However, other reports have indicated that ErbB-2 expression is not correlated with prognosis [84, 85]. While the combined expression profile of ErbB-1 and ErbB-2 has been suggested to be a better outcome predictor than each marker alone, this finding has also not been corroborated [86, 87].

Variable expression of sex steroid hormone receptors has been postulated as a potential cause for differential behavior of UCB between genders, although direct evidence to this effect is lacking [88]. Across both genders, decreased estrogen receptor-β expression has been associated with better progression-free survival rates in patients with noninvasive UCB [89]. A meta-analysis of 2,049 patients with bladder cancer showed that estrogen receptor-β positive rates were significantly higher in high-grade and muscle-invasive tumors [90]. Androgen receptor (AR) is a nuclear receptor and ligand-dependent transcription factor that mediates biologic effects of androgens. Its expression is inversely correlated with pathological stage; a study noted that 75 and 21.4% of non-muscle-invasive and muscle-invasive UCB, respectively, expressed AR [91]. Another study noted that loss of AR expression was associated with higher-grade and invasive tumors; however, no association was found with patient outcomes [89]. In contrast, a study of 472 UCB patients failed to find any association between AR expression and disease stage, grade, or outcomes [92].

Janus kinase (JAK) constitutes a family of tyrosine kinases that is activated by cytokine and growth receptors and mediates multiple signaling pathways. Following JAK activation, the most well-characterized molecular events include activation of the signal transducer and activator of transcription (STAT) pathway, which control transcription of several important genes. STAT1 can reduce Bcl-2 expression, and STAT3 has the opposite effect [93]. In combination with other markers, *STAT3* expression can predict risk of recurrence and survival in patients with UCB [94].

MRE11 is a nuclear protein with exo- and endonuclease activity that is responsible for telomere length maintenance and DNA double-strand break repair in conjunction with a DNA ligase. MRE11 underexpression in primary tumors has been associated with worse cancer-specific survival; high MRE11 expression in patients undergoing radical radiotherapy for muscle-invasive UCB has been associated with better outcomes [95, 96]. This predictive effect has been postulated to be under the control of post-transcriptional regulatory mechanisms [97]. Certain germline *MRE11* variants have also been identified as markers of radiotherapy outcomes in muscle-invasive UCB [98]. However, the prognostic impact of MRE11 on post-radiotherapy outcomes has not been validated by other studies [99].

3.4 Inflammation and Immune Modulation

Modulation of the host's immune mechanisms is an important way by which bladder cancer progresses. Interleukin-6 (IL-6) is a cytokine that modulates the immune system presumably via increased JAK signaling, leading to proliferation and activation of cytotoxic T cells, proliferation and differentiation of B cells, and production of acute-phase proteins. IL-6 signaling is initiated when it binds to its non-signaling receptor IL-6R, which also exists in soluble form (IL-6sR). Elevated IL-6 and IL-6sR levels were associated with advanced pathological stage, lymphovascular invasion, and nodal metastases in UCB patients [100]. Both biomarkers were also independent predictors of disease recurrence, and cancer-specific mortality after adjusting for stage and grade.

NF-κB is another important transcription factor that plays an important role in inflammation, autoimmune response, cell proliferation, and apoptosis by regulating the expression of genes involved in these processes. Bacillus Calmette–Guérin-induced IL-6 expression by UCB occurs as an immediate–early gene pathway that requires NF-κB [101]. A study examining a functional insertion/deletion polymorphism in the promoter region of *NFKB1* showed that non-muscle-invasive UCB patients with the homozygous deletion had a higher risk of recurrence than those with the homozygous insertion [102]. *NFKBIA*, a gene encoding for a member of the NF-κB inhibitor family, was one of the key markers identified by a machine-learning algorithm that could predict recurrence in patients with non-muscle-invasive UCB at first presentation [103].

C-reactive protein (CRP) is an acute-phase protein of hepatic origin that increases following IL-6 secretion by macrophages and T cells. As the most widely studied serum marker for inflammation in bladder cancer, elevated CRP levels have been associated with adverse outcome [104]. Although variables for adjustment have varied among studies, CRP has been shown to be an independent prognostic factor for cancer-specific and overall mortality [105–109]

3.5 Modulation of Tumor Angiogenesis

Angiogenesis involves production tumor cell-derived factors that interact with stromal elements to recruit endothelial cells to the site of malignancy and establish a vascular supply, which provides the required nutrients for growth of the cancer cells. Angiogenesis is histologically measured by microvessel density, which may be associated with disease-free and overall survival in UCB [110]. Microvessel density quantification may also provide additional prognostic information in UCB patients with p53-altered tumors [111]. While the prognostic association of microvessel density has not been confirmed by other studies, it has been shown to be higher in patients with lymph node metastasis [112, 113].

VEGFs are strong angiogenesis-promoting signaling proteins that stimulate nitric oxide synthase, which in turn stimulates nitric oxide formation and tumor vascularization. In a study of 204 patients treated with radical cystectomy and bilateral pelvic lymphadenectomy, VEGF was overexpressed in 86% of patients, supporting its role in bladder tumorigenesis and identifying it as a potential target for therapy [113]. Increased expression of VEGF in non-muscle-invasive UCB is associated with early recurrence and progression [114]. High serum levels of VEGF are associated with advanced UCB stage and grade, vascular invasion, CIS, metastases, and poor disease-free survival [115]. VEGF overexpression in primary tumors has been associated with advanced stage and grade, lymphovascular invasion, nodal metastasis, disease recurrence, and shorter disease-free survival [116, 117].

VEGF stimulates cellular responses by binding to its corresponding receptors (VEGFRs). VEGFR2 (KDR/Flk-1) mediates most of the known cellular responses to VEGF. VEGFR2 expression has been associated with advanced bladder cancer stage and muscle invasion [118]. Another study has also shown that *VEGFR2* expression may be an important determinant for nodal metastasis in UCB patients [119].

VEGF also induces the formation of urokinase-type plasminogen activator (uPA), which degrades the extracellular matrix, thereby facilitating endothelial cell migration and invasion. uPA generates plasmin that stimulates production of basic and acidic fibroblast growth factors (bFGF and aFGF, respectively). Preoperative plasma uPA levels have been associated with lymphovascular invasion, nodal metastasis, disease progression, and death from UCB [120]. The proangiogenic bFGF has been associated with established features of biologically aggressive disease including higher pathologic stage, lymphovascular invasion, lymph node metastasis, and disease recurrence [113]. Urine bFGF levels have been correlated with UCB stage and local disease recurrence [121, 122]. Urinary aFGF levels in invasive UCB patients also show correlation with disease stage [123].

In addition to regulating the cell cycle, p53 plays an important role in angiogenesis by upregulating TSP-1, a potent inhibitor of angiogenesis. Tumors with p53 alterations are associated with decreased TSP-1 expression, and such tumors demonstrate higher microvessel density [124]. TSP-1 underexpression has been associated with lower probabilities of recurrence-free and overall survival in UCB. A combination of angiogenesis-related biomarkers including VEGF, bFGF, and TSP-1 has also been associated with established clinicopathologic features of biologically aggressive disease in patients who underwent radical cystectomy for muscle-invasive UCB [113]. On multivariable analyses that adjusted for standard pathological features, bFGF and TSP-1 were identified as independent predictors of disease recurrence and cancer-specific mortality.

3.6 Regulation of Tumor Cell Invasion

The ability of urothelial carcinoma cells to invade the vasculature and lymphatics determines their potential to spread to adjacent structures and metastasize to distant sites. Ubiquitous to all tissues, cadherins are prime mediators of intercellular adhesion. E-cadherin is the prototypic member of the cadherin family, and it plays a critical role in epithelial cell–cell adhesion. Decreased E-cadherin expression has been significantly correlated with higher risk of tumor recurrence and progression, as well as with shorter survival in UCB patients [70, 125–128]. A whole transcriptome analysis of 199 patients with invasive UCB who underwent radical cystectomy with extended pelvic lymphadenectomy identified protocadherin 19 (*PCDH19*), which encodes for a member of the cadherin superfamily, as one of the most important members of a 51-feature classifier for predicting lymph node metastasis [129].

A tumor's ability to degrade the matrix and invade the basement membrane is facilitated by the actions of several protease families including uPAs and MMPs. Expression levels of transcripts encoding thymidine phosphorylase, an enzyme that promotes MMP production, is 33-fold higher in muscle-invasive UCB than in non-muscle-invasive tumors, and 260-fold higher than in normal bladder [130].

The corresponding protein levels in muscle-invasive tumors are eightfold higher than in non-muscle-invasive tumors and 15-fold higher than in normal bladder tissue [131]. Increased nuclear reactivity of thymidine phosphorylase has been associated with a higher risk of non-muscle-invasive UCB recurrence [132, 133]. Increased MMP-2 and MMP-9 expression have been associated with higher UCB stage and grade [134, 135]. MMP-2 overexpression can also predict poor relapse-free and disease-specific survival [136]. The MMP-9/E-cadherin ratio is also reportedly prognostic for disease-specific survival in UCB patients [137]. Increased MMP-9 serum levels have been found in patients with advanced stage and grade, and distant metastasis [138]. Elevated serum MMP-7 levels have also been associated with metastatic disease and are predictors of metastasis-free, disease-specific, and overall survival in bladder cancer [139]. These findings have been validated in an independent cohort [140].

Integrins are transmembrane glycoproteins which, when altered, can promote tumor progression, invasion, and metastasis. They are receptors for proteins such as adhesion molecules and collagen. Intercellular adhesion molecule 1 (ICAM1) is a member of the immunoglobulin superfamily that binds to certain integrin classes. Immunohistochemical studies in UCB have shown that ICAM1 expression is closely associated with an infiltrative histological phenotype [141]. Serum ICAM1 levels have also been correlated with the presence, grade, and size of bladder tumors [142]. *ICAM1* is a member of multimarker models that can predict nodal status in patients with UCB [143]. In normal urothelial cells, the α6β4 integrin is in close relationship with collagen VII, and it restricts cell migration. Loss of polarity of α6β4 expression has been noted in non-muscle-invasive UCB, and muscle-invasive tumors show either a loss of α6β4 and/or collagen VII expression or a lack of colocalization of the two proteins [144]. Patients with tumors that show weak α6β4 immunoreactivity have better outcomes than those with either no expression or strong overexpression [145].

CA 19-9, a member of the carbohydrate antigen family, is a common tumor marker for pancreatic cancer. Carcinoembryonic antigen (CEA) describes a set of highly related glycoproteins involved in cell adhesion. Elevated precystectomy serum levels of CA 19-9 and CEA have been shown to be independent predictors of worse overall survival in patients with bladder cancer [146]. Elevated serum CA 19-9 levels have also been associated with poor recurrence-free survival and can potentially identify patients who may respond to neoadjuvant chemotherapy [147]. Overall, molecular markers of invasion are therefore relatively reliable predictors of patient outcome in UCB.

4 Prognostic Value of Multimarker Assessment

Alterations in several molecular pathways can, in tandem, influence the pathogenesis of bladder tumors and their ultimate clinical behavior. Analyzing these alterations in combination may therefore provide deeper insight into the pathobiology of the disease, while also generating marker panels that may be able to better predict patient outcome and treatment response. Such panels can be generated across all strata of functional cellular processing—at the epigenetic, genetic, transcriptomic, proteomic, and metabolomic levels.

Gene-level profiling and transcriptome-level profiling are the most commonly used approaches in UCB, and these have been used to identify markers that characterize various subsets of patients with bladder cancer [148]. The advent of technologies that can assess multiple markers in a reliable, efficient, and cost-effective way have led to their adoption for development of prognostic panels. Several studies have assessed carefully selected molecular targets across several UCB-associated cellular pathways in an attempt to define prognostic signatures [149].

This strategy was used to develop an objective method for predicting recurrence and progression in patients with noninvasive tumors at first presentation to potentially allow for treatment individualization [74]. A 24-gene panel spanning across relevant cancer pathways was used to profile patients who initially presented with Ta grade 2–3 tumors who belonged to one of three outcome-based groups: those with no recurrence, recurrence, or progression within 5 years of follow-up. A multivariable model based on *CCND3* expression showed 97% sensitivity and 63% specificity for identifying patients who recurred. A similar model based on *HRAS*, *VEGFR2,* and *VEGF* identified patients who progressed with 81% sensitivity and 94% specificity.

This approach was also used to identify molecular alterations associated with disease progression across all UCB stages, which could potentially supplement traditional staging in predicting outcomes [94]. The expressions of 69 genes involved in different cancer pathways were assessed on primary UCB specimens to identify a panel of four markers (*JUN*, *MAP2K6*, *STAT3,* and *ICAM1*) that were associated with disease recurrence and overall survival. Differences in 5-year probabilities for recurrence and survival based on a favorable versus unfavorable profile using this panel were 41 versus 88% and 61 versus 5%, respectively (both, $P < 0.001$). The prognostic potential of this panel was confirmed on an independent external dataset (disease-specific survival, $P = 0.039$).

Efforts to profile the entire coding region of the bladder cancer genome by interrogating thousands of genes using high-throughput array-based technologies have led to deeper understanding of the molecular alterations that are associated with the disease. In one effort, 105 bladder tumors were analyzed using oligonucleotide arrays, and support vector machine algorithms were used to test the prognostic abilities of the profiled genes [150]. For predicting overall survival, resulting accuracies were 82 and 90% when considering all UCB patients or only those with muscle-invasive disease, respectively. A 174-probe signature was also attributed to patients with node-positive disease and poor survival.

Investigators from Chungbuk National University (Chungbuk, South Korea) have also employed high-throughput profiling strategies to identify several markers associated with progression of non-muscle-invasive bladder cancer. The group initially identified an eight-gene signature (comprising *S100A8*, *CELSR3*, *PFKFB4*,

HMOX1, *MTAP*, *MGC17624*, *KIF1A,* and *COCH*) that was associated with disease progression in this patient subgroup [151]. Interestingly, *S100A8* in combination with *IL1B*, *S100A9,* and *EGFR* was also identified as important mediators of progression for muscle-invasive bladder cancer in a separate analysis [152]. The group also identified an expression signature of *S100A8*-correlated genes as being a strong predictor of progression in patients with non-muscle-invasive disease [153]. A multivariable Cox regression model using a subset of three genes from the original signature (*CELSR3*, *KIF1A,* and *COCH*) was also shown to be an independent predictor of non-muscle-invasive bladder cancer progression [154]. Decreased *MGC17624* expression was correlated with disease progression in the original analysis, and its association with *RUNX3* promoter methylation was shown to be associated with poor prognosis in patients with non-muscle-invasive tumors [155]. Hypermethylation of three other genes (*HOXA9*, *ISL1,* and *ALDH1A3*) was also shown to be an independent predictor of non-muscle-invasive disease recurrence and progression [156].

Examination of methylation profiles of other markers have also resulted in identification of prognostic panels. An investigation of the methylation status of 20 cancer-associated genes in microdissected tumor samples from 105 patients with non-muscle-invasive UCB resulted in a panel of six genes, where methylation was associated with disease recurrence [157]. *TIMP-3* methylation was noted to be associated with prolonged recurrence-free survival. Another study looked at methylation levels of six markers in 368 urine sediment samples collected from 90 patients with noninvasive UCB [158]. This identified a panel of three markers (*SOX1*, *IRAK3*, and *L1-MET*) that discriminated between patients with and without recurrence with sensitivity and specificity of 80 and 97%, respectively, in the validation set.

Decision models based on clinicopathologic metrics can provide reasonable prognostic value to influence patient management [159, 160]. Recent studies have focused on combining such clinical models with biomarkers to improve prognostic performance. When employed with microarray technology that can interrogate the entire coding region of the human genome while also accounting for splice variants and non-protein-coding transcripts, the resulting combination has the potential to greatly broaden the realm of transcriptomic profiling in UCB [161]. A large effort to discover and validate a prognostic genomic signature for clinically high-risk bladder cancer used transcriptome-wide profiling of patients with muscle-invasive and/or node-positive UCB, resulting in the identification of a 15-feature genomic classifier that had a prognostic value of 77% on blinded independent validation [162]. The genomic classifier also uniquely reported on the prognostic potential of certain non-protein-coding transcripts, which have recently been shown to play important regulatory roles in cancer development [163]. While the prognostic accuracy of a model that comprised clinical variables alone was 78% in the validation set, it improved to 86% when the genomic classifier was added (Fig. 2). Performance of the 15-feature genomic classifier was also validated on four independent datasets that confirmed its prognostic potential.

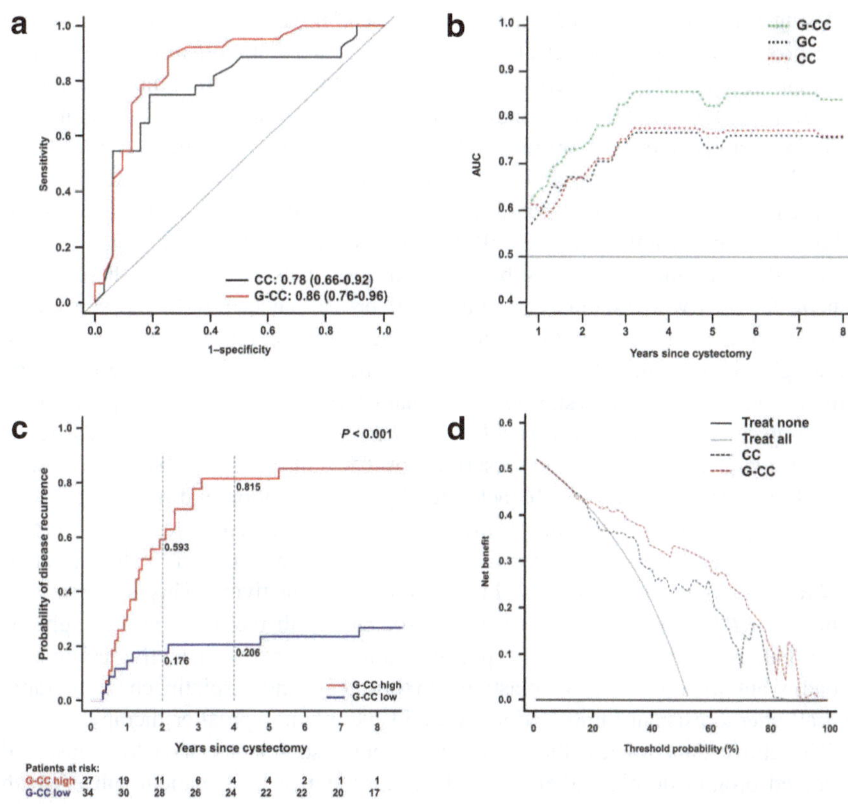

Fig. 2 Comparative performance of a clinical classifier model (CC), a 15-feature genomic classifier (GC), and both in combination (G-CC) for predicting recurrence in a validation set of patients who underwent radical cystectomy for bladder cancer. **a** Receiver operating characteristic curves show that G-CC had higher area under curve (AUC) compared with CC. AUCs and associated 95% confidence intervals are shown at the bottom right of the panel. **b** Survival AUCs plotted over a range of time points following cystectomy show that G-CC has superior performance compared with GC and CC. **c** Cumulative incidence plot for recurrence-free survival indicates significantly elevated recurrence probabilities for patients with high G-CC scores. **d** Decision curve analysis indicates higher net benefit of G-CC over CC over a wide range of decision-to-treat thresholds Adapted and reproduced with permission from Mitra et al. [162]

Another study has further examined the prognostic importance of a nine-biomarker panel across all UCB stages [70]. In this study, the addition of smoking history to a clinical model improved its prognostic accuracy from 76 to 81%. The prognostic accuracy increased to 85% when information from the biomarker panel was added, which was significantly higher than the clinical model alone ($P < 0.001$) or when combined with clinical and patient smoking variables ($P = 0.018$). Subsequent studies have confirmed that combining smoking information with molecular markers can improve prognostication in UCB patients [164].

Using primary tumor gene expression datasets, novel UCB subtypes have also been proposed by Volkmer et al. based on molecular determinants of tumor differentiation states: basal, intermediate, and differentiated [165]. This study noted that each subtype harbored a unique tumor-initiating population, and keratin 14 (*KRT14*) marked the most primitive differentiation state that preceded *KRT5* and *KRT20* expression. The basal UCB differentiation subtype was associated with significantly worse overall survival compared with intermediate and differentiated subtypes. Using whole genome mRNA expression profiling, Choi et al. documented three unique molecular subtypes of muscle-invasive UCB that shared some genetic features with established subtypes of breast cancer [166]. The study designated these subtypes as basal, luminal, and p53-like muscle-invasive tumors. Although this basal subset had a distinct molecular signature from that described by Volkmer et al., both these subsets were characterized by increased expression of high molecular weight keratins (*KRT14* and *KRT5*). In addition, the basal subset of muscle-invasive bladder tumors described by Choi et al. shared biomarkers with basal breast cancers and was characterized by p63 activation and more aggressive disease at presentation. Tumors in the luminal subset contained features of active PPARγ and estrogen receptor transcription and were enriched with activating *FGFR3* mutations and potential FGFR inhibitor sensitivity. This subtype also exhibited *KRT20* upregulation that was associated with the differentiated subtype described by Volkmer et al. The p53-like tumors were consistently resistant to neoadjuvant methotrexate, vinblastine, doxorubicin, and cisplatin chemotherapy, and all chemoresistant tumors adopted a p53-like phenotype after therapy.

The above data suggest that high-throughput assessment can yield robust and validated prognostic biomarker panels that can identify UCB patient subsets with varying outcomes. Their performance may be enhanced in combination with clinical and epidemiologic variables, thereby identifying candidates who may need more aggressive management.

5 Conclusions

Bladder cancer is now being recognized as a disease that cannot be treated exclusively on the basis of pathologic staging; therapeutic strategies need to also account for the molecular alterations in individual tumors. The availability of sophisticated profiling strategies has allowed for increased understanding of the molecular events that lead to urothelial tumorigenesis and progression. Future UCB management will employ consensus marker panels that can provide accurate predictions of prognosis and therapeutic response in individual patients. Recent efforts toward characterizing the bladder cancer genome have laid the roadmap toward identifying the potential therapeutic roles for several targeted agents [167]. However, the use of prognostic markers in clinical decision-making algorithms has thus far not gained universal traction in UCB management. Barriers to incorporation of biomarkers in clinical practice include inadequate independent validation, lack of consensus on reference standards, limited evidence of analytic and clinical validity of standardized assays, and limited validation in prospective randomized trials. Efforts are now underway to define best practice standards for prognostic and therapeutic biomarker reporting, and development of quality systems for theranostic implementation [168–170]. Risk-stratifying patients based on validated standardized prognostic marker panels followed by optimal surgical treatment and interrupting crucial pathway checkpoints through employment of therapeutic agents that target multiple molecular pathways will be crucial toward effective management of this disease.

Funding Acknowledgement This research was not sponsored by any funding agency in the public, commercial, or not-for-profit sectors.

References

1. Daneshmand S, Patel S, Lotan Y et al (2018) Efficacy and safety of blue light flexible cystoscopy with hexaminolevulinate (HAL) in the surveillance of bladder cancer: a phase III, comparative, multi-center study. J Urol 199:1158
2. Zlatev DV, Altobelli E, Liao JC (2015) Advances in imaging technologies in the evaluation of high-grade bladder cancer. Urol Clin North Am 42:147
3. Birkhahn M, Mitra AP, Williams AJ et al (2013) A novel precision-engineered microfiltration device for capture and characterisation of bladder cancer cells in urine. Eur J Cancer 49:3159
4. Mitra AP, Cote RJ (2010) Molecular screening for bladder cancer: progress and potential. Nat Rev Urol 7:11
5. Advanced Bladder Cancer (ABC) Meta-analysis Collaboration (2005) Neoadjuvant chemotherapy in invasive bladder cancer: update of a systematic review and meta-analysis of individual patient data. Eur Urol 48:202
6. Daneshmand S, Ahmadi H, Schuckman AK et al (2014) Enhanced recovery protocol after radical cystectomy for bladder cancer. J Urol 192:50
7. Zehnder P, Studer UE, Skinner EC et al (2013) Unaltered oncological outcomes of radical cystectomy with extended lymphadenectomy over three decades. BJU Int 112:E51
8. Siegel RL, Miller KD, Jemal A (2018) Cancer statistics, 2018. CA Cancer J Clin 68:7
9. Torre LA, Bray F, Siegel RL et al (2015) Global cancer statistics, 2012. CA Cancer J Clin 65:87
10. Mitra AP, Bartsch G, Cote RJ (2018) Risk factors and molecular features associated with bladder cancer development. In: Hansel DE, Lerner SP (eds) Precision molecular pathology of bladder cancer. Springer Nature, Cham, Switzerland, pp 3–28
11. Mitra AP (2016) Molecular substratification of bladder cancer: moving towards individualized patient management. Ther Adv Urol 8:215
12. Mitra AP, Jordà M, Cote RJ (2012) Pathological possibilities and pitfalls in detecting aggressive bladder cancer. Curr Opin Urol 22:397
13. Zehnder P, Moltzahn F, Daneshmand S et al (2014) Outcome in patients with exclusive carcinoma in situ (CIS) after radical cystectomy. BJU Int 113:65
14. Wu XR (2005) Urothelial tumorigenesis: a tale of divergent pathways. Nat Rev Cancer 5:713
15. Knowles MA (2006) Molecular subtypes of bladder cancer: Jekyll and Hyde or chalk and cheese? Carcinogenesis 27:361

16. Rieger-Christ KM, Mourtzinos A, Lee PJ et al (2003) Identification of fibroblast growth factor receptor 3 mutations in urine sediment DNA samples complements cytology in bladder tumor detection. Cancer 98:737
17. van Rhijn BW, van der Kwast TH, Vis AN et al (2004) *FGFR3* and *P53* characterize alternative genetic pathways in the pathogenesis of urothelial cell carcinoma. Cancer Res 64:1911
18. Bakkar AA, Wallerand H, Radvanyi F et al (2003) *FGFR3* and *TP53* gene mutations define two distinct pathways in urothelial cell carcinoma of the bladder. Cancer Res 63:8108
19. Orlow I, LaRue H, Osman I et al (1999) Deletions of the INK4A gene in superficial bladder tumors. Association with recurrence. Am J Pathol 155:105
20. Mitra AP, Datar RH, Cote RJ (2006) Molecular pathways in invasive bladder cancer: new insights into mechanisms, progression, and target identification. J Clin Oncol 24:5552
21. Spruck CH III, Ohneseit PF, Gonzalez-Zulueta M et al (1994) Two molecular pathways to transitional cell carcinoma of the bladder. Cancer Res 54:784
22. Hartmann A, Schlake G, Zaak D et al (2002) Occurrence of chromosome 9 and p53 alterations in multifocal dysplasia and carcinoma in situ of human urinary bladder. Cancer Res 62:809
23. Korkolopoulou P, Christodoulou P, Lazaris A et al (2001) Prognostic implications of aberrations in p16/pRb pathway in urothelial bladder carcinomas: a multivariate analysis including p53 expression and proliferation markers. Eur Urol 39:167
24. Mitra AP, Quinn DI, Dorff TB et al (2012) Factors influencing post-recurrence survival in bladder cancer following radical cystectomy. BJU Int 109:846
25. The Cancer Genome Atlas Research Network (2014) Comprehensive molecular characterization of urothelial bladder carcinoma. Nature 507:315
26. Nordentoft I, Lamy P, Birkenkamp-Demtröder K et al (2014) Mutational context and diverse clonal development in early and late bladder cancer. Cell Rep 7:1649
27. Mitra AP, Cote RJ (2009) Molecular pathogenesis and diagnostics of bladder cancer. Annu Rev Pathol 4:251
28. Mitra AP, Cote RJ (2007) Searching for novel therapeutics and targets: insights from clinical trials. Urol Oncol 25:341
29. Youssef RF, Mitra AP, Bartsch G Jr et al (2009) Molecular targets and targeted therapies in bladder cancer management. World J Urol 27:9
30. Mitra AP, Hansel DE, Cote RJ (2012) Prognostic value of cell-cycle regulation biomarkers in bladder cancer. Semin Oncol 39:524
31. Mitra AP, Birkhahn M, Cote RJ (2007) p53 and retinoblastoma pathways in bladder cancer. World J Urol 25:563
32. Mitra AP, Datar RH, Cote RJ (2005) Molecular staging of bladder cancer. BJU Int 96:7
33. Mitra AP, Lin H, Cote RJ et al (2005) Biomarker profiling for cancer diagnosis, prognosis and therapeutic management. Natl Med J India 18:304
34. Esrig D, Elmajian D, Groshen S et al (1994) Accumulation of nuclear p53 and tumor progression in bladder cancer. N Engl J Med 331:1259
35. Sarkis AS, Dalbagni G, Cordon-Cardo C et al (1993) Nuclear overexpression of p53 protein in transitional cell bladder carcinoma: a marker for disease progression. J Natl Cancer Inst 85:53
36. Serth J, Kuczyk MA, Bokemeyer C et al (1995) p53 immunohistochemistry as an independent prognostic factor for superficial transitional cell carcinoma of the bladder. Br J Cancer 71:201
37. Chatterjee SJ, Datar R, Youssefzadeh D et al (2004) Combined effects of p53, p21, and pRb expression in the progression of bladder transitional cell carcinoma. J Clin Oncol 22:1007
38. Shariat SF, Tokunaga H, Zhou J et al (2004) p53, p21, pRB, and p16 expression predict clinical outcome in cystectomy with bladder cancer. J Clin Oncol 22:1014
39. Shariat SF, Lotan Y, Karakiewicz PI et al (2009) p53 predictive value for pT1-2 N0 disease at radical cystectomy. J Urol 182:907

40. Shariat SF, Zlotta AR, Ashfaq R et al (2007) Cooperative effect of cell-cycle regulators expression on bladder cancer development and biologic aggressiveness. Mod Pathol 20:445
41. Shariat SF, Bolenz C, Karakiewicz PI et al (2010) p53 expression in patients with advanced urothelial cancer of the urinary bladder. BJU Int 105:489
42. Shariat SF, Chade DC, Karakiewicz PI et al (2010) Combination of multiple molecular markers can improve prognostication in patients with locally advanced and lymph node positive bladder cancer. J Urol 183:68
43. George B, Datar RH, Wu L et al (2007) *p53* gene and protein status: The role of *p53* alterations in predicting outcome in patients with bladder cancer. J Clin Oncol 25:5352
44. Malats N, Bustos A, Nascimento CM et al (2005) P53 as a prognostic marker for bladder cancer: a meta-analysis and review. Lancet Oncol 6:678
45. Stadler WM, Lerner SP, Groshen S et al (2011) Phase III study of molecularly targeted adjuvant therapy in locally advanced urothelial cancer of the bladder based on p53 status. J Clin Oncol 29:3443
46. Stein JP, Ginsberg DA, Grossfeld GD et al (1998) Effect of $p21^{WAF1/CIP1}$ expression on tumor progression in bladder cancer. J Natl Cancer Inst 90:1072
47. Simon R, Struckmann K, Schraml P et al (2002) Amplification pattern of 12q13-q15 genes (*MDM2*, *CDK4*, *GLI*) in urinary bladder cancer. Oncogene 21:2476
48. Bates S, Phillips AC, Clark PA et al (1998) $p14^{ARF}$ links the tumour suppressors RB and p53. Nature 395:124
49. Rebouissou S, Herault A, Letouze E et al (2012) *CDKN2A* homozygous deletion is associated with muscle invasion in *FGFR3*-mutated urothelial bladder carcinoma. J Pathol 227:315
50. Miyamoto H, Shuin T, Torigoe S et al (1995) Retinoblastoma gene mutations in primary human bladder cancer. Br J Cancer 71:831
51. Kapur P, Lotan Y, King E et al (2011) Primary adenocarcinoma of the urinary bladder: value of cell cycle biomarkers. Am J Clin Pathol 135:822
52. Kamai T, Takagi K, Asami H et al (2001) Decreasing of $p27^{Kip1}$ and cyclin E protein levels is associated with progression from superficial into invasive bladder cancer. Br J Cancer 84:1242
53. Shariat SF, Bolenz C, Godoy G et al (2009) Predictive value of combined immunohistochemical markers in patients with pT1 urothelial carcinoma at radical cystectomy. J Urol 182:78
54. Shariat SF, Karakiewicz PI, Ashfaq R et al (2008) Multiple biomarkers improve prediction of bladder cancer recurrence and mortality in patients undergoing cystectomy. Cancer 112:315
55. Shariat SF, Chromecki TF, Cha EK et al (2012) Risk stratification of organ confined bladder cancer after radical cystectomy using cell cycle related biomarkers. J Urol 187:457
56. Koga S, Hirohata S, Kondo Y et al (2000) A novel telomerase-specific gene therapy: gene transfer of caspase-8 utilizing the human telomerase catalytic subunit gene promoter. Hum Gene Ther 11:1397
57. Karam JA, Lotan Y, Karakiewicz PI et al (2007) Use of combined apoptosis biomarkers for prediction of bladder cancer recurrence and mortality after radical cystectomy. Lancet Oncol 8:128
58. Shariat SF, Ashfaq R, Karakiewicz PI et al (2007) Survivin expression is associated with bladder cancer presence, stage, progression, and mortality. Cancer 109:1106
59. Shariat SF, Karakiewicz PI, Godoy G et al (2009) Survivin as a prognostic marker for urothelial carcinoma of the bladder: a multicenter external validation study. Clin Cancer Res 15:7012
60. Ong F, Moonen LM, Gallee MP et al (2001) Prognostic factors in transitional cell cancer of the bladder: an emerging role for Bcl-2 and p53. Radiother Oncol 61:169

61. Hussain SA, Ganesan R, Hiller L et al (2003) BCL2 expression predicts survival in patients receiving synchronous chemoradiotherapy in advanced transitional cell carcinoma of the bladder. Oncol Rep 10:571
62. Cooke PW, James ND, Ganesan R et al (2000) Bcl-2 expression identifies patients with advanced bladder cancer treated by radiotherapy who benefit from neoadjuvant chemotherapy. BJU Int 85:829
63. Kong G, Shin KY, Oh YH et al (1998) Bcl-2 and p53 expressions in invasive bladder cancers. Acta Oncol 37:715
64. Wolf HK, Stober C, Hohenfellner R et al (2001) Prognostic value of p53, p21/WAF1, Bcl-2, Bax, Bak and Ki-67 immunoreactivity in pT1 G3 urothelial bladder carcinomas. Tumour Biol 22:328
65. Gonzalez-Campora R, Davalos-Casanova G, Beato-Moreno A et al (2007) BCL-2, TP53 and BAX protein expression in superficial urothelial bladder carcinoma. Cancer Lett 250:292
66. Maluf FC, Cordon-Cardo C, Verbel DA et al (2006) Assessing interactions between mdm-2, p53, and bcl-2 as prognostic variables in muscle-invasive bladder cancer treated with neo-adjuvant chemotherapy followed by locoregional surgical treatment. Ann Oncol 17:1677
67. Giannopoulou I, Nakopoulou L, Zervas A et al (2002) Immunohistochemical study of pro-apoptotic factors Bax, Fas and CPP32 in urinary bladder cancer: prognostic implications. Urol Res 30:342
68. Korkolopoulou P, Lazaris A, Konstantinidou AE et al (2002) Differential expression of bcl-2 family proteins in bladder carcinomas. Relationship with apoptotic rate and survival. Eur Urol 41:274
69. Mitra AP, Lin H, Datar RH et al (2006) Molecular biology of bladder cancer: prognostic and clinical implications. Clin Genitourin Cancer 5:67
70. Mitra AP, Castelao JE, Hawes D et al (2013) Combination of molecular alterations and smoking intensity predicts bladder cancer outcome: a report from the Los Angeles Cancer Surveillance Program. Cancer 119:756
71. Pasin E, Josephson DY, Mitra AP et al (2008) Superficial bladder cancer: an update on etiology, molecular development, classification, and natural history. Rev Urol 10:31
72. van Rhijn BW, Zuiverloon TC, Vis AN et al (2010) Molecular grade (*FGFR3*/MIB-1) and EORTC risk scores are predictive in primary non-muscle-invasive bladder cancer. Eur Urol 58:433
73. Jebar AH, Hurst CD, Tomlinson DC et al (2005) *FGFR3* and Ras gene mutations are mutually exclusive genetic events in urothelial cell carcinoma. Oncogene 24:5218
74. Birkhahn M, Mitra AP, Williams AJ et al (2010) Predicting recurrence and progression of noninvasive papillary bladder cancer at initial presentation based on quantitative gene expression profiles. Eur Urol 57:12
75. Wright C, Mellon K, Johnston P et al (1991) Expression of mutant p53, c-erbB-2 and the epidermal growth factor receptor in transitional cell carcinoma of the human urinary bladder. Br J Cancer 63:967
76. Korkolopoulou P, Christodoulou P, Kapralos P et al (1997) The role of p53, MDM2 and c-erb B-2 oncoproteins, epidermal growth factor receptor and proliferation markers in the prognosis of urinary bladder cancer. Pathol Res Pract 193:767
77. Mellon JK, Lunec J, Wright C et al (1996) c-erbB-2 in bladder cancer: Molecular biology, correlation with epidermal growth factor receptors and prognostic value. J Urol 155:321
78. Liukkonen T, Rajala P, Raitanen M et al (1999) Prognostic value of MIB-1 score, p53, EGFr, mitotic index and papillary status in primary superficial (Stage pTa/T1) bladder cancer: a prospective comparative study. Eur Urol 36:393
79. Kramer C, Klasmeyer K, Bojar H et al (2007) Heparin-binding epidermal growth factor-like growth factor isoforms and epidermal growth factor receptor/ErbB1 expression in bladder cancer and their relation to clinical outcome. Cancer 109:2016

80. Lipponen P, Eskelinen M (1994) Expression of epidermal growth factor receptor in bladder cancer as related to established prognostic factors, oncoprotein (c-erbB-2, p53) expression and long-term prognosis. Br J Cancer 69:1120
81. Kruger S, Weitsch G, Buttner H et al (2002) Overexpression of c-erbB-2 oncoprotein in muscle-invasive bladder carcinoma: relationship with gene amplification, clinicopathological parameters and prognostic outcome. Int J Oncol 21:981
82. Kruger S, Weitsch G, Buttner H et al (2002) HER2 overexpression in muscle-invasive urothelial carcinoma of the bladder: prognostic implications. Int J Cancer 102:514
83. Bolenz C, Shariat SF, Karakiewicz PI et al (2010) Human epidermal growth factor receptor 2 expression status provides independent prognostic information in patients with urothelial carcinoma of the urinary bladder. BJU Int 106:1216
84. Kassouf W, Black PC, Tuziak T et al (2008) Distinctive expression pattern of ErbB family receptors signifies an aggressive variant of bladder cancer. J Urol 179:353
85. Jimenez RE, Hussain M, Bianco FJ Jr et al (2001) Her-2/neu overexpression in muscle-invasive urothelial carcinoma of the bladder: prognostic significance and comparative analysis in primary and metastatic tumors. Clin Cancer Res 7:2440
86. Chow NH, Chan SH, Tzai TS et al (2001) Expression profiles of ErbB family receptors and prognosis in primary transitional cell carcinoma of the urinary bladder. Clin Cancer Res 7:1957
87. Memon AA, Sorensen BS, Meldgaard P et al (2006) The relation between survival and expression of HER1 and HER2 depends on the expression of HER3 and HER4: a study in bladder cancer patients. Br J Cancer 94:1703
88. Mitra AP, Skinner EC, Schuckman AK et al (2014) Effect of gender on outcomes following radical cystectomy for urothelial carcinoma of the bladder: a critical analysis of 1,994 patients. Urol Oncol 32:52.e1
89. Tuygun C, Kankaya D, Imamoglu A et al (2011) Sex-specific hormone receptors in urothelial carcinomas of the human urinary bladder: a comparative analysis of clinicopathological features and survival outcomes according to receptor expression. Urol Oncol 29:43
90. Ide H, Inoue S, Miyamoto H (2017) Histopathological and prognostic significance of the expression of sex hormone receptors in bladder cancer: a meta-analysis of immunohistochemical studies. PLoS ONE 12:e0174746
91. Boorjian S, Ugras S, Mongan NP et al (2004) Androgen receptor expression is inversely correlated with pathologic tumor stage in bladder cancer. Urology 64:383
92. Mir C, Shariat SF, van der Kwast TH et al (2011) Loss of androgen receptor expression is not associated with pathological stage, grade, gender or outcome in bladder cancer: a large multi-institutional study. BJU Int 108:24
93. Stephanou A, Brar BK, Knight RA et al (2000) Opposing actions of STAT-1 and STAT-3 on the Bcl-2 and Bcl-x promoters. Cell Death Differ 7:329
94. Mitra AP, Pagliarulo V, Yang D et al (2009) Generation of a concise gene panel for outcome prediction in urinary bladder cancer. J Clin Oncol 27:3929
95. Choudhury A, Nelson LD, Teo MT et al (2010) MRE11 expression is predictive of cause-specific survival following radical radiotherapy for muscle-invasive bladder cancer. Cancer Res 70:7017
96. Laurberg JR, Brems-Eskildsen AS, Nordentoft I et al (2012) Expression of TIP60 (tat-interactive protein) and MRE11 (meiotic recombination 11 homolog) predict treatment-specific outcome of localised invasive bladder cancer. BJU Int 110:E1228
97. Martin RM, Kerr M, Teo MT et al (2014) Post-transcriptional regulation of MRE11 expression in muscle-invasive bladder tumours. Oncotarget 5:993
98. Teo MT, Dyrskjøt L, Nsengimana J et al (2014) Next-generation sequencing identifies germline *MRE11A* variants as markers of radiotherapy outcomes in muscle-invasive bladder cancer. Ann Oncol 25:877

99. Desai NB, Scott SN, Zabor EC et al (2016) Genomic characterization of response to chemoradiation in urothelial bladder cancer. Cancer 122:3715
100. Andrews B, Shariat SF, Kim JH et al (2002) Preoperative plasma levels of interleukin-6 and its soluble receptor predict disease recurrence and survival of patients with bladder cancer. J Urol 167:1475
101. Chen FH, Crist SA, Zhang GJ et al (2002) Interleukin-6 production by human bladder tumor cell lines is up-regulated by bacillus Calmette-Guerin through nuclear factor-kappaB and Ap-1 via an immediate early pathway. J Urol 168:786
102. Riemann K, Becker L, Struwe H et al (2007) Insertion/deletion polymorphism in the promoter of NFKB1 as a potential molecular marker for the risk of recurrence in superficial bladder cancer. Int J Clin Pharmacol Ther 45:423
103. Bartsch G Jr, Mitra AP, Mitra SA et al (2016) Use of artificial intelligence and machine learning algorithms with gene expression profiling to predict recurrent nonmuscle invasive urothelial carcinoma of the bladder. J Urol 195:493
104. Masson-Lecomte A, Rava M, Real FX et al (2014) Inflammatory biomarkers and bladder cancer prognosis: a systematic review. Eur Urol 66:1078
105. Hilmy M, Campbell R, Bartlett JM et al (2006) The relationship between the systemic inflammatory response, tumour proliferative activity, T-lymphocytic infiltration and COX-2 expression and survival in patients with transitional cell carcinoma of the urinary bladder. Br J Cancer 95:1234
106. Gakis G, Todenhöfer T, Renninger M et al (2011) Development of a new outcome prediction model in carcinoma invading the bladder based on preoperative serum C-reactive protein and standard pathological risk factors: the TNR-C score. BJU Int 108:1800
107. Yoshida S, Saito K, Koga F et al (2008) C-reactive protein level predicts prognosis in patients with muscle-invasive bladder cancer treated with chemoradiotherapy. BJU Int 101:978
108. Ishioka J, Saito K, Sakura M et al (2012) Development of a nomogram incorporating serum C-reactive protein level to predict overall survival of patients with advanced urothelial carcinoma and its evaluation by decision curve analysis. Br J Cancer 107:1031
109. Nakagawa T, Hara T, Kawahara T et al (2013) Prognostic risk stratification of patients with urothelial carcinoma of the bladder with recurrence after radical cystectomy. J Urol 189:1275
110. Bochner BH, Cote RJ, Weidner N et al (1995) Angiogenesis in bladder cancer: relationship between microvessel density and tumor prognosis. J Natl Cancer Inst 87:1603
111. Bochner BH, Esrig D, Groshen S et al (1997) Relationship of tumor angiogenesis and nuclear p53 accumulation in invasive bladder cancer. Clin Cancer Res 3:1615
112. Jaeger TM, Weidner N, Chew K et al (1995) Tumor angiogenesis correlates with lymph node metastases in invasive bladder cancer. J Urol 154:69
113. Shariat SF, Youssef RF, Gupta A et al (2010) Association of angiogenesis related markers with bladder cancer outcomes and other molecular markers. J Urol 183:1744
114. Crew JP, O'Brien T, Bradburn M et al (1997) Vascular endothelial growth factor is a predictor of relapse and stage progression in superficial bladder cancer. Cancer Res 57:5281
115. Bernardini S, Fauconnet S, Chabannes E et al (2001) Serum levels of vascular endothelial growth factor as a prognostic factor in bladder cancer. J Urol 166:1275
116. Zu X, Tang Z, Li Y et al (2006) Vascular endothelial growth factor-C expression in bladder transitional cell cancer and its relationship to lymph node metastasis. BJU Int 98:1090
117. Herrmann E, Eltze E, Bierer S et al (2007) VEGF-C, VEGF-D and Flt-4 in transitional bladder cancer: relationships to clinicopathological parameters and long-term survival. Anticancer Res 27:3127
118. Xia G, Kumar SR, Hawes D et al (2006) Expression and significance of vascular endothelial growth factor receptor 2 in bladder cancer. J Urol 175:1245

119. Mitra AP, Almal AA, George B et al (2006) The use of genetic programming in the analysis of quantitative gene expression profiles for identification of nodal status in bladder cancer. BMC Cancer 6:159
120. Shariat SF, Monoski MA, Andrews B et al (2003) Association of plasma urokinase-type plasminogen activator and its receptor with clinical outcome in patients undergoing radical cystectomy for transitional cell carcinoma of the bladder. Urology 61:1053
121. Nguyen M, Watanabe H, Budson AE et al (1993) Elevated levels of the angiogenic peptide basic fibroblast growth factor in urine of bladder cancer patients. J Natl Cancer Inst 85:241
122. Gazzaniga P, Gandini O, Gradilone A et al (1999) Detection of basic fibroblast growth factor mRNA in urinary bladder cancer: correlation with local relapses. Int J Oncol 14:1123
123. Chopin DK, Caruelle JP, Colombel M et al (1993) Increased immunodetection of acidic fibroblast growth factor in bladder cancer, detectable in urine. J Urol 150:1126
124. Grossfeld GD, Ginsberg DA, Stein JP et al (1997) Thrombospondin-1 expression in bladder cancer: Association with p53 alterations, tumor angiogenesis, and tumor progression. J Natl Cancer Inst 89:219
125. Mahnken A, Kausch I, Feller AC et al (2005) E-cadherin immunoreactivity correlates with recurrence and progression of minimally invasive transitional cell carcinomas of the urinary bladder. Oncol Rep 14:1065
126. Mhawech-Fauceglia P, Fischer G, Beck A et al (2006) Raf1, Aurora-A/STK15 and E-cadherin biomarkers expression in patients with pTa/pT1 urothelial bladder carcinoma; a retrospective TMA study of 246 patients with long-term follow-up. Eur J Surg Oncol 32:439
127. Byrne RR, Shariat SF, Brown R et al (2001) E-cadherin immunostaining of bladder transitional cell carcinoma, carcinoma in situ and lymph node metastases with long-term followup. J Urol 165:1473
128. Bringuier PP, Umbas R, Schaafsma HE et al (1993) Decreased E-cadherin immunoreactivity correlates with poor survival in patients with bladder tumors. Cancer Res 53:3241
129. Seiler R, Lam LL, Erho N et al (2016) Prediction of lymph node metastasis in patients with bladder cancer using whole transcriptome gene expression signatures. J Urol 196:1036
130. O'Brien T, Cranston D, Fuggle S et al (1995) Different angiogenic pathways characterize superficial and invasive bladder cancer. Cancer Res 55:510
131. O'Brien TS, Fox SB, Dickinson AJ et al (1996) Expression of the angiogenic factor thymidine phosphorylase/platelet-derived endothelial cell growth factor in primary bladder cancers. Cancer Res 56:4799
132. Aoki S, Yamada Y, Nakamura K et al (2006) Thymidine phosphorylase expression as a prognostic marker for predicting recurrence in primary superficial bladder cancer. Oncol Rep 16:279
133. Nonomura N, Nakai Y, Nakayama M et al (2006) The expression of thymidine phosphorylase is a prognostic predictor for the intravesical recurrence of superficial bladder cancer. Int J Clin Oncol 11:297
134. Davies B, Waxman J, Wasan H et al (1993) Levels of matrix metalloproteases in bladder cancer correlate with tumor grade and invasion. Cancer Res 53:5365
135. Gerhards S, Jung K, Koenig F et al (2001) Excretion of matrix metalloproteinases 2 and 9 in urine is associated with a high stage and grade of bladder carcinoma. Urology 57:675
136. Vasala K, Paakko P, Turpeenniemi-Hujanen T (2003) Matrix metalloproteinase-2 immunoreactive protein as a prognostic marker in bladder cancer. Urology 62:952
137. Slaton JW, Millikan R, Inoue K et al (2004) Correlation of metastasis related gene expression and relapse-free survival in patients with locally advanced bladder cancer treated with cystectomy and chemotherapy. J Urol 171:570
138. Guan KP, Ye HY, Yan Z et al (2003) Serum levels of endostatin and matrix metalloproteinase-9 associated with high stage and grade primary transitional cell carcinoma of the bladder. Urology 61:719
139. Szarvas T, Becker M, vom Dorp F et al (2010) Matrix metalloproteinase-7 as a marker of metastasis and predictor of poor survival in bladder cancer. Cancer Sci 101:1300

140. Szarvas T, Jäger T, Becker M et al (2011) Validation of circulating MMP-7 level as an independent prognostic marker of poor survival in urinary bladder cancer. Pathol Oncol Res 17:325
141. Roche Y, Pasquier D, Rambeaud JJ et al (2003) Fibrinogen mediates bladder cancer cell migration in an ICAM-1-dependent pathway. Thromb Haemost 89:1089
142. Ozer G, Altinel M, Kocak B et al (2003) Potential value of soluble intercellular adhesion molecule-1 in the serum of patients with bladder cancer. Urol Int 70:167
143. Mitra AP, Cote RJ (2011) Molecular signatures that predict nodal metastasis in bladder cancer: does the primary tumor tell tales? Expert Rev Anticancer Ther 11:849
144. Liebert M, Washington R, Wedemeyer G et al (1994) Loss of co-localization of a6b4 integrin and collagen VII in bladder cancer. Am J Pathol 144:787
145. Grossman HB, Lee C, Bromberg J et al (2000) Expression of the a6b4 integrin provides prognostic information in bladder cancer. Oncol Rep 7:13
146. Ahmadi H, Djaladat H, Cai J et al (2014) Precystectomy serum levels of carbohydrate antigen 19-9, carbohydrate antigen 125, and carcinoembryonic antigen: prognostic value in invasive urothelial carcinoma of the bladder. Urol Oncol 32:648
147. Bazargani ST, Clifford T, Djaladat H et al (2017) Association between epithelial tumor markers' trends during the course of treatment and oncological outcomes in urothelial bladder cancer. Urol Oncol 35:609
148. Bartsch G, Mitra AP, Cote RJ (2010) Expression profiling for bladder cancer: strategies to uncover prognostic factors. Expert Rev Anticancer Ther 10:1945
149. Birkhahn M, Mitra AP, Cote RJ (2007) Molecular markers for bladder cancer: the road to a multimarker approach. Expert Rev Anticancer Ther 7:1717
150. Sanchez-Carbayo M, Socci ND, Lozano J et al (2006) Defining molecular profiles of poor outcome in patients with invasive bladder cancer using oligonucleotide microarrays. J Clin Oncol 24:778
151. Kim WJ, Kim EJ, Kim SK et al (2010) Predictive value of progression-related gene classifier in primary non-muscle invasive bladder cancer. Mol Cancer 9:3
152. Kim WJ, Kim SK, Jeong P et al (2011) A four-gene signature predicts disease progression in muscle invasive bladder cancer. Mol Med 17:478
153. Kim SK, Kim EJ, Leem SH et al (2010) Identification of *S100A8*-correlated genes for prediction of disease progression in non-muscle invasive bladder cancer. BMC Cancer 10:21
154. Jeong P, Ha YS, Cho IC et al (2011) Three-gene signature predicts disease progression of non-muscle invasive bladder cancer. Oncol Lett 2:679
155. Ha YS, Kim JS, Yoon HY et al (2012) Novel combination markers for predicting progression of nonmuscle invasive bladder cancer. Int J Cancer 131:E501
156. Kim YJ, Yoon HY, Kim JS et al (2013) *HOXA9*, *ISL1* and *ALDH1A3* methylation patterns as prognostic markers for nonmuscle invasive bladder cancer: Array-based DNA methylation and expression profiling. Int J Cancer 133:1135
157. Friedrich MG, Chandrasoma S, Siegmund KD et al (2005) Prognostic relevance of methylation markers in patients with non-muscle invasive bladder carcinoma. Eur J Cancer 41:2769
158. Su SF, de Castro Abreu AL, Chihara Y et al (2014) A panel of three markers hyper- and hypomethylated in urine sediments accurately predicts bladder cancer recurrence. Clin Cancer Res 20:1978
159. Mitra AP, Skinner EC, Miranda G et al (2013) A precystectomy decision model to predict pathological upstaging and oncological outcomes in clinical stage T2 bladder cancer. BJU Int 111:240
160. Ahmadi H, Mitra AP, Abdelsayed GA et al (2013) Principal component analysis based pre-cystectomy model to predict pathological stage in patients with clinical organ-confined bladder cancer. BJU Int 111:E167
161. Mitra AP, Bartsch CC, Cote RJ (2009) Strategies for molecular expression profiling in bladder cancer. Cancer Metastasis Rev 28:317

162. Mitra AP, Lam LL, Ghadessi M et al (2014) Discovery and validation of novel expression signature for postcystectomy recurrence in high-risk bladder cancer. J Natl Cancer Inst 106: dju290
163. Mitra SA, Mitra AP, Triche TJ (2012) A central role for long non-coding RNA in cancer. Front Genet 3:17
164. Wang LC, Xylinas E, Kent MT et al (2014) Combining smoking information and molecular markers improves prognostication in patients with urothelial carcinoma of the bladder. Urol Oncol 32:433
165. Volkmer JP, Sahoo D, Chin RK et al (2012) Three differentiation states risk-stratify bladder cancer into distinct subtypes. Proc Natl Acad Sci U S A 109:2078
166. Choi W, Porten S, Kim S et al (2014) Identification of distinct basal and luminal subtypes of muscle-invasive bladder cancer with different sensitivities to frontline chemotherapy. Cancer Cell 25:152
167. Mitra AP, Lerner SP (2015) Potential role for targeted therapy in muscle-invasive bladder cancer: lessons from the Cancer Genome Atlas and beyond. Urol Clin North Am 42:201
168. Srivastava S, Gray JW, Reid BJ et al (2008) Translational Research Working Group developmental pathway for biospecimen-based assessment modalities. Clin Cancer Res 14:5672
169. Khleif SN, Doroshow JH, Hait WN (2010) AACR-FDA-NCI Cancer Biomarkers Collaborative consensus report: advancing the use of biomarkers in cancer drug development. Clin Cancer Res 16:3299
170. Kattan MW, Hess KR, Amin MB et al (2016) American Joint Committee on Cancer acceptance criteria for inclusion of risk models for individualized prognosis in the practice of precision medicine. CA Cancer J Clin 66:370

The Role and Importance of Timely Radical Cystectomy for High-Risk Non-muscle-Invasive Bladder Cancer

Daniel J. Lee and Sam S. Chang

Contents

Abstract

Non-muscle-invasive bladder cancer accounts for the majority of incident bladder cancers but is a heterogeneous disease with variation in clinical presentation, course, and outcomes. Risk stratification techniques have attempted to identify those at highest risk of cancer recurrence and progression to help personalize and individualize treatment options. Radical cystectomy during the optimal window of curability could improve cancer outcomes; however, identifying the disease and patient characteristics as well as the correct timing

D. J. Lee · S. S. Chang (✉)
Department of Urologic Surgery, Vanderbilt University Medical Center, Nashville, TN, USA
e-mail: sam.chang@Vanderbilt.Edu

S. Daneshmand and K. G. Chan (eds.), *Genitourinary Cancers*, Cancer Treatment and Research 175, https://doi.org/10.1007/978-3-319-93339-9_9

to intervene remains difficult. We review the natural history of non-muscle-invasive bladder cancer, discuss different risk-stratification techniques and how they can help identify those most likely to benefit from radical treatment, and examine the evidence supporting the benefit of timely cystectomy.

Keywords

Non-muscle-invasive bladder cancer · Timely cystectomy · Early cystectomy Micropapillary bladder cancer · High-risk bladder cancer

1 Introduction

Urothelial carcinoma of the bladder (UCB) is a common, costly, and complex disease and is the 6th most commonly diagnosed malignancy in the USA with more than 79,000 new diagnoses expected in 2017 [120]. Bladder cancer has the highest lifetime treatment cost of all cancers [106] and cost approximately $4 billion to treat in 2010 [80]. A large portion of this cost is due to necessary prolonged surveillance, as the natural history of UCB is marked by high rates of recurrence and progression. At the time of diagnosis, approximately 75% of UCB are non-muscle-invasive bladder cancer (NMIBC) [90] and up to 70% of patients with NMIBC will recur within the first year after transurethral resection of the bladder tumor (TURBT). Ten to twenty percent of patients eventually experience progression to muscle-invasive bladder cancer (MIBC) [134].

In the USA, the historical accepted standard therapy for MIBC has been radical cystectomy and lymph node dissection [128]; neoadjuvant chemotherapy more recently has become integrated [103, 110]. However, the relative benefit of radical cystectomy for NMIBC, especially for those who are considered at high risk for progression or recurrence, has not been well characterized or adopted. In one survey, 80% of American urologists would not recommend cystectomy for patients with NMIBC that was refractory to two courses of intravesical Bacillus Calmette–Guerin (BCG) [66]; these patients have an approximately 80% risk of treatment failure or progression with continued intravesical therapy [18, 42]. Radical cystectomy for patients with NMIBC has often been termed “early,” “immediate,” or “up-front” cystectomy, with the implication that extirpative surgery is offered and performed before evidence of muscle invasion or shortly after development of muscle invasion. However, with evidence highlighting the risk of underestimating disease status and tools to help improve prediction of high-risk features in NMIBC, we consider the description and terminology of a “timely cystectomy” during the window of curability, rather than waiting for pathologic and/or radiologic evidence of muscle invasion, as the most appropriate course [19, 21].

In this review, we characterize the role of radical cystectomy in the management of high-risk NMIBC. We examine recent strategies in risk stratification, including molecular and genomic subclassification, discuss the natural history of high-risk NMIBC and the prognostic impact of variant histology, and compare the evidence for a "timely" cystectomy versus a "delayed" cystectomy.

2 Risk Stratification

The clinical course and treatment outcomes with NMIBC are often variable and reflect biological and genetic diversity [37]. With this inherent heterogeneity, the identification of predictive and prognostic clinical and biological parameters is crucial to identify patients who can be safely managed with local therapy (e.g., TURBT with intravesical therapy) versus patients who would benefit and need timely radical cystectomy. Accurate risk stratification is essential to maximize benefits and minimize potential treatment harms. This is especially important for bladder cancer, as radical cystectomy is associated with potentially significant risks of postoperative complications [26, 73, 126, 128, 129], mortality rates up to 10% [34, 109, 129], and significant impact on quality of life [139, 152]. Current risk stratification relies on pathological features from a TURBT [20], where the presence of any of the following usually confers a high risk of progression or recurrence: lamina propria invasion (i.e., cT1), multifocality, tumor size >3 cm, any recurrent high-grade Ta disease, any CIS, any lymphovascular invasion (LVI), high-grade prostatic urethral involvement, any BCG failure with high-grade disease, or any variant histology [20, 31] (Table 1).

Table 1 AUA risk stratification for non-muscle-invasive bladder cancer

Low risk	Low-grade solitary Ta <3 cm
	Papillary urothelial neoplasm of low malignant potential
Intermediate risk	Recurrence within 1 year, low-grade Ta
	Solitary low-grade Ta >3 cm
	Low-grade Ta, multifocal
	High-grade Ta, <3 cm
	Low-grade T1
High risk	High-grade T1
	Any recurrent, high-grade Ta
	Any high-grade Ta, >3 cm (or multifocal)
	Any CIS
	Any BCG failure in high-grade case
	Any variant histology
	Any LVI
	Any high-grade prostatic urethral involvement

*Adapted from AUA/SUO guidelines, Chang et al. [20]

2.1 Predictive Models

In an effort to improve risk stratification, several prognostic tools have been developed. The European Organization for Research and Treatment of Cancer (EORTC) risk calculator was created from a pooled analysis of 7 EORTC trials of 2596 patients with NMIBC [134]. A separate risk-stratification tool was developed by the Club Urologico Espanol de Tratamiento Oncologico (CUETO) that included 1062 patients from 4 trials who underwent BCG treatment for NMIBC [42, 43]. Both the EORTC and CUETO risk calculators can improve risk stratification by utilizing different clinical and pathological features to calculate the probability of recurrence and progression at one and five years. These efforts should be lauded; however, several important limitations should be considered. The cohorts used to construct the prognostic models inevitably do not reflect contemporary practices and limit the clinical application. In the EORTC prognostic model, less than 10% received BCG treatment, 10% received single-dose postoperative mitomycin C, re-staging TURBT were not routinely performed, and certain pathological features that have been found to be closely associated with recurrence and progression, such as LVI or variant histology, were not captured [134]. In comparison, the CUETO model included patients who underwent BCG; however, about a third of the patients received 9 or fewer instillations, only 10% of the patients had CIS, re-staging TURBT was not performed, and LVI or variant histology status were not captured [42]. With the utilization of these historical cohorts to construct the predictive models, the value of both tools may be limited for today's patient. In a multi-institutional external validation study, both the EORTC and CUETO risk calculators had poor discrimination for disease recurrence and progression (c-index 0.52–0.66), low positive predictive value (21–24%), and overestimated the risk of disease progression in high-risk NMIBC [151]. A recent update of the EORTC prognostic model attempted to address the lack of maintenance BCG in the cohort; however, the utility of the updated model is again limited by the absence of patients with CIS and lack of routine re-resection [16].

2.2 Pathological Substaging and Lymphovascular Invasion

Over the past two decades, pathological subclassification of T1 NMIBC according to the depth of invasion relative to the muscularis mucosa-vascular plexus has been proposed as an approach to improve risk stratification. These subclassifications would separate T1 tumors into T1a, T1b, or T1c tumors depending on the depth of invasion above, into, and beyond the muscularis mucosa, respectively. Several studies support the depth of invasion as an adverse prognostic risk factor and is significantly associated with progression and cancer-specific survival [6, 9, 40, 58, 81, 92, 108, 155]. In a large meta-analysis of 15,215 patients with NMIBC from 73 studies, the depth of invasion into the lamina propria (T1b/c) had the highest impact on progression and cancer-specific survival (HR 3.3 and 2.2, respectively) compared to other pathological risk factors [81].

However, the detection of the muscularis mucosa within the lamina propria is extremely inconsistent. The muscularis mucosa is often scattered and discontinuous in about 90% of TURBT specimens and is not detectable in 6–75% of cases [9, 107]. There may also be a significant learning curve in the detection rate of the muscularis mucosa, as some have found an approximately 30% increase in the detection rate after 8 years [92]. One way to utilize the prognostic information of the depth of invasion without depending on the presence of muscularis mucosa is to measure the depth of invasion and dichotomize the substaging system into microinvasive (i.e., depth $\leq$ 0.5 mm) or extensive (depth > 0.5 mm). Utilization of this substaging system was found to be superior to the EORTC risk calculator in predicting progression [142]. Because of the uneven thickness of the lamina propria, many pathologists consider the 0.5-mm margin to be an unreliable cut-off [22, 96]. More recent investigations utilizing different invasion depth cut-off (1 mm) have found a more reliable association with progression-free survival [96]. Pathologic substaging techniques may therefore help improve existing risk-stratification techniques, but have not been widely adopted.

2.3 Lymphovascular Invasion

Lymphovascular invasion (LVI) has the potential to be an important prognostic indicator for NMIBC. The association of LVI with outcomes in MIBC has been established and has been associated with adverse pathological features such as increased T stage, tumor grade, and lymph node metastasis [7, 8, 83, 124, 125]. Patients with LVI had twice the odds of extravesical bladder cancer (pT3-4 or node positive) [8], and the presence of LVI in the TURBT specimen can predict the presence of extravesical disease at cystectomy [50, 150]. LVI has also been found to be associated with recurrence-free survival, cancer-specific survival, and overall survival [7, 8, 83, 124, 125]. The association between LVI and outcomes in NMIBC has not been as consistent. In smaller series, there was no association between LVI and progression or recurrence in NMIBC [12, 86, 114]; however, in larger multi-institutional cohorts, there has been a significant association between LVI and recurrence-free survival, progression-free survival, and cancer-specific survival [23, 46, 91, 138]. In a meta-analysis of over 3900 patients, LVI in the TURBT specimens was associated with recurrence-free survival (pooled HR 2.3) and progression-free survival (pooled HR 2.3) [72].

Despite its prognostic ability, there are several limitations to the utilization of LVI in clinical decision-making for NMIBC. Artifacts such as tissue retraction can mimic vascular invasion, the TURBT specimens may only represent a small sample of the actual tumor burden, and distinguishing between lymphatics and blood vessels can be difficult [114, 136]. With these factors influencing the sampling ability of TURBT for LVI, it is not surprising that the concordance in LVI presence between TURBT and cystectomy specimens can be variable, with sensitivity rates that range from 18 to 79% and a negative predictive value around 50–70% [47, 76, 105, 130].

In one study, among the patients with no evidence of LVI at TURBT, more than 30% of the patients had subsequent LVI at radical cystectomy [105].

2.4 Presence of Carcinoma In Situ

Carcinoma in situ (CIS) is a distinct form of NMIBC that can present in isolation or synchronously with UCB, but the presence of CIS increases the risk of recurrence and progression of UCB [17]. The risk of upstaging and occult disease in CIS is high; detection of occult nodal micrometastasis is around 6% in most studies [137], and synchronous presence of CIS with high-grade T1 disease led to a pathological upstaging in 55% of the patients, compared to an upstaging of 6% with high-grade T1 alone [82]. CIS also portends a high risk of progression, as about 40–80% of NMIBC with CIS will progress to muscle-invasive disease [3, 27, 41, 60, 101]. In a study of patients with only pathological CIS at the time of cystectomy, 4% were found with positive nodes, and about 12% developed metastases over a mean follow-up of 3 years [54]. In addition, the presence of CIS increases the risk of extravesical recurrences of urothelial carcinoma, especially in the upper tracts [27]. In their guidelines statement for NMIBC management [20], the American Urological Association and Society for Urologic Oncology created a risk-stratification table and treatment algorithm to help clinicians determine the appropriate evidence-based management according to risk strata based on pathologic criteria as described but also included how patients responded to therapy.

2.5 Molecular Markers

In light of the limitations of current risk-stratification tools and techniques, there has been a growing effort to identify clinically relevant molecular and genomic classifications in bladder cancer. The presence of certain biomarkers such as p53, pRB, and Ki-67 have been found to have a significant association with increased recurrence and decreased survival after radical cystectomy [116, 141]. The addition of these biomarkers to previously used prognostic nomograms improved the predictive accuracy of recurrence and survival rates after cystectomy [115]. In NMIBC, however, the utility of biomarkers has been inconsistent. Numerous biomarkers have been investigated with conflicting results [28, 38, 74, 95, 114, 127]. Subsequent multi-institutional studies that investigated multiple biomarkers and gene expression signatures found no association with recurrence and did not improve the predictive ability of existing risk prognostication models [39, 94, 95].

In contrast, a wide variety of molecular alterations, such as oncogene activation, chromosomal alterations, tumor suppressor loss, and changes to cell-cycle regulators, have been found to be associated with tumor progression [11, 45, 74, 112, 113, 127, 143, 144, 153] and show promise as prognostic indicators. Mutations or overexpression of p53, the most commonly studied biomarker in bladder cancer, have been found to be associated with tumor progression in most studies

[49, 78, 87, 113, 143], but not consistently in all studies [48, 117]. Another commonly studied mutation in NMIBC, fibroblast growth factor receptor 3 (FGFR3), appears to be associated with a lower rate of progression [14, 59, 144] and has been found in up to 90% of low-grade Ta lesions compared to about 20% of high-grade T1 tumors [143].

Given the biological heterogeneity of NMIBC, several studies have attempted to investigate whether certain panels or combinations of molecular markers can be used to improve risk stratification for NMIBC. Combining FGFR3 mutation status with Ki-67 expression to form a molecular grade was found to be significantly associated with progression [14] and, when added to the EORTC risk models for progression, was able to significantly improve the accuracy and discrimination [144]. Two separate biomarker studies using tissue microarrays, one investigating p53, pRB, p21, and p27 [113], with the other studying cyclin D1, MCM7, TRIM29, and UBE2C [45], reported significant associations between not only between the presence of the biomarker and the risk of tumor progression, but the number of alterations in these panels with progression [113].

Improvements in genetic sequencing technology have improved our understanding of bladder tumor biology and the potential for classifying NMIBC into risk-stratified molecular subclasses. Genomic classifiers were independently associated with progression [39] and able to improve on the accuracy of predictive models for progression. Epigenetic alterations have also been found to be associated with progression-free survival and cancer-specific survival in high-grade T1 tumors [4] and progression in Ta tumors [70]. Although these molecular and genomic markers have promise in risk prognostication and individualizing patient care, none of these markers are routinely available at the point of care currently.

Combining gene expression and molecular markers has allowed for the identification of distinct molecular subtypes within NMIBC into basal or luminal subtypes [2, 24, 30, 84, 88, 97, 104, 121]. Luminal bladder cancers tend to have papillary features and mutations common to NMIBC such as FGFR3, whereas basal subtypes are enriched with squamous and sarcomatoid features, express biomarkers that are associated with epithelial to mesenchymal transition, and are often metastatic at diagnosis [24, 30, 88]. These subtypes have differential responses to various agents and can help provide improved prognostic information and help tailor individualized management strategies [24, 51, 98]. For example, basal bladder cancers are enriched with programmed death ligand 1 (PD-L1) T cells, epidermal growth factor receptor (EGFR), and hypoxia-inducible factor 1, with early evidence suggesting a good response with atezolizumab [100], EGFR inhibitors [104], and bevacizumab in combination with cisplatin-based chemotherapy [85]. The basal-like subtypes are significantly associated with the risk of progression, and the use of the combined molecular and genomic subtypes accurately identified more than 80% of the patients who progressed within 3 years. There are several markers and molecular subclassifications that have the potential to be valuable to improve the risk stratification and predictive ability of these prognostic models for NMIBC. However, continued investigations are necessary to validate the utilization of these markers and refine how pathological and molecular information is combined to individualize patient management.

2.6 Variant Histology

Bladder cancer can undergo divergent differentiation resulting in a wide variety of histologic variants [148] that is often under-recognized; one study found that up to 44% of variant histology was missed by community pathologists [111]. A large bladder cancer registry of about 30,000 people in the Netherlands found that about 8% had variant histology, of whom only about a quarter of those with variant histology presented with NMIBC [99]. Although each divergent histology represents a different tumor biology, they are currently considered a high-risk group in NMIBC for progression [20]. A key factor in managing NMIBC with variant histology is the increased risk of understaging compared to those with pure urothelial histology, as up to 30–60% of patients with NMIBC and variant histology were then upstaged on subsequent cystectomy [69, 146]. In addition, patients with variant histology has also been associated with higher rates of locally advanced disease at presentation [149], and higher rates of occult metastatic disease, as up to 30% of micropapillary bladder cancer was found to have occult nodal disease at cystectomy [68], and has been independently associated with nodal metastasis and decreased survival [36, 71]. These findings indicate that even with non-muscle-invasive disease, variant histology may be associated with high rates of occult metastatic disease that could be understaged at the point of treatment decision. The American Urological Association (AUA) and Society of Urologic Oncology (SUO) guidelines recommend cystectomy for these histologic variants such as micropapillary, plasmacytoid, or sarcomatoid that have been found to be aggressive, have higher rates of upstaging and occult metastatic disease, and have unclear responses to intravesical therapy [20]. The one major exception is small cell carcinoma of the bladder, which is often metastatic at presentation, and is usually treated with chemotherapy with agents such as etoposide and cisplatin, or a combination of chemoradiation [25].

3 Treatment Strategies by Risk Stratification

For low-risk NMIBC, a single immediate instillation of intravesical chemotherapy, such as mitomycin, epirubicin, or gemcitabine, is recommended within 24 h of a TURBT [20]. A meta-analysis of the randomized trials showed a 35% decreased risk of recurrence in patients with low- or intermediate-risk NMIBC receiving intravesical chemotherapy [132]. For intermediate-risk NMIBC, another meta-analysis of randomized trials showed that a 1-year course of intravesical chemotherapy after TURBT also showed a 44% decreased risk of recurrence [64]. For high-risk NMIBC, multiple randomized controlled trials and meta-analyses have supported the effectiveness of BCG over TUR alone or TUR with mitomycin C in reducing progression and recurrence in NMIBC [15, 53, 79, 118, 119, 133]. Use of BCG has been shown to reduce recurrence by about 39–70% and progression by 27–34% in NMIBC [15, 53, 79, 118, 119, 133]. However, about 20–50% of patients with NMIBC will still progress to muscle-invasive disease despite intravesical therapy [27, 140], with a long-term disease-specific survival of 63% (median 15-year follow-up) [27].

3.1 BCG Failure

Instances of progression or recurrence on intravesical BCG therapy can now be stratified into BCG responsive or non-responsive [65]. Patients with evidence of a rapid recurrence, recurrence despite adequate BCG treatment, or signs of worsening and progressive disease have a high likelihood of invasive or metastatic disease [18, 62, 77], and significant delays in radical cystectomy have been associated with worse survival outcomes [63].

4 Evidence for Timely Cystectomy

With all high-risk NMIBC, a balance must be made between the risks of overtreatment with radical cystectomy versus the risks of treatment delay and disease progression with TURBT and intravesical therapies. There have been no randomized trials comparing radical cystectomy versus bladder preservation strategies with intravesical therapies, and most of the retrospective studies comparing the treatment modalities suffer from selection bias. However, evidence from multiple studies has provided support for a timely cystectomy.

First, patients with high-risk NMIBC have improved survival with a timely, early cystectomy compared to a deferred cystectomy after progression of disease or failure of BCG intravesical therapy [33, 35, 56, 63, 67, 131, 135] (see Table 2). Although the definitions of "early" and "deferred" cystectomy were different for each trial, the cancer-specific survival rates for almost all the studies were significantly higher for those who had an immediate cystectomy (10-year rates around 80%) compared to those who had deferred cystectomy (10-year rates around 51–61%) [33, 35, 56, 63, 67, 131, 135]. The two studies that did not find a significant survival advantage to a timely cystectomy [33, 135] compared those who had an immediate cystectomy after diagnosis to those who had intravesical treatment. The intravesical treatment arm included those who responded to BCG maintenance therapy and not just those who progressed and required cystectomy, which likely explains why these studies found no difference in cancer-specific survival. In addition, local rates of recurrence and progression were relatively high at around 30%, with a higher progression rate than in those who underwent immediate cystectomy [135]. Despite the differences in time points in the studies, the importance of avoiding lengthy delays to cystectomy in high-risk NMIBC can be clearly seen; in the study by Herr et al. [63], the 15-year cancer-specific survival was significantly higher when the delayed cystectomy occurred after 1 year (34%) compared to 2 years after the initial BCG treatment (26%). In a follow-up study comparing the same historical cohort of NMIBC, where cystectomy was reserved for evidence of progression to muscle-invasive disease, to a more contemporary cohort, where immediate cystectomy occurred in about 50% of the patients that had recurrence with cT1 disease, Raj et al. [102] found that the 5-year cancer-specific survival was significantly higher (69%) in the contemporary cohort compared to 52% in the historical cohort. Likewise, those who were upstaged from NMIBC to pathological T2 disease had significantly worse 5-year recurrence-free survival rates (61%) than those who were accurately staged as muscle-invasive (74%) and proceeded to a radical cystectomy [52]. Furthermore, in a retrospective review of 46 patients with high-risk NMIBC that was refractory to intravesical therapy, the progression-free survival rate was only 54% at an average of about 5-year follow-up and no different from patients undergoing cystectomy for muscle-invasive bladder cancer [123]. Therefore, the timing of cystectomy is essential before the development of non-organ-confined disease that could develop during local treatment.

The second reason for a timely cystectomy in NMIBC is the ability to stage accurately and evaluate the extent of disease. An inherent problem in the diagnosis and staging of UCB is the inability to identify muscle invasion. Anywhere from 20 to 60% of clinical T1 (cT1) bladder tumors are incorrectly staged [5, 44, 93, 122, 128, 154]; among patients with presumed cT1 NMIBC who undergo a cystectomy, 25–50% are found to have MIBC on pathology [13, 21, 128], and up to 15% are found with micro-metastatic disease to the lymph nodes [10, 89, 123, 128, 147, 154]. Re-staging TURBT is essential to mitigate the risk of understaging [61]; however, it does not eliminate it. A retrospective single institutional review of 84 patients who underwent immediate cystectomy after a re-staging TURBT confirmed NMIBC found that 20% of the patients were upstaged to MIBC [29].

This is particularly important for NMIBC with variant histology, such as micropapillary disease, where understaging and occult metastatic disease can be more frequent [69, 146]. Many of these variants including pure squamous cell [1], sarcomatoid [145], plasmacytoid [32], and micropapillary [68] will present with advanced staged, local progression, or distant metastasis at presentation. Because of their aggressive nature, if a histologic variant is noninvasive at TURBT, a timely cystectomy during the window of opportunity for cure would be strongly recommended [20]. In a single-institution review of patients with non-muscle-invasive micropapillary bladder cancer, Kamat et al. [69] found that 22% of the patients initially treated with BCG developed metastases, and that those treated with an immediate cystectomy had a 10-year disease-specific survival of 72%, compared to a median disease-specific survival of approximately 5 years for those who had delayed cystectomy (10-year disease-specific survival rate of 0%).

Table 2 Comparison of early and delayed cystectomy

					Early cystectomy	Delayed cystectomy	*p*-value
Author	Ref	N	Cohort	Definitions	Cancer-specific survival	Cancer-specific survival	
Herr and Sogani [63]	121	90	High-risk NMIBC who underwent at least one course of BCG	Early RC: within 2 years of initial BCG	15 yr: 69%	15 yr: 26%	0.001
				Delayed RC: after 2 years of initial BCG			
				Early RC: within 1 year of initial BCG	15 yr: 75%	15 yr: 34%	0.001
				Delayed RC: after 1 year of initial BCG			
Denzinger et al. [35]	122	105	High-grade T1	Early RC: average 4 weeks after initial TURBT	1o yr: 78%	10 yr: 51%	<0.01
				Delayed RC: after induction BCG, on average 11 months after initial TURBT			
Hautmann et al. [56]	123	223	High-grade T1	Early RC: within 90 days of initial TURBT	10 yr: 79%	10 yr: 65%	NA
				Delayed RC: if progression after induction BCG			
De Berardinis et al. [33]	124	152	High-risk NMIBC	Early RC: within 60 days of re-TURBT	10 yr: 78%	10 yr: 78%*	0.98
				Delayed RC: after induction and maintenance BCG, with signs of progression			
Stöckle et al. [131]	125	73	High-grade T1	Early RC: immediately following initial TURBT	5 yr: 90%	5 yr: 62%	0.001
				Delayed RC: after recurrence			

(continued)

Table 2 (continued)

					Early cystectomy	Delayed cystectomy	*p*-value
Author	Ref	N	Cohort	Definitions	Cancer-specific survival	Cancer-specific survival	
Jäger et al. [67]	126	278	High-grade T1	Early RC: within 5–12 months of initial TURBT	10 yr: 79%	10 yr: 61%	NA
				Delayed RC: after 12 months of initial TURBT			
Thalmann et al. [135]		121	High-grade T1	Early RC: within 3 months of initial TURBT	5 yr: 69%	5 yr: 80%*	0.3
				Delayed RC: after induction BCG, with signs of recurrence, median time to RC of 13 months			

*Comparison of early cystectomy versus those treated with BCG (deferred cystectomy and including those who did not progress)

Abbreviations: *RC* radical cystectomy, *TURBT* transurethral resection of bladder tumor, *BCG* Bacillus Calmette–Guerin

A third reason for a timely cystectomy for high-risk NMIBC is the excellent cancer outcomes associated with radical cystectomy. For all patients undergoing cystectomy for high-grade T1 disease at TURBT, the 5-year cancer-specific survival rates are almost 90% [81], with 5-year overall survival for organ-confined disease on pathological review around 80% [128]. In addition, the increasing utilization of orthotopic continent diversions have led to improvements in the quality of life outcomes with cystectomies; one study found that the well-being and quality of life outcomes of patients who underwent a cystectomy with orthotopic diversion were similar to a matched control population [57]. The ability to offer an orthotopic diversion may reduce the reluctance of physicians to recommend a cystectomy, especially to younger patients, and therefore help decrease the time to surgery. In one study, Hautmann et al. [55] found that orthotopic diversions were performed much sooner after diagnosis than ileal conduits (4 vs. 15 months) and that patients with the orthotopic diversions had higher cancer-specific survival rates even after adjusting for stage (77% vs. 28%). Likewise, in a modeling study of patients with high-risk NMIBC, Kulkarni et al. [75] found that young patients had a higher-quality adjusted life expectancy with immediate cystectomy compared to conservative therapy with repeated cystoscopies and BCG treatments. Furthermore, improvements in surgical technique and innovations in perioperative management, such as the use of enhanced recovery after surgery protocols [139], have helped improve the postoperative outcomes and length of stay after a cystectomy [26].

5 Conclusion

The accurate identification of high-risk disease and delivery of timely treatment are essential components of individualized care for NMIBC. Current strategies for risk stratification and treatment are not optimal. However, improvements in prognostic models, pathological staging techniques, and tumor markers will continue to refine and personalize risk stratification strategies. Patients with high-risk NMIBC should be counseled early in their presentation about the risks of progression and possible benefit of a cystectomy in a timely fashion. Continued engagement of patients in understanding the risks and possible benefits involved in the decision-making process may help avoid any potential delays in treatment and help improve outcomes with NMIBC.

References

1. Abdollah F, Sun M, Jeldres C, Schmitges J, Thuret R, Djahangirian O et al (2012) Survival after radical cystectomy of non-bilharzial squamous cell carcinoma versus urothelial carcinoma: a competing-risks analysis. BJU Int 109(4):564–569
2. Aine M, Eriksson P, Liedberg F, Sjödahl G, Höglund M (2015) Biological determinants of bladder cancer gene expression subtypes. Sci Rep 5:10957
3. Althausen AF, Prout GR, Daly JJ (1976) Non-invasive papillary carcinoma of the bladder associated with carcinoma in situ. J Urol 116(5):575–580
4. Alvarez-Múgica M, Cebrian V, Fernández-Gómez JM, Fresno F, Escaf S, Sánchez-Carbayo M (2010) Myopodin methylation is associated with clinical outcome in patients with T1G3 bladder cancer. J Urol 184(4):1507–1513
5. Amling CL, Thrasher JB, Frazier HA, Dodge RK, Robertson JE, Paulson DF (1994) Radical cystectomy for stages Ta, Tis and T1 transitional cell carcinoma of the bladder. J Urol 151(1):31–35 discussion 35–36
6. Angulo JC, Lopez JI, Grignon DJ, Sanchez-Chapado M (1995) Muscularis mucosa differentiates two populations with different prognosis in stage T1 bladder cancer. Urology 45(1):47–53
7. Aziz A, Shariat SF, Roghmann F, Brookman-May S, Stief CG, Rink M et al (2016) Prediction of cancer-specific survival after radical cystectomy in pT4a urothelial carcinoma of the bladder: development of a tool for clinical decision-making. BJU Int 117(2):272–279
8. Berman DM, Kawashima A, Peng Y, Mackillop WJ, Siemens DR, Booth CM (2015) Reporting trends and prognostic significance of lymphovascular invasion in muscle-invasive urothelial carcinoma: a population-based study. Int J Urol 22(2):163–170
9. Bernardini S, Billerey C, Martin M, Adessi GL, Wallerand H, Bittard H (2001) The predictive value of muscularis mucosae invasion and p 53 over expression on progression of stage T1 bladder carcinoma. J Urol 165(1):42–46 discussion 46

10. Bianco FJ, Justa D, Grignon DJ, Sakr WA, Pontes JE, Wood DP (2004) Management of clinical T1 bladder transitional cell carcinoma by radical cystectomy. Urol Oncol 22(4): 290–294
11. Breyer J, Otto W, Wirtz RM, Wullich B, Keck B, Erben P, et al (2016) ERBB2 Expression as potential risk-stratification for early cystectomy in patients with pT1 bladder cancer and concomitant carcinoma in situ. Urol Int
12. Brimo F, Wu C, Zeizafoun N, Tanguay S, Aprikian A, Mansure JJ et al (2013) Prognostic factors in T1 bladder urothelial carcinoma: the value of recording millimetric depth of invasion, diameter of invasive carcinoma, and muscularis mucosa invasion. Hum Pathol 44(1):95–102
13. Bruins HM, Skinner EC, Dorin RP, Ahmadi H, Djaladat H, Miranda G et al (2014) Incidence and location of lymph node metastases in patients undergoing radical cystectomy for clinical non-muscle invasive bladder cancer: results from a prospective lymph node mapping study. Urol Oncol 32(1):24.e13–24.e19
14. Burger M, van der Aa MN, van Oers JM, Brinkmann A, van der Kwast TH, Steyerberg EC et al (2008) Prediction of progression of non-muscle-invasive bladder cancer by WHO 1973 and 2004 grading and by FGFR3 mutation status: a prospective study. Eur Urol 54(4):835–843
15. Böhle A, Jocham D, Bock PR (2003) Intravesical bacillus Calmette-Guerin versus mitomycin C for superficial bladder cancer: a formal meta-analysis of comparative studies on recurrence and toxicity. J Urol 169(1):90–95
16. Cambier S, Sylvester RJ, Collette L, Gontero P, Brausi MA, van Andel G et al (2016) EORTC nomograms and risk groups for predicting recurrence, progression, and disease-specific and overall survival in non-muscle-invasive stage Ta-T1 urothelial bladder cancer patients treated with 1–3 years of maintenance bacillus calmette-guérin. Eur Urol 69(1):60–69
17. Casey RG, Catto JW, Cheng L, Cookson MS, Herr H, Shariat S et al (2015) Diagnosis and management of urothelial carcinoma in situ of the lower urinary tract: a systematic review. Eur Urol 67(5):876–888
18. Catalona WJ, Hudson MA, Gillen DP, Andriole GL, Ratliff TL (1987) Risks and benefits of repeated courses of intravesical bacillus Calmette-Guerin therapy for superficial bladder cancer. J Urol 137(2):220–224
19. Chang SS (2006) The adverse consequences of delaying radical cystectomy. Nat Clin Pract Urol 3(6):300–301
20. Chang SS, Boorjian SA, Chou R, Clark PE, Daneshmand S, Konety BR et al (2016) Diagnosis and treatment of non-muscle invasive bladder cancer: AUA/SUO guideline. J Urol 196(4):1021–1029
21. Chang SS, Cookson MS (2005) Non-muscle-invasive bladder cancer: the role of radical cystectomy. Urology 66(5):917–922
22. Chang WC, Chang YH, Pan CC (2012) Prognostic significance in substaging of T1 urinary bladder urothelial carcinoma on transurethral resection. Am J Surg Pathol 36(3):454–461
23. Cho KS, Seo HK, Joung JY, Park WS, Ro JY, Han KS et al (2009) Lymphovascular invasion in transurethral resection specimens as predictor of progression and metastasis in patients with newly diagnosed T1 bladder urothelial cancer. J Urol 182(6):2625–2630
24. Choi W, Porten S, Kim S, Willis D, Plimack ER, Hoffman-Censits J et al (2014) Identification of distinct basal and luminal subtypes of muscle-invasive bladder cancer with different sensitivities to frontline chemotherapy. Cancer Cell 25(2):152–165
25. Choong NW, Quevedo JF, Kaur JS (2005) Small cell carcinoma of the urinary bladder. The Mayo Clinic experience. Cancer 103(6):1172–1178
26. Cookson MS, Chang SS, Wells N, Parekh DJ, Smith JA (2003) Complications of radical cystectomy for nonmuscle invasive disease: comparison with muscle invasive disease. J Urol 169(1):101–104
27. Cookson MS, Herr HW, Zhang ZF, Soloway S, Sogani PC, Fair WR (1997) The treated natural history of high risk superficial bladder cancer: 15-year outcome. J Urol 158(1):62–67

28. Dalbagni G, Parekh DJ, Ben-Porat L, Potenzoni M, Herr HW, Reuter VE (2007) Prospective evaluation of p53 as a prognostic marker in T1 transitional cell carcinoma of the bladder. BJU Int 99(2):281–285
29. Dalbagni G, Vora K, Kaag M, Cronin A, Bochner B, Donat SM et al (2009) Clinical outcome in a contemporary series of restaged patients with clinical T1 bladder cancer. Eur Urol 56(6):903–910
30. Damrauer JS, Hoadley KA, Chism DD, Fan C, Tiganelli CJ, Wobker SE et al (2014) Intrinsic subtypes of high-grade bladder cancer reflect the hallmarks of breast cancer biology. Proc Natl Acad Sci U S A 111(8):3110–3115
31. Daneshmand S (2013) Determining the role of cystectomy for high-grade T1 urothelial carcinoma. Urol Clin North Am 40(2):233–247
32. Dayyani F, Czerniak BA, Sircar K, Munsell MF, Millikan RE, Dinney CP et al (2013) Plasmacytoid urothelial carcinoma, a chemosensitive cancer with poor prognosis, and peritoneal carcinomatosis. J Urol 189(5):1656–1661
33. De Berardinis E, Busetto GM, Antonini G, Giovannone R, Gentile V (2011) T1G3 high-risk NMIBC (non-muscle invasive bladder cancer): conservative treatment versus immediate cystectomy. Int Urol Nephrol 43(4):1047–1057
34. Dell'Oglio P, Tian Z, Leyh-Bannurah SR, Trudeau V, Larcher A, Moschini M et al (2017) Short-form charlson comorbidity index for assessment of perioperative mortality after radical cystectomy. J Natl Compr Canc Netw 15(3):327–333
35. Denzinger S, Fritsche HM, Otto W, Blana A, Wieland WF, Burger M (2008) Early versus deferred cystectomy for initial high-risk pT1G3 urothelial carcinoma of the bladder: do risk factors define feasibility of bladder-sparing approach? Eur Urol 53(1):146–152
36. Domanowska E, Jozwicki W, Domaniewski J, Golda R, Skok Z, Wiśniewska H et al (2007) Muscle-invasive urothelial cell carcinoma of the human bladder: multidirectional differentiation and ability to metastasize. Hum Pathol 38(5):741–746
37. Droller MJ (2005) Biological considerations in the assessment of urothelial cancer: a retrospective. Urology 66(5 Suppl):66–75
38. Duggan BJ, McKnight JJ, Williamson KE, Loughrey M, O'Rourke D, Hamilton PW et al (2003) The need to embrace molecular profiling of tumor cells in prostate and bladder cancer. Clin Cancer Res 9(4):1240–1247
39. Dyrskjøt L, Zieger K, Real FX, Malats N, Carrato A, Hurst C et al (2007) Gene expression signatures predict outcome in non-muscle-invasive bladder carcinoma: a multicenter validation study. Clin Cancer Res 13(12):3545–3551
40. Faivre d'Arcier B, Celhay O, Safsaf A, Zairi A, Pfister C, Soulié M et al (2010) T1 bladder carcinoma: prognostic value of the muscularis mucosae invasion (T1a/T1b). A multicenter study by the French Urological Association (CCAFU). Prog Urol 20(6):440–449
41. Farrow GM, Utz DC, Rife CC, Greene LF (1977) Clinical observations on sixty-nine cases of in situ carcinoma of the urinary bladder. Cancer Res 37(8 Pt 2):2794–2798
42. Fernandez-Gomez J, Madero R, Solsona E, Unda M, Martinez-Pineiro L, Gonzalez M et al (2009) Predicting nonmuscle invasive bladder cancer recurrence and progression in patients treated with bacillus Calmette-Guerin: the CUETO scoring model. J Urol 182(5):2195–2203
43. Fernandez-Gomez J, Solsona E, Unda M, Martinez-Piñeiro L, Gonzalez M, Hernandez R et al (2008) Prognostic factors in patients with non-muscle-invasive bladder cancer treated with bacillus Calmette-Guérin: multivariate analysis of data from four randomized CUETO trials. Eur Urol 53(5):992–1001
44. Freeman JA, Esrig D, Stein JP, Simoneau AR, Skinner EC, Chen SC et al (1995) Radical cystectomy for high risk patients with superficial bladder cancer in the era of orthotopic urinary reconstruction. Cancer 76(5):833–839
45. Fristrup N, Birkenkamp-Demtröder K, Reinert T, Sanchez-Carbayo M, Segersten U, Malmström PU et al (2013) Multicenter validation of cyclin D1, MCM7, TRIM29, and UBE2C as prognostic protein markers in non-muscle-invasive bladder cancer. Am J Pathol 182(2):339–349

46. Fritsche HM, Burger M, Svatek RS, Jeldres C, Karakiewicz PI, Novara G et al (2010) Characteristics and outcomes of patients with clinical T1 grade 3 urothelial carcinoma treated with radical cystectomy: results from an international cohort. Eur Urol 57(2): 300–309
47. Gakis G, Todenhöfer T, Braun M, Fend F, Stenzl A, Perner S (2015) Immunohistochemical assessment of lymphatic and blood vessel invasion in T1 urothelial carcinoma of the bladder. Scand J Urol 49(5):382–387
48. Gardiner RA, Walsh MD, Allen V, Rahman S, Samaratunga ML, Seymour GJ et al (1994) Immunohistological expression of p53 in primary pT1 transitional cell bladder cancer in relation to tumour progression. Br J Urol 73(5):526–532
49. Goebell PJ, Groshen SG, Schmitz-Dräger BJ (2010) p53 immunohistochemistry in bladder cancer–a new approach to an old question. Urol Oncol 28(4):377–388
50. Green DA, Rink M, Hansen J, Cha EK, Robinson B, Tian Z et al (2013) Accurate preoperative prediction of non-organ-confined bladder urothelial carcinoma at cystectomy. BJU Int 111(3):404–411
51. Groenendijk FH, de Jong J, Fransen van de Putte EE, Michaut M, Schlicker A, Peters D et al (2016) ERBB2 mutations characterize a subgroup of muscle-invasive bladder cancers with excellent response to neoadjuvant chemotherapy. Eur Urol 69(3):384–388
52. Guzzo TJ, Magheli A, Bivalacqua TJ, Nielsen ME, Attenello FJ, Schoenberg MP et al (2009) Pathological upstaging during radical cystectomy is associated with worse recurrence-free survival in patients with bacillus Calmette-Guerin-refractory bladder cancer. Urology 74(6):1276–1280
53. Han RF, Pan JG (2006) Can intravesical bacillus Calmette-Guérin reduce recurrence in patients with superficial bladder cancer? A meta-analysis of randomized trials. Urology 67(6):1216–1223
54. Hassan JM, Cookson MS, Smith JA, Johnson DL, Chang SS (2004) Outcomes in patients with pathological carcinoma in situ only disease at radical cystectomy. J Urol 172(3): 882–884
55. Hautmann RE, Paiss T (1998) Does the option of the ileal neobladder stimulate patient and physician decision toward earlier cystectomy? J Urol 159(6):1845–1850
56. Hautmann RE, Volkmer BG, Gust K (2009) Quantification of the survival benefit of early versus deferred cystectomy in high-risk non-muscle invasive bladder cancer (T1 G3). World J Urol 27(3):347–351
57. Henningsohn L, Steven K, Kallestrup EB, Steineck G (2002) Distressful symptoms and well-being after radical cystectomy and orthotopic bladder substitution compared with a matched control population. J Urol 168(1):168–174 discussion 174–165
58. Hermann GG, Horn T, Steven K (1998) The influence of the level of lamina propria invasion and the prevalence of p53 nuclear accumulation on survival in stage T1 transitional cell bladder cancer. J Urol 159(1):91–94
59. Hernández S, López-Knowles E, Lloreta J, Kogevinas M, Amorós A, Tardón A et al (2006) Prospective study of FGFR3 mutations as a prognostic factor in nonmuscle invasive urothelial bladder carcinomas. J Clin Oncol 24(22):3664–3671
60. Herr HW (1983) Carcinoma in situ of the bladder. Semin Urol 1(1):15–22
61. Herr HW (1999) The value of a second transurethral resection in evaluating patients with bladder tumors. J Urol 162(1):74–76
62. Herr HW (2000) Timing of cystectomy for superficial bladder tumors. Urol Oncol 5(4): 162–165
63. Herr HW, Sogani PC (2001) Does early cystectomy improve the survival of patients with high risk superficial bladder tumors? J Urol 166(4):1296–1299
64. Huncharek M, Geschwind JF, Witherspoon B, McGarry R, Adcock D (2000) Intravesical chemotherapy prophylaxis in primary superficial bladder cancer: a meta-analysis of 3703 patients from 11 randomized trials. J Clin Epidemiol 53(7):676–680

65. Jarow JP, Lerner SP, Kluetz PG, Liu K, Sridhara R, Bajorin D et al (2014) Clinical trial design for the development of new therapies for nonmuscle-invasive bladder cancer: report of a Food and Drug Administration and American Urological Association Public Workshop. Urology 83(2):262–264
66. Joudi FN, Smith BJ, O'Donnell MA, Konety BR (2003) Contemporary management of superficial bladder cancer in the United States: a pattern of care analysis. Urology 62(6): 1083–1088
67. Jäger W, Thomas C, Haag S, Hampel C, Salzer A, Thüroff JW et al (2011) Early versus delayed radical cystectomy for 'high-risk' carcinoma not invading bladder muscle: delay of cystectomy reduces cancer-specific survival. BJU Int 108(8 Pt 2):E284–E288
68. Kamat AM, Dinney CP, Gee JR, Grossman HB, Siefker-Radtke AO, Tamboli P et al (2007) Micropapillary bladder cancer: a review of the University of Texas M. D. Anderson Cancer Center experience with 100 consecutive patients. Cancer 110(1):62–67
69. Kamat AM, Gee JR, Dinney CP, Grossman HB, Swanson DA, Millikan RE et al (2006) The case for early cystectomy in the treatment of nonmuscle invasive micropapillary bladder carcinoma. J Urol 175(3 Pt 1):881–885
70. Kandimalla R, van Tilborg AA, Kompier LC, Stumpel DJ, Stam RW, Bangma CH et al (2012) Genome-wide analysis of CpG island methylation in bladder cancer identified TBX2, TBX3, GATA2, and ZIC4 as pTa-specific prognostic markers. Eur Urol 61(6):1245–1256
71. Kassouf W, Agarwal PK, Grossman HB, Leibovici D, Munsell MF, Siefker-Radtke A et al (2009) Outcome of patients with bladder cancer with pN+ disease after preoperative chemotherapy and radical cystectomy. Urology 73(1):147–152
72. Kim HS, Kim M, Jeong CW, Kwak C, Kim HH, Ku JH (2014) Presence of lymphovascular invasion in urothelial bladder cancer specimens after transurethral resections correlates with risk of upstaging and survival: a systematic review and meta-analysis. Urol Oncol 32(8): 1191–1199
73. Kim SP, Boorjian SA, Shah ND, Karnes RJ, Weight CJ, Moriarty JP et al (2012) Contemporary trends of in-hospital complications and mortality for radical cystectomy. BJU Int 110(8):1163–1168
74. Knowles MA (2006) Molecular subtypes of bladder cancer: Jekyll and Hyde or chalk and cheese? Carcinogenesis 27(3):361–373
75. Kulkarni GS, Finelli A, Fleshner NE, Jewett MA, Lopushinsky SR, Alibhai SM (2007) Optimal management of high-risk T1G3 bladder cancer: a decision analysis. PLoS Med 4(9): e284
76. Kunju LP, You L, Zhang Y, Daignault S, Montie JE, Lee CT (2008) Lymphovascular invasion of urothelial cancer in matched transurethral bladder tumor resection and radical cystectomy specimens. J Urol 180(5):1928–1932 discussion 1932
77. Lerner SP, Tangen CM, Sucharew H, Wood D, Crawford ED (2009) Failure to achieve a complete response to induction BCG therapy is associated with increased risk of disease worsening and death in patients with high risk non-muscle invasive bladder cancer. Urol Oncol 27(2):155–159
78. Malats N, Bustos A, Nascimento CM, Fernandez F, Rivas M, Puente D et al (2005) P53 as a prognostic marker for bladder cancer: a meta-analysis and review. Lancet Oncol 6(9): 678–686
79. Malmström PU, Sylvester RJ, Crawford DE, Friedrich M, Krege S, Rintala E et al (2009) An individual patient data meta-analysis of the long-term outcome of randomised studies comparing intravesical mitomycin C versus bacillus Calmette-Guérin for non-muscle-invasive bladder cancer. Eur Urol 56(2):247–256
80. Mariotto AB, Yabroff KR, Shao Y, Feuer EJ, Brown ML (2011) Projections of the cost of cancer care in the United States: 2010–2020. J Natl Cancer Inst 103(2):117–128
81. Martin-Doyle W, Leow JJ, Orsola A, Chang SL, Bellmunt J (2015) Improving selection criteria for early cystectomy in high-grade t1 bladder cancer: a meta-analysis of 15,215 patients. J Clin Oncol 33(6):643–650

82. Masood S, Sriprasad S, Palmer JH, Mufti GR (2004) T1G3 bladder cancer–indications for early cystectomy. Int Urol Nephrol 36(1):41–44
83. Mathieu R, Lucca I, Rouprêt M, Briganti A, Shariat SF (2016) The prognostic role of lymphovascular invasion in urothelial carcinoma of the bladder. Nat Rev Urol 13(8):471–479
84. McConkey DJ, Choi W, Dinney CP (2014) New insights into subtypes of invasive bladder cancer: considerations of the clinician. Eur Urol 66(4):609–610
85. McConkey DJ, Choi W, Ochoa A, Siefker-Radtke A, Czerniak B, Dinney CP (2015) Therapeutic opportunities in the intrinsic subtypes of muscle-invasive bladder cancer. Hematol Oncol Clin North Am 29(2):377–394 x–xi
86. Miyake M, Gotoh D, Shimada K, Tatsumi Y, Nakai Y, Anai S et al (2015) Exploration of risk factors predicting outcomes for primary T1 high-grade bladder cancer and validation of the Spanish Urological Club for oncological treatment scoring model: long-term follow-up experience at a single institute. Int J Urol 22(6):541–547
87. Moonen PM, van Balken-Ory B, Kiemeney LA, Schalken JA, Witjes JA (2007) Prognostic value of p53 for high risk superficial bladder cancer with long-term followup. J Urol 177(1): 80–83
88. Network CGAR (2014) Comprehensive molecular characterization of urothelial bladder carcinoma. Nature 507(7492):315–322
89. Nieder AM, Simon MA, Kim SS, Manoharan M, Soloway MS (2006) Radical cystectomy after bacillus Calmette-Guérin for high-risk Ta, T1, and carcinoma in situ: defining the risk of initial bladder preservation. Urology 67(4):737–741
90. Nielsen ME, Smith AB, Meyer AM, Kuo TM, Tyree S, Kim WY et al (2014) Trends in stage-specific incidence rates for urothelial carcinoma of the bladder in the United States: 1988–2006. Cancer 120(1):86–95
91. Olsson H, Hultman P, Rosell J, Jahnson S (2013) Population-based study on prognostic factors for recurrence and progression in primary stage T1 bladder tumours. Scand J Urol 47(3):188–195
92. Orsola A, Trias I, Raventós CX, Español I, Cecchini L, Búcar S et al (2005) Initial high-grade T1 urothelial cell carcinoma: feasibility and prognostic significance of lamina propria invasion microstaging (T1a/b/c) in BCG-treated and BCG-non-treated patients. Eur Urol 48(2):231–238 discussion 238
93. Pagano F, Bassi P, Galetti TP, Meneghini A, Milani C, Artibani W et al (1991) Results of contemporary radical cystectomy for invasive bladder cancer: a clinicopathological study with an emphasis on the inadequacy of the tumor, nodes and metastases classification. J Urol 145(1):45–50
94. Park J, Song C, Shin E, Hong JH, Kim CS, Ahn H (2013) Do molecular biomarkers have prognostic value in primary T1G3 bladder cancer treated with bacillus Calmette-Guerin intravesical therapy? Urol Oncol 31(6):849–856
95. Passoni N, Gayed B, Kapur P, Sagalowsky AI, Shariat SF, Lotan Y (2016) Cell-cycle markers do not improve discrimination of EORTC and CUETO risk models in predicting recurrence and progression of non-muscle-invasive high-grade bladder cancer. Urol Oncol 34(11):485.e487–485.e414
96. Patriarca C, Hurle R, Moschini M, Freschi M, Colombo P, Colecchia M et al (2016) Usefulness of pT1 substaging in papillary urothelial bladder carcinoma. Diagn Pathol 11:6
97. Patschan O, Sjödahl G, Chebil G, Lövgren K, Lauss M, Gudjonsson S et al (2015) A Molecular pathologic framework for risk stratification of stage T1 urothelial carcinoma. Eur Urol 68(5):824–832 discussion 835–826
98. Plimack ER, Dunbrack RL, Brennan TA, Andrake MD, Zhou Y, Serebriiskii IG et al (2015) Defects in DNA repair genes predict response to neoadjuvant cisplatin-based chemotherapy in muscle-invasive bladder cancer. Eur Urol 68(6):959–967
99. Ploeg M, Aben KK, Hulsbergen-van de Kaa CA, Schoenberg MP, Witjes JA, Kiemeney LA (2010) Clinical epidemiology of nonurothelial bladder cancer: analysis of the Netherlands Cancer Registry. J Urol 183(3):915–920

100. Powles T, Eder JP, Fine GD, Braiteh FS, Loriot Y, Cruz C et al (2014) MPDL3280A (anti-PD-L1) treatment leads to clinical activity in metastatic bladder cancer. Nature 515(7528):558–562
101. Prout GR, Griffin PP, Daly JJ (1987) The outcome of conservative treatment of carcinoma in situ of the bladder. J Urol 138(4):766–770
102. Raj GV, Herr H, Serio AM, Donat SM, Bochner BH, Vickers AJ et al (2007) Treatment paradigm shift may improve survival of patients with high risk superficial bladder cancer. J Urol 177(4):1283–1286 discussion 1286
103. Reardon ZD, Patel SG, Zaid HB, Stimson CJ, Resnick MJ, Keegan KA et al (2015) Trends in the use of perioperative chemotherapy for localized and locally advanced muscle-invasive bladder cancer: a sign of changing tides. Eur Urol 67(1):165–170
104. Rebouissou S, Bernard-Pierrot I, de Reyniès A, Lepage ML, Krucker C, Chapeaublanc E et al (2014) EGFR as a potential therapeutic target for a subset of muscle-invasive bladder cancers presenting a basal-like phenotype. Sci Transl Med 6(244):244ra291
105. Resnick MJ, Bergey M, Magerfleisch L, Tomaszewski JE, Malkowicz SB, Guzzo TJ (2011) Longitudinal evaluation of the concordance and prognostic value of lymphovascular invasion in transurethral resection and radical cystectomy specimens. BJU Int 107(1):46–52
106. Riley GF, Potosky AL, Lubitz JD, Kessler LG (1995) Medicare payments from diagnosis to death for elderly cancer patients by stage at diagnosis. Med Care 33(8):828–841
107. Ro JY, Ayala AG, el-Naggar A (1987) Muscularis mucosa of urinary bladder. Importance for staging and treatment. Am J Surg Pathol 11(9):668–673
108. Rouprêt M, Seisen T, Compérat E, Larré S, Mazerolles C, Gobet F et al (2013) Prognostic interest in discriminating muscularis mucosa invasion (T1a vs. T1b) in nonmuscle invasive bladder carcinoma: French national multicenter study with central pathology review. J Urol 189(6):2069–2076
109. Schiffmann J, Gandaglia G, Larcher A, Sun M, Tian Z, Shariat SF et al (2014) Contemporary 90-day mortality rates after radical cystectomy in the elderly. Eur J Surg Oncol 40(12):1738–1745
110. Sfakianos JP, Galsky MD (2015) Neoadjuvant chemotherapy in the management of muscle-invasive bladder cancer: bridging the gap between evidence and practice. Urol Clin North Am 42(2):181–187 viii
111. Shah RB, Montgomery JS, Montie JE, Kunju LP (2013) Variant (divergent) histologic differentiation in urothelial carcinoma is under-recognized in community practice: impact of mandatory central pathology review at a large referral hospital. Urol Oncol 31(8):1650–1655
112. Shariat SF, Ashfaq R, Sagalowsky AI, Lotan Y (2007) Association of cyclin D1 and E1 expression with disease progression and biomarkers in patients with nonmuscle-invasive urothelial cell carcinoma of the bladder. Urol Oncol 25(6):468–475
113. Shariat SF, Ashfaq R, Sagalowsky AI, Lotan Y (2007) Predictive value of cell cycle biomarkers in nonmuscle invasive bladder transitional cell carcinoma. J Urol 177(2):481–487 discussion 487
114. Shariat SF, Bolenz C, Godoy G, Fradet Y, Ashfaq R, Karakiewicz PI et al (2009) Predictive value of combined immunohistochemical markers in patients with pT1 urothelial carcinoma at radical cystectomy. J Urol 182(1):78–84 discussion 84
115. Shariat SF, Chromecki TF, Cha EK, Karakiewicz PI, Sun M, Fradet Y et al (2012) Risk stratification of organ confined bladder cancer after radical cystectomy using cell cycle related biomarkers. J Urol 187(2):457–462
116. Shariat SF, Tokunaga H, Zhou J, Kim J, Ayala GE, Benedict WF et al (2004) p53, p21, pRB, and p16 expression predict clinical outcome in cystectomy with bladder cancer. J Clin Oncol 22(6):1014–1024
117. Shariat SF, Weizer AZ, Green A, Laucirica R, Frolov A, Wheeler TM et al (2000) Prognostic value of P53 nuclear accumulation and histopathologic features in T1 transitional cell carcinoma of the urinary bladder. Urology 56(5):735–740

118. Shelley MD, Kynaston H, Court J, Wilt TJ, Coles B, Burgon K et al (2001) A systematic review of intravesical bacillus Calmette-Guerin plus transurethral resection versus transurethral resection alone in Ta and T1 bladder cancer. BJU Int 88(3):209–216
119. Shelley MD, Wilt TJ, Court J, Coles B, Kynaston H, Mason MD (2004) Intravesical bacillus Calmette-Guérin is superior to mitomycin C in reducing tumour recurrence in high-risk superficial bladder cancer: a meta-analysis of randomized trials. BJU Int 93(4):485–490
120. Siegel RL, Miller KD, Jemal A (2017) Cancer statistics, 2017. CA Cancer J Clin 67(1):7–30
121. Sjödahl G, Lauss M, Lövgren K, Chebil G, Gudjonsson S, Veerla S et al (2012) A molecular taxonomy for urothelial carcinoma. Clin Cancer Res 18(12):3377–3386
122. Soloway MS, Lopez AE, Patel J, Lu Y (1994) Results of radical cystectomy for transitional cell carcinoma of the bladder and the effect of chemotherapy. Cancer 73(7):1926–1931
123. Solsona E, Iborra I, Rubio J, Casanova J, Almenar S (2004) The optimum timing of radical cystectomy for patients with recurrent high-risk superficial bladder tumour. BJU Int 94(9): 1258–1262
124. Sonpavde G, Khan MM, Svatek RS, Lee R, Novara G, Tilki D et al (2011) Prognostic risk stratification of pathological stage T2N0 bladder cancer after radical cystectomy. BJU Int 108(5):687–692
125. Sonpavde G, Khan MM, Svatek RS, Lee R, Novara G, Tilki D et al (2011) Prognostic risk stratification of pathological stage T3N0 bladder cancer after radical cystectomy. J Urol 185(4):1216–1221
126. Sood A, Kachroo N, Abdollah F, Sammon JD, Löppenberg B, Jindal T et al (2017) An evaluation of the timing of surgical complications following radical cystectomy: data from the american college of surgeons national surgical quality improvement program. Urology
127. Stein JP, Grossfeld GD, Ginsberg DA, Esrig D, Freeman JA, Figueroa AJ et al (1998) Prognostic markers in bladder cancer: a contemporary review of the literature. J Urol 160(3 Pt 1):645–659
128. Stein JP, Lieskovsky G, Cote R, Groshen S, Feng AC, Boyd S et al (2001) Radical cystectomy in the treatment of invasive bladder cancer: long-term results in 1,054 patients. J Clin Oncol 19(3):666–675
129. Stimson CJ, Chang SS, Barocas DA, Humphrey JE, Patel SG, Clark PE et al (2010) Early and late perioperative outcomes following radical cystectomy: 90-day readmissions, morbidity and mortality in a contemporary series. J Urol 184(4):1296–1300
130. Streeper NM, Simons CM, Konety BR, Muirhead DM, Williams RD, O'Donnell MA et al (2009) The significance of lymphovascular invasion in transurethral resection of bladder tumour and cystectomy specimens on the survival of patients with urothelial bladder cancer. BJU Int 103(4):475–479
131. Stöckle M, Alken P, Engelmann U, Jacobi GH, Riedmiller H, Hohenfellner R (1987) Radical cystectomy–often too late? Eur Urol 13(6):361–367
132. Sylvester RJ, Oosterlinck W, Holmang S, Sydes MR, Birtle A, Gudjonsson S et al (2016) Systematic review and individual patient data meta-analysis of randomized trials comparing a single immediate instillation of chemotherapy after transurethral resection with transurethral resection alone in patients with stage pTa-pT1 urothelial carcinoma of the bladder: which patients benefit from the instillation? Eur Urol 69(2):231–244
133. Sylvester RJ, van der Meijden AP, Lamm DL (2002) Intravesical bacillus Calmette-Guerin reduces the risk of progression in patients with superficial bladder cancer: a meta-analysis of the published results of randomized clinical trials. J Urol 168(5):1964–1970
134. Sylvester RJ, van der Meijden AP, Oosterlinck W, Witjes JA, Bouffioux C, Denis L et al (2006) Predicting recurrence and progression in individual patients with stage Ta T1 bladder cancer using EORTC risk tables: a combined analysis of 2596 patients from seven EORTC trials. Eur Urol 49(3):466–465 discussion 475–467
135. Thalmann GN, Markwalder R, Shahin O, Burkhard FC, Hochreiter WW, Studer UE (2004) Primary T1G3 bladder cancer: organ preserving approach or immediate cystectomy? J Urol 172(1):70–75

136. Thompson IM, Tangen C, Basler J, Crawford ED (2002) Impact of previous local treatment for prostate cancer on subsequent metastatic disease. J Urol 168(3):1008–1012
137. Tilki D, Reich O, Svatek RS, Karakiewicz PI, Kassouf W, Novara G et al (2010) Characteristics and outcomes of patients with clinical carcinoma in situ only treated with radical cystectomy: an international study of 243 patients. J Urol 183(5):1757–1763
138. Tilki D, Shariat SF, Lotan Y, Rink M, Karakiewicz PI, Schoenberg MP et al (2013) Lymphovascular invasion is independently associated with bladder cancer recurrence and survival in patients with final stage T1 disease and negative lymph nodes after radical cystectomy. BJU Int 111(8):1215–1221
139. Tyson MD, Chang SS (2016) Enhanced recovery pathways versus standard care after cystectomy: a meta-analysis of the effect on perioperative outcomes. Eur Urol 70(6):995–1003
140. van den Bosch S, Alfred Witjes J (2011) Long-term cancer-specific survival in patients with high-risk, non-muscle-invasive bladder cancer and tumour progression: a systematic review. Eur Urol 60(3):493–500
141. van Rhijn BW, Catto JW, Goebell PJ, Knüchel R, Shariat SF, van der Poel HG et al (2014) Molecular markers for urothelial bladder cancer prognosis: toward implementation in clinical practice. Urol Oncol 32(7):1078–1087
142. van Rhijn BW, Liu L, Vis AN, Bostrom PJ, Zuiverloon TC, Fleshner NE et al (2012) Prognostic value of molecular markers, sub-stage and European Organisation for the Research and Treatment of Cancer risk scores in primary T1 bladder cancer. BJU Int 110(8):1169–1176
143. van Rhijn BW, Vis AN, van der Kwast TH, Kirkels WJ, Radvanyi F, Ooms EC et al (2003) Molecular grading of urothelial cell carcinoma with fibroblast growth factor receptor 3 and MIB-1 is superior to pathologic grade for the prediction of clinical outcome. J Clin Oncol 21(10):1912–1921
144. van Rhijn BW, Zuiverloon TC, Vis AN, Radvanyi F, van Leenders GJ, Ooms BC et al (2010) Molecular grade (FGFR3/MIB-1) and EORTC risk scores are predictive in primary non-muscle-invasive bladder cancer. Eur Urol 58(3):433–441
145. Wang J, Wang FW, Lagrange CA, Hemstreet III GP, Kessinger A (2010) Clinical features of sarcomatoid carcinoma (carcinosarcoma) of the urinary bladder: analysis of 221 cases. Sarcoma
146. Weizer AZ, Wasco MJ, Wang R, Daignault S, Lee CT, Shah RB (2009) Multiple adverse histological features increase the odds of under staging T1 bladder cancer. J Urol 182(1):59–65 discussion 65
147. Wiesner C, Pfitzenmaier J, Faldum A, Gillitzer R, Melchior SW, Thüroff JW (2005) Lymph node metastases in non-muscle invasive bladder cancer are correlated with the number of transurethral resections and tumour upstaging at radical cystectomy. BJU Int 95(3):301–305
148. Willis D, Kamat AM (2015) Nonurothelial bladder cancer and rare variant histologies. Hematol Oncol Clin North Am 29(2):237–252 viii
149. Willis DL, Porten SP, Kamat AM (2013) Should histologic variants alter definitive treatment of bladder cancer? Curr Opin Urol 23(5):435–443
150. Xie HY, Zhu Y, Yao XD, Zhang SL, Dai B, Zhang HL et al (2012) Development of a nomogram to predict non-organ-confined bladder urothelial cancer before radical cystectomy. Int Urol Nephrol 44(6):1711–1719
151. Xylinas E, Kent M, Kluth L, Pycha A, Comploj E, Svatek RS et al (2013) Accuracy of the EORTC risk tables and of the CUETO scoring model to predict outcomes in non-muscle-invasive urothelial carcinoma of the bladder. Br J Cancer
152. Yang LS, Shan BL, Shan LL, Chin P, Murray S, Ahmadi N et al (2016) A systematic review and meta-analysis of quality of life outcomes after radical cystectomy for bladder cancer. Surg Oncol 25(3):281–297

153. Yates DR, Rehman I, Abbod MF, Meuth M, Cross SS, Linkens DA et al (2007) Promoter hypermethylation identifies progression risk in bladder cancer. Clin Cancer Res 13(7): 2046–2053
154. Yiou R, Patard JJ, Benhard H, Abbou CC, Chopin DK (2002) Outcome of radical cystectomy for bladder cancer according to the disease type at presentation. BJU Int 89(4): 374–378
155. Younes M, Sussman J, True LD (1990) The usefulness of the level of the muscularis mucosae in the staging of invasive transitional cell carcinoma of the urinary bladder. Cancer 66(3):543–548

Enhanced Recovery After Surgery for Radical Cystectomy

Avinash Chenam and Kevin G. Chan

Contents

A. Chenam · K. G. Chan (✉)
Department of Surgery, Division of Urology and Urologic Oncology, City of Hope National Medical Center, 1500 E. Duarte Rd, MOB L002H, Duarte, CA 91010, USA
e-mail: kchan@coh.org

A. Chenam
e-mail: achenam@coh.org

S. Daneshmand and K. G. Chan (eds.), *Genitourinary Cancers*, Cancer Treatment and Research 175, https://doi.org/10.1007/978-3-319-93339-9_10

Abstract

Even with advances in perioperative medical care, anesthetic management, and surgical techniques, radical cystectomy (RC) continues to be associated with a high morbidity rate as well as a prolonged length of hospital stay. In recent years, there has been great interest in identifying multimodal and interdisciplinary strategies that help accelerate postoperative convalescence by reducing variation in perioperative care of patients undergoing complex surgeries. Enhanced recovery after surgery (ERAS) attempts to evaluate and incorporate scientific evidence for modifying as many of the factors contributing to the morbidity of RC as possible, and optimize how patients are cared for before and after surgery. In this chapter, we review the preoperative, intraoperative and postoperative elements of using an ERAS protocol for RC.

Keywords

Enhanced recovery after surgery · Radical cystectomy · Bladder cancer

1 Introduction

Bladder cancer is currently the fourth most common cancer and the eighth leading cause of cancer death among men in the USA [1]. It is predominantly a disease of the aging population, with a peaking incidence in the seventh decade when comorbid conditions are frequently present [1–3]. The overwhelming majority of bladder carcinomas (90%) are urothelial carcinomas, with 20% of this group presenting with muscle-invasive disease [4]. The gold standard treatment for muscle-invasive bladder cancer as well as high-risk non-muscle-invasive bladder cancers is radical cystectomy (RC).

Every year, approximately 10,000 RC operations are performed across the USA, [5]. The procedure along with pelvic lymph node dissection (PLND) and intestinal urinary diversion is among the most complex urological operations with many potential complications including postoperative cardiorespiratory failure, deep vein thrombosis, ileus, and metabolic derangement. Although advances in perioperative medical care, anesthetic management, and surgical techniques have lowered mortality to less than 3%, postoperative complications occur in 30–64% of patients and readmission are necessary in up to 30% of patients after RC [6–10]. Greater mortality and morbidity are observed in the elderly [11, 12]. Further, patients who undergo such a radical intervention are often admitted for long hospital stays as RC continues to be associated with a length of stay (LOS) of 8–11 days [7, 13]. Given the prolonged LOS, the high complication and readmission rates, there is much room for improvement in current RC care.

In recent years, there has been great interest in identifying multimodal and interdisciplinary strategies that help accelerate postoperative convalescence by reducing variation in perioperative care of patients undergoing complex surgeries. In the literature, multiple terms have been used to describe this concept: enhanced recovery after surgery (ERAS), enhanced recovery program (ERP), enhanced recovery after cystectomy (ERAC), fast-track surgery, accelerated recovery pathway, and care coordination pathway. However, common to all these approaches is the attempt to evaluate and incorporate scientific evidence for modifying as many of the factors contributing to the morbidity of RC as possible and optimize how patients are cared for before and after surgery [14].

Originating in the 1990s, the concept of fast-track surgery was created by Danish surgeon Henrik Kehlet, who studied the physiological stress response after colorectal surgery to determine if patients could easily be discharged much earlier than was traditionally practiced [15]. A separate group formally coined the term ERAS, describing it as a multimodal, perioperative approach that applies evidence-based interventions (including elimination of unnecessary measures) to modify the surgical stress response and shorten patient recovery time [16, 17]. Delivered by a team of professionals—anesthesia, surgeons, physiotherapists, and nurses—the concept has since been rolled out across many surgical specialties, creating procedure specific protocols in the fields of colorectal, urological, gynecological, vascular, and orthopedic surgery. The four keys to any ERAS protocol include: (1) appropriate preoperative assessment, patient identification and preparation prior to admission, (2) reducing physical stress of the operation—through a series of modifications to surgical and anesthesia intraoperative care, (3) a structured approach to the immediate postoperative care, including pain relief and nutrition, and (4) early mobilization.

Within the urologic literature, ERAS for RC has faced criticism for overreliance on retrospective evidence, use of higher level but not necessarily applicable colorectal data, and inconsistent application of enhanced recovery principles across protocols [14]. Most studies examining enhanced recovery for RC have been nonrandomized, small, and retrospective. In this chapter, we review the current evidence for using an enhanced recovery protocol for RC.

Table 1 Preoperative aspects of ERAS for radical cystectomy

Preoperative ERAS elements
Patient counseling and education • Provide leaflets or multimedia information • Set expectations • Discharge planning • Stoma education
Preoperative medical optimization • Optimize medical diseases • Encourage smoking and alcohol cessation • Physical conditioning (prehab) • Improve nutritional status
Avoid mechanical bowel preparation
Avoid fasting
Carbohydrate loading
Alvimopan administration
Pre-anesthetic medication • Avoid long active sedatives
Thromboembolic prophylaxis • Low-molecular weight or unfragmented heparin • Compression stockings and intermittent pneumatic compression devices

2 Preoperative ERAS Elements

At the core of any ERAS protocol is good communication between the patient, urologist, urology stoma nurse specialist, anesthetist, and general practitioner. Before proceeding with RC with any patient, it is important to identify patients at high risk of postoperative morbidity, as it helps guide the risk versus benefit ratio of operative intervention and furthermore determine their postoperative care requirements. One should perform a thorough history and identify preexisting cardiovascular and respiratory disease by simple self-assessment questionnaires. These can be used to measure a patient's functional capacity and get a rough estimate of a patient's peak oxygen uptake. One metabolic equivalent (MET) represents the oxygen consumption of an adult at rest (i.e., 3.5 ml/kg/min), and varying degrees of exercise are designated a number of METs. Patients being considered for major surgery should be able to perform >4 METs, which is roughly the equivalent exertion of climbing one flight of stairs [18] (Table 1).

2.1 Preoperative Counseling and Education

There is no evidence that preoperative patient information and counseling improves outcomes after RC [17]. However, detailed information given to patients preoperatively may diminish fear and anxiety and enhance postoperative recovery and accelerate hospital discharge [19, 20]. Personal counseling, leaflets, or multimedia information containing explanations of the procedure along with tasks that the patient should be encouraged to fulfill may improve perioperative feeding, early postoperative mobilization, pain control, and respiratory physiotherapy [21–24]. In the colorectal literature, lack of adequate preoperative stoma education has been shown to be an independent risk factor for delayed discharge in patients on ERAS pathways [25]. Additionally, the patient should be actively engaged by preoperatively meeting members of the entire surgical team [26].

2.2 Preoperative Medical Optimization

Optimization of medical diseases (diabetes, hypertension, and anemia) along with physical exercise and cessation of smoking, drugs, or alcohol are preoperative conditioning measures that have been identified as reducing post RC complication [12, 27]. Alcohol abusers have a two-to-threefold increase in postoperative morbidity with the most frequent complications being bleeding, wound complications, and cardiopulmonary complications. One month of preoperative abstinence reduces postoperative morbidity by improving organ function [28, 29]. Another patient factor that has a negative influence on recovery is smoking. Current smokers have an increased risk for postoperative pulmonary and wound complications [30]. One month of abstinence from smoking is required to reduce the incidence of complications [30, 31]. However, aside from a retrospective cohort analysis identifying most of these risk factors, there is no other available evidence in urologic literature showing that their correction improves outcome [12, 17].

Physical conditioning (prehab) and muscle training may improve recovery rates. Several randomized controlled trials across various surgical fields (general abdominal surgery, cardiothoracic surgery, and orthopedic surgery) have investigated the role of preoperative physical conditioning on surgical outcomes [32–38]. Although there were varying degrees of improvement in physiological function and surgical recovery, only one study found improvement in physiological function that correlated with improved surgical recovery [24].

Studies have also demonstrated correlation between markers of malnutrition and adverse outcomes in RC [39]. In a dataset of patients undergoing gastrointestinal cancer surgery, poor nutritional status was directly correlated with extended LOS and increased risk of complications [40]. In RC patients, Gregg et al. reported nutritional deficiencies in almost 20% of patients and suggested severely malnourished patients should be treated for 10–14 days prior to surgery in order to decrease complications, even if surgical delay is implied [39]. Treatment to improve preoperative nutrition status includes nutritional supplements and immune-enhancing nutritional supplements (arginine, glutamine, nucleic acid, omega-3 fatty acids, antioxidants), which allow for the up-regulation of pro- and anti-inflammatory compounds. Bertrand and colleagues demonstrated that seven days of oral immune nutritional support intake preoperatively reduced postoperative complications, LOS, postoperative ileus, and pyelonephritis in RC patients [41].

2.3 Oral Mechanical Bowel Preparation

In colonic surgery, mechanical bowel preparation can dehydrate patients and cause electrolyte imbalance, physiological stress, and prolonged ileus. A meta-analysis including 5000 patients undergoing elective colorectal surgery identified no benefits for performing mechanical bowel preparation, concluding mechanical bowel preparation may be associated with greater morbidity, particularly anastomotic leakage and wound complications [42].

In the urologic literature, Tahibi and colleagues prospectively found no difference in morbidity or LOS when comparing 32 RC without bowel prep to 30 patients that had undergone standard 3-day mechanical bowel prep [43]. Similarly, Xu et al. found no statistical difference in morbidity, LOS, or time to first bowel movement by randomizing 86 patients [44]. Other randomized controlled trials in urologic literature have shown no differences in recovery of bowel function, time to discharge, or overall complication rates despite differences in design and heterogeneity of the "no bowel prep" arm (no bowel prep versus limited bowel versus enema only) [45, 46]. Currently, there is a lack of evidence from large randomized controlled trials to support using bowel preparation in RC patients.

2.4 Preoperative Fasting

Fasting from midnight has been standard practice in the belief that this secures an empty stomach and thereby reduces the risk of pulmonary aspiration in elective surgery. However, there has never been any scientific evidence behind this dogma. A Cochrane review of 22 RCTs showed that fasting from midnight neither reduce gastric content nor raises the pH of gastric fluid compared with patients allowed free intake of clear fluids until 2 h before anesthesia for surgery [47]. Equally, intake of clear fluids >2 h before surgery does not increase the prevalence of complications. Based on available evidence, the European Anesthesia Guidelines state that clear fluids are permitted up to 2 h and solids foods up to 6 h before the induction of anesthesia [48].

2.5 Preoperative Carbohydrate Loading

While there is no study evaluating carbohydrate loading in RC patients, it has been shown that such preoperative loading decreases thirst, reduces insulin resistance, and helps maintain lean body mass and muscle strength in colorectal surgery [27]. A meta-analysis of preoperative liquid carbohydrate treatment in open abdominal surgery patients revealed a significant reduction in LOS compared with controls [49]. In a double-blinded randomized controlled trial, Hausel and colleagues demonstrated reduced incidence of postoperative nausea and vomiting in patients receiving carbohydrate loading [50]. In summary, carbohydrate loading is a standard-of-care technique in ERAS programs that is safe in diabetic populations and can be given up to 2 h before surgery [51].

2.6 Preoperative Alvimopan Administration

As the most common complication following RC, postoperative ileus is a particular focus of ERAS protocols. Postoperative ileus can impair a patient's nutritional status, increase the probability of morbidity, and increase LOS as well as costs [6, 7, 12, 52, 53]. The use of alvimopan has been associated with a reduced LOS and faster recovery of bowel function after abdominal surgery and RC [54, 55]. In the urologic literature, one of the few randomized controlled trials evaluating an individual component of enhanced recovery following cystectomy was recently published by Lee et al. regarding the use of alvimopan (a peripherally acting μ-opioid receptor antagonist) and its impact on bowel recovery [55]. In this multicenter randomized controlled trial, the alvimopan cohort had a shorter LOS (7.4 vs. 10.1 days), passed a bowel movement more quickly (5.5 vs. 6.8 days), and had 20% fewer episodes of postoperative ileus-related morbidity (nasogastric tube reinsertion, prolonged stay, or readmission due to ileus). It should be noted that the study included a high proportion of patients who underwent open RC, as minimally invasive surgery using multimodal analgesia has shown lower morphine requirements than open surgery [56, 57]. However, positive effects of alvimopan administration in minimally invasive surgery have also been demonstrated. In a series of 117 patients undergoing robotic RC, Tobis and colleagues showed alvimopan administration appeared to reduce the time to return of bowel function (5 vs. 6 days) and initiation of diet (6 vs. 7 days) following robotic RC [58].

2.7 Pre-anesthetic Medication

A large proportion of patients are undergoing RC experience perioperative psychological distress [59]. Preoperative education can reduce patient anxiety to an acceptable level without the need for anxiolytic medication. However if pre-medication with anxiolytics is required, long-acting sedative pre-medication should be avoided, especially in elderly patients, for up to 4 h post-surgery as it affects immediate postoperative recovery by impairing mobility and oral intake [17, 27]. Short-acting benzodiazepines such as midazolam are preferred, if necessary, to reduce anxiety and facilitate patient positioning [17, 27].

2.8 Thromboembolic Prophylaxis

Currently, no randomized control trial or prospective study has compared complication rates with and without deep vein thrombosis prophylaxis in RC patients. However, as the incidence of clinically significant deep vein thrombosis after cystectomy is estimated at 4%, thromboembolic prophylaxis using low-molecular weight or unfragmented heparin should be used to reduce the risk of symptomatic thrombosis [60]. Additionally, compressive stockings and intermittent pneumatic compression devices can further decrease this risk.

Regarding the duration of thromboembolic prophylaxis in the postoperative setting, Bergqvist and colleagues observed a significant decrease in the post-hospitalization venous thromboembolism rate among abdominal and pelvic surgical oncology cases in which low-molecular-weight heparin prophylaxis was continued for 19–21 days after a standard in-house anticoagulation regimen compared with placebo [61].

3 Intraoperative ERAS Elements

The intraoperative period is a critical time in the ERAS pathway, with specific considerations from both the anesthetic and surgical perspectives (Table 2).

3.1 Antimicrobial Prophylaxis and Skin Preparation

As cystectomy is considered a "clean-contaminated" surgery, antibiotic prophylaxis for patients undergoing RC should cover against aerobic and anaerobic organisms. The European Association of Urology guidelines suggest that antibiotics should be administered no earlier than 1 h before surgery and continued for up to 24 h and extending to 72 h for patients with specific infection risk factors or prolonged operations (>3 h). The National Surgical Infection Prevention Project also advised that antibiotics should be administered before skin incision and less than 1 h before surgery [62]. Although the best antibiotic regimen is unclear and likely depends on local antibiotic-resistance profiles, the American Urological Association guidelines recommend a second-generation or third-generation cephalosporin or a combination of gentamicin and metronidazole for 24 h perioperatively if there are no patient risk factors.

Regarding the optimal skin preparation, several ERAS guidelines recommend skin preparation prior to surgery using a chlorhexidine–alcohol scrub to prevent surgical site infections (SSIs) [17, 27]. A study comparing different types of skin

Table 2 Intraoperative aspects of ERAS for radical cystectomy

Intraoperative ERAS elements
Antibiotic prophylaxis and skin preparation
Anesthetic protocols • Use of thoracic epidural • Neural blockade • Minimal opioid use • Prevention of intraoperative hypothermia • Individualized goal-directed fluid therapy
Minimize incision (minimally invasive approach)
Drain strategy

cleansing showed that the overall prevalence of surgical site infection was 40% lower in a concentrated chlorhexidine–alcohol group than in a povidone-iodine group [63]. However, there is a risk of fire-based injuries and burn injuries if diathermy is used in the presence of alcohol-based skin solutions [64].

3.2 Anesthetic Protocols

Evidence from colorectal and RC studies suggest that ERAS anesthetic protocols should encompass the use of thoracic epidural (T9-11), minimal opioid use, replacing it with fentanyl-based short-acting opioids, and strategies for prevention of hypothermia, hypoxemia, and hypovolemia [65].

No prospective single-intervention study has been conducted to assess epidural analgesia in the perioperative management of RC; however, there has been strong evidence shown in open colorectal surgery that epidural analgesia reduces the stress response to surgery, provides superior pain relief, reduces postoperative complications, and accelerates functional recovery [66]. In colorectal surgery, the administration of thoracic epidural anesthesia is widely recommended to reduce LOS and postoperative ileus compared with patient-controlled analgesia [27] (Table 3).

Recent ERAS society cystectomy recommendations strongly encourage the use of a thoracic epidural for 72 h after surgery, as the benefits listed are key components in delivering an effective ERAS protocol [17]. Epidural analgesia in combination with paracetamol and nonsteroidal anti-inflammatories (where there are no contraindications) reduces and often removes the need for systemic opioid analgesia, and its associated side effects of bowel dysfunction, respiratory depression, and nausea [18]. In open RC, various studies have demonstrated the successful use of epidural anesthesia or patient-controlled analgesia and rectus sheath catheters; however, no prospective studies have compared these anesthetic protocols in RC surgeries [26, 67–69].

Table 3 Postoperative aspects of ERAS for radical cystectomy

Postoperative ERAS elements
Avoid postoperative nasogastric intubation
Early oral intake
Early mobilization
Ureteral stenting
Gum chewing
Multimodal opioid-sparing analgesia combined with regional or local anesthesia
Discharge planning

3.3 Prevention of Intraoperative Hypothermia

Perioperative hypothermia (core body temperature of less than 36 °C), which is common during major surgery, may promote surgical wound infection by triggering thermoregulatory vasoconstriction [70]. This subsequently decreases subcutaneous oxygen tension and reduces the strength of the healing wound by reducing the deposition of collagen. Hypothermia also directly impairs immune function. In colorectal surgery, avoiding intraoperative hypothermia has shown to decrease the incidence of infectious complications, help protect against perioperative coagulopathy, and reduce LOS [26, 70]. Given the similar physiopathology resulting in impaired thermoregulation in cystectomy procedures, maintaining normothermia is strongly warranted [17]. The most effective warming strategies are forced-air warming blankets and warmed IV fluids [70].

3.4 Perioperative Fluid Management

Fluid management in patients undergoing RC can be challenging as urine output is often not measurable intraoperatively. Both fluid excess and hypovolemia can provoke splanchnic hypoperfusion, which can then result in ileus, increased morbidity and longer LOS [71]. Primary research efforts in perioperative care have focused on determination of what constitutes optimal fluid management during surgery.

Goal-directed fluid therapy (GDFT) using cardiac output monitors, such as a transesophageal Doppler device to guide fluid and inotropic therapy, is one such strategy. Used in conjunction with invasive arterial pressure monitoring and central mixed venous oxygen saturation from a central venous pressure line, intraoperative individualized fluid therapy aims to optimize cardiac output, and therefore tissue perfusion and oxygenation. By optimizing blood flow to tissues, GDFT aims to improve gut perfusion thereby reducing the incidence of hypoperfusion and therefore occult bowel ischemia and postoperative ileus and allows the anesthetists a better guide as to how the patient is responding to the significant fluid shifts that occur during major surgery [71].

In colorectal surgery, GDFT has been shown to improve outcomes and reduce complication rates and LOS [71, 72]. However, these studies evaluated GDFT against standard fluid management techniques, and the comparison groups often had fluid overload or unwarranted restrictions [71, 72]. In a small randomized controlled trial, Pillai and colleagues investigated the effects of GDFT in RC patients and concluded that patients who underwent GDFT had a reduced incidence of ileus and of nausea and vomiting at 24 and 48 h [73]. Large prospective studies are needed in urology to compare restricted, balanced, and GDFT in patients undergoing RC. However, it is reasonable to assume that patients undergoing major or high-risk surgery need a dedicated, individualized goal-directed fluid management run by an experienced anesthetist to ensure adequate tissue perfusion, and a Doppler-guided strategy may prove a valuable adjunct in these cases [17].

3.5 Minimally Invasive Approach

Another factor contributing to the morbidity of RC is the complexity of the procedure itself. It involves multiple surgeries in one: deep pelvic dissection to remove the bladder, lymphadenectomy, and extensive bowel manipulation for the urinary diversion. With the majority of RC being performed by high-volume surgeons, innovation in surgical performance has focused on operative approach (robotic versus open). By offering a minimally invasive surgery over an open approach, the hope is to decrease the patients' inflammatory response and reduce the risk of postoperative ileus, complications, and duration of hospital stay. Robotic surgery, however, is not without its physiological challenges. It requires a prolonged period of steep Trendelenburg position, together with pneumoperitoneum, **and** can produce dramatic physiological derangement, particularly in the elderly populations with multiple comorbidities who present for RC.

First reported in 2003 as a feasible approach, robotic RC requires smaller incisions, reduces analgesic use, reduces bowel handling, and decreases blood loss [57, 74]. A recent meta-analysis comparing open to robotic RC found robotic RC was associated with less blood loss and shorter LOS [75]. However, open RC demonstrated a clear advantage to robotic RC in terms of reduced operating time. The International Robotic Cystectomy Consortium reported on over 1000 patients and demonstrated 30-day complication rate of 41% (61% were low-grade complications) with similar oncological outcomes to the open approach and dependent on surgeon's experience [76]. Three randomized trials have been published comparing open RC with robotic RC, with strikingly similar results to each other [57, 77, 78]. Robotic RC has been shown to improve some perioperative parameters such as estimated blood loss and LOS, but in all three studies no significant differences were found in complication rates. A systematic review comparing RARC with ORC similarly concluded that although RARC can be performed safely, complication rates remain significant [79].

When looking at oncologic outcomes of the minimally invasive approach, Yuh and colleagues performed a systematic review of over 100 papers and found 5-year oncologic outcomes similar between robotic RC and open RC [80]. Additionally, Snow-Lisy and colleagues reported on a cohort of 120 patients with 10-year follow-up and proved no differences in overall survival, cancer-specific survival, and recurrence-free survival when comparing the minimally invasive RC approach to the open approach [81].

Another variable often thought to contribute to complications and readmissions of RC is the type of urinary diversion the patients receives. Choice of urinary diversion depends largely on oncological eligibility, patient comorbidities, surgeon preference, and patient preference. Nazmy and colleagues stratified complications by urinary diversion type in robotic RC patients, and despite the selection of a more comorbid population for ileal conduit diversion, patients with ileal conduit diversion had a decreased likelihood of complications compared to patients with Indiana pouch and orthotopic bladder substitute diversion [82]. However, other studies have shown comparable rates of 90-day complication rates between ileal conduits and neobladders, suggesting the choice of diversion may contribute less to the morbidity of the procedure than previously thought [83–85]. However, the impact of the choice of urinary diversion remains to be completely defined.

It aims to further reduce the invasiveness of the procedure, intracorporeal urinary diversion (ICUD) has been performed in certain centers. Early, small studies comparing ICUD with extracorporeal urinary diversion have it to be safe and suggest less gastrointestinal complications and less overall 90-day complications [86]. However, the consortium paper had notable limitations including its retrospective, non-uniform data collection; lack of complication/readmission data in 118 patients (12.6%); and that the majority of ICUDs were ileal conduits which may have confounded results with regard to gastrointestinal and overall complications. Overall, ICUD remains a challenging aspect of the robotic RC procedure and should remain in the hands of a few very high-volume centers.

Despite the inclusion of the minimally invasive approach in the ERAS Society guidelines published by Cerantola and colleagues [17], the superiority of robotic versus open cystectomy remains to be demonstrated definitively. Future high-quality, high-volume randomized, controlled studies such as the prospective randomized open versus robotic cystectomy (RAZOR) trial examining this question is accruing and should help in reaching definitive conclusions on the role of robotic RC [87].

3.6 Resection Site Drainage

Regardless of the surgical approach, the use of intraabdominal drains continues to be debated. In colorectal surgery, meta-analyses have concluded that intraabdominal drains confer no benefits in terms of anastomotic dehiscence, wound infection, reoperation, extra-abdominal complications, or mortality [88]. For RC and urinary reconstruction, even though observational studies have shown no detriment to omission or early removal of the drain, or to shortening the drain into a stoma bag [4, 89, 90], the subject remains controversial given the risk of urinary leakage within the peritoneal cavity.

4 Postoperative ERAS Elements

Historically, RC patients were kept nothing by mouth, with a nasogastric tube (NGT), bedbound, and had a prolonged hospital stay. However, with ERAS, almost the direct opposite has become the standard of care, owing to the consideration of a number of postoperative factors.

4.1 Urinary Drainage

In a small randomized controlled trial, Mattei and colleagues investigated the effect of time-to-stent removal in ileal bladder substitute and ileal conduit patients [91]. The study compared patients whose stents were removed directly following ureteroileal anastomosis with those whose stents were removed 5–10 days after surgery. Stenting was associated with improved upper tract drainage, lower postoperative ileus, and reduced rate of metabolic acidosis [91]. However, the best time for removal of a ureteric drain/stent after RC has not been clearly established [26].

4.2 Nasogastric Intubation

Many centers now remove NGTs at the end of surgery in RC cases, to avoid delayed gastric emptying, nausea, and vomiting that would otherwise delay patient mobilization and therefore participation in an ERAS protocol. Extrapolation is possible from level 1a evidence relating to colorectal surgery to show NGTs are not only unnecessary, but also detrimental. In a meta-analysis of 33 randomized controlled trials including 5240 patients on the use of NGT decompression after abdominal surgery, patients not having routine NGT use had an earlier return of bowel function ($p < 0.00001$) and decrease in pulmonary complications ($p = 0.01$). [92] Although most data are associated with colorectal surgery, numerous reports suggest relevance to urological procedures [93, 94].

4.3 Prevention of Postoperative Ileus

With respect to the prevention of postoperative ileus, specific treatments such as preoperative alvimopan, fluid monitoring, performing a minimally invasive approach, and ureteral stenting have already been discussed in this review. Gum chewing is a form of sham feeding that has been studied specifically in the context of open and robotic RC in two trials that showed a significantly decreased time to flatus and first bowel motion in both open and robotic groups with gum chewing [95, 96]. Despite these findings, there was no significant difference in LOS and postoperative complications. Nonetheless, gum chewing should be started on postoperative day 1 and continued through the hospital course in order to reduce postoperative ileus.

Prokinetic agents, such as erythromycin and metoclopramide, have shown no benefit in decreasing time to flatus or first bowel movement [97, 98]. However, in light of this evidence, metoclopramide was removed from one of the most established ERAS protocols for RC, resulting in a significant increase in postoperative nausea and vomiting and prompting its reinstitution to facilitate tolerance of early enteral intake [99, 100].

Prophylactic oral laxatives have been recommended after surgery, as they are associated with an earlier return to normal bowel function and a reduction in time to defecation [17, 27, 101]. However, no prospective studies have systematically evaluated the benefits of oral laxatives in colorectal or urological surgery with or without the use of ERAS pathways [26].

4.4 Early Feeding

Contrary to conventional surgical dogma that feeding should begin only after the return of bowel function (passage of flatus or stool), early feeding can reduce insulin resistance, with beneficial effects on muscle function, wound healing, and sepsis [102]. Although no evidence supporting an early oral diet exists for RC specifically, Behrns and colleagues found that beginning an oral diet with clear liquids on postoperative day 2 and progressing quickly to a regular diet decreased LOS without increasing postoperative morbidity in elective intestinal surgery [103]. Similarly, Fearon and colleagues used a multimodal approach, including early oral feeding postoperatively, carbohydrate and fluid loading preoperatively, and decreased LOS from 10 days to 7 days in patients undergoing elective colorectal surgery [104]. Additionally, a meta-analysis of major abdominal surgery (not including RC) concluded that pneumonia, anastomotic dehiscence, wound infection, and mortality were all less likely with early feeding. Secondary end points, including time to flatus, time to bowel motion, and LOS, were all also improved by early feeding [105]. Given the evidence presented above, prevalence of malnutrition in patients undergoing RC, and lack of evidence against it, early oral feeding should be encouraged postoperatively. However, a risk of early postoperative oral intake is vomiting, and active interventions, such as scheduled anti-emetics, chewing gum, cholinergic stimulants, laxatives, prokinetic agents, and limitations on narcotic administration, must be instituted alongside early oral intake to prevent postoperative nausea and vomiting.

In addition to early feeding, postoperatively intravenous fluid should be minimized to prevent fluid overload and bowel edema [100]. If normovolemic hypotension is seen with thoracic epidural anesthesia, it should be corrected with vasopressors instead of intravenous fluid [106]. However, if parenteral fluids are needed, balanced crystalloid such as Ringer's lactate solution should be used instead of normal saline to protect against electrolyte disruption (i.e., hyperchloremic metabolic acidosis) [107].

4.5 Postoperative Analgesia

With the aim of providing effective pain relief and minimizing adverse effects, especially those that are associated with opioids, multimodal opioid-sparing analgesia combined with regional or local anesthesia is a key component of ERAS. The use of thoracic epidural analgesia with wound infiltration or rectus sheath cannulas is recommended for 24–72 h post-surgery [108]. Ventham and colleagues reported that subfascial wound catheter placement significantly improved analgesia and diminished opioid requirements [109].

The use of regular intravenous or oral paracetamol as well as nonsteroid anti-inflammatories (NSAIDs) have been a well-documented aspect of many RC ERAS protocols [67–69]. Specifically, the NSAID ketorolac, when used in conjunction with morphine, has been found to decrease the rate of postoperative ileus by over fivefold in a series of colorectal surgery patients [104]. However, concerns exist regarding the cardiac toxicity and anastomotic dehiscence with NSAID use [110, 111].

Overall, few studies (and no prospective studies) have examined the adaptation of multimodal opioid-sparing analgesia to RC, and in the future, randomized controlled trials are needed to compare the effects of these pain medications on RC patients.

4.6 Early Mobility

Appropriate analgesia facilitates early postoperative mobility, which in turn may counteract insulin resistance, reduce thromboembolic events and chest infection rates, increase muscle strength, and possibly reduce ileus [27, 112]. In an ERAS series of laparoscopic colorectal surgery patients, it was shown that early mobilization was associated with improved outcomes and lack of adherence to early mobilization protocols was associated with longer LOS [113]. Recently, Jensen and colleagues showed that in a population of 57 RC patients, increased mobilization can improve the ability of patients to perform activities of daily living [114]. However, no ERAS studies on exclusively RC patients suggest that early mobilization plays a role in decreased morbidity or LOS following surgery. Nonetheless, early ambulation is widely practiced in established RC ERAS protocols. In a review of 10 single-center studies, early mobilization was the only intervention unanimously used by the reviewed centers [14].

4.7 Discharge Criteria

ERAS programs recommend that discharge should only occur when patients have resumed adequate oral intake and normal bowel function with effective oral pain management and when no other clinical or biochemical concerns remain, including stoma or neobladder competency [26]. In regard to stoma care, nurse specialists play a key role in engaging patient participation in the initial perioperative period. One center reported that early visits, from day one, ensure patients feel supported in coming to terms with the appearance of their stoma, and from day two, patients are encouraged to engage in their stoma care, for example changing the stoma pouch

[115]. After discharge, patients should feel well supported and routine telephone consultation, as well as the provision of an emergency patient hotline, has been suggested as a standard of care [89, 90].

4.8 Quality of Life

Quality of life measures have not always been documented with conventional care. Within ERAS protocols, some have evaluated their impact on quality of life [116, 117]. In a systematic review of various abdominal surgeries (not including cystectomy), Stowers et al. observed no improvements in quality of life, between ERAS and standard of care [116]. However, Karl and colleagues randomized patients to conventional care or ERAS for RC patients and assessed outcomes according to European Organization for Research and Treatment of Cancer (EORTC) quality of life (QLQ-30) questionnaires [117]. When analyzing the emotional functioning score exclusively, they found a stable score during hospitalization in the conventional care group, whereas continuous improvement was found in the ERAS group. In RC patients, this study was the first of its kind demonstrating an emotional benefit for patients undergoing an ERAS protocol [117].

5 Future Considerations for ERAS

As previously mentioned, ERAS for RC has faced criticism for overreliance on retrospective evidence, use of higher level but not necessarily applicable colorectal data, and inconsistent application of enhanced recovery principles across protocols [14]. In a summary of the current evidence behind ERAS for RC, Cerantola and colleagues proposed 22 core ERAS elements, and of those 22 elements, the highest quality evidence came from the colorectal literature [17]. Given the oncological, procedural (prolonged extent and duration of spillage of urine as well bowel contents within the peritoneal cavity), and morbidity differences between colorectal and cystectomy surgery, there is an urgent need to evaluate ERAS pathways in patients undergoing urological surgery, specifically RC.

Several groups have published the results of their proposed ERAS protocols in RC (Table 4) [4, 52, 69, 90, 99, 117–126]. Although most demonstrate improved postoperative recovery for patients, the ERAS protocols themselves are quite varied with only a small portion of series implementing more than 50% of the 22 recommended ERAS principles. The inconsistency in enhanced recovery protocols in urology has led to some confusion as to which elements of these protocols are truly necessary and which make the biggest difference for patients' recoveries after RC. Nonetheless, the interventions used most frequently (in >50% of studies) in most published series includes the circumvention of mechanical bowel preparation and routine NGT placement, preoperative carbohydrates loading, the use of epidural

Table 4 Recent publications on enhanced recovery after surgery (ERAS) protocols for radical cystectomy (RC)

Series	Year	Study type	Comparative control group included	Number of ERAS patients	Robotic RC included	Number of ERAS items
Maffezzini et al. [52]	2007	Retrospective	No	68	No	9
Arumainayagam et al. [119]	2008	Retrospective	Yes	56	No	9
Pruthi et al. [100]	2010	Retrospective	No	100	No	8
Saar et al. [120]	2013	Prospective	Yes	31	Yes	9
Mukhtar et al. [4]	2013	Prospective	Yes	51	No	14
Daneshmand et al. [69]	2014	Prospective	Yes (Historical)	110	No	11
Dutton et al. [90]	2014	Retrospective	No	165	No	19
Guan et al. [121]	2014	Retrospective	Yes	60	No	7
Karl et al. [118]	2014	Prospective	Yes (RCT)	62	No	7
Smith et al. [91]	2014	Retrospective	Yes	64	No	7
Cerruto et al. [122]	2014	Prospective	No	31	No	17
Persson et al. [123]	2015	Retrospective	Yes	31	No	13
Koupparis et al. [124]	2015	Retrospective	Yes	102	Yes	10
Xu et al. [125]	2015	Retrospective	Yes	124	No	17
Collins et al. [126]	2016	Prospective	Yes	135	Yes	20
Chipollini et al. [127]	2017	Retrospective	Yes	112	No	11

RCT—randomized controlled trial

analgesia, thromboembolic and antimicrobial prophylaxis, opioid-sparing analgesia, judicious fluid management, prevention of intraoperative hypothermia, early mobilization and early oral feeding. In addition, several protocols require a fair measure of coordination on the part of the clinical care team to ensure compliance. For example, Daneshmand and colleagues were able to decrease LOS from 8 to 4 days without impacting complication rates (65% vs. 64%) or readmissions (21% vs. 18%) in a series of 126 ERAS patients after RC. However, the protocol involved measures such as paraincisional subfascial catheters for continuous local anesthesia, and coordination for patients to receive 1 L intravenous fluid every other day after hospital discharge to preempt dehydration (a common cause for readmission after RC). Such elements may be difficult to reproduce with 100% compliance.

ERAS protocols have been adopted in many surgical specialties, particularly colorectal surgery, with improvements in mortality and morbidity. However, urologists have been slower to embrace ERAS than other surgical subspecialties. A survey was sent to Society of Urologic Oncology members with a self-identified special interest in bladder cancer, asking whether they consider themselves ERAS adapters and inquiring specifically about adherence to seven components of virtually all ERAS protocols (comprehensive preoperative education, bowel preparation avoidance, NGT avoidance, intraoperative normothermia, opioid avoidance, early ambulation, and early feeding) [127]. While nearly half of the bladder cancer surgeons contacted responded to the survey, and 64% of respondents considered themselves to adhere to ERAS principles for RC, only 20% practiced all 7 interventions. The most commonly cited reasons for non-adopting ERAS protocols were the lack of convincing evidence, the belief that ERAS does not work, and lack of institutional support. With the exception of specific medications whose availability or ease of use may differ by hospital, adopting ERAS principles (like omitting a bowel preparation or avoiding opioid analgesics) requires a change in practice patterns. The successful implementation of an ERAS program requires full commitment and support of the involved parties and to convince urologists to change their long-established ways for taking care of some of their sickest patients. There will need to be a high-quality, prospective study to provide convincing evidence of the utility of ERAS for RC [14].

6 Conclusion

In summary, even with the limitations of ERAS regarding the generalizability of urologic evidence, a tipping point is being reached where it is hard to deny the growing evidence showing that ERAS protocols have a positive impact on patient recovery. However, it remains to be determined exactly which elements of ERAS have the most substantial impact. In the future, high-quality prospective, randomized controlled multicenter studies where components can be isolated or added sequentially are needed to validate the different elements of ERAS protocols.

References

1. Siegel R, Naishadham D, Jemal A (2013) Cancer statistics. CA Cancer J Clin 63:11–30
2. Gellert C, Scho B (2015) Smoking and all-cause mortality in older people. Arch Intern Med 172:837–844
3. Skeldon SC, Goldenberg SL (2015) Bladder cancer: a portal into men's health. Urol Oncol 33:40–44
4. Mukhtar S, Ayres BE, Issa R, Swinn MJ, Perry MJA (2013) Challenging boundaries: an enhanced recovery program for radical cystectomy. Ann R Coll Surg Engl 95:200–206

5. HCUP Nationwide Inpatient Sample (NIS). Healthcare Cost and Utilization Project (HCUP). Rockville, MD: Agency for Healthcare Research and Quality, 2011. www.hcup-us.ahrq.gov/nisoverview.jsp
6. Chang SS, Cookson MS, Baumgartner RG, Wells N, Smith JA Jr (2002) Analysis of early complications after radical cystectomy: results of a collaborative care pathway. J Urol 167:2012–2016
7. Shabsigh A, Korets R, Vora KC et al (2009) Defining early morbidity of radical cystectomy for subjects with bladder cancer using a standardized reporting methodology. Eur Urol 55:164–174
8. Yuh BE, Nazmy M, Ruel NH et al (2012) Standardized analysis of frequency and severity of complications after robot-assisted radical cystectomy. Eur Urol 6:806–813
9. Musch M, Janowski M, Steves A et al (2014) Comparison of early postoperative morbidity after robot-assisted and open radical cystectomy: results of a prospective observational study. Brit J Urol 113:458–467
10. Stimson CJ, Chang SS, Barocas DA et al (2010) Early and late perioperative outcomes follow radical cystectomy: 90-day readmissions, morbidity and mortality in a contemporary series. J Urol 184:1296–1300
11. Clark PE, Stein PJ, Groshen SG et al (2005) Radical cystectomy in the elderly. Cancer 103:546–552
12. Hollembeck BK, Miller DC, Taub D et al (2005) Identifying risk factors for potentially avoidable complications following radical cystectomy. J Urol 174:1231–1237
13. Kim SP, Shah ND, Karnes J et al (2012) The implications of hospital acquired adverse events on mortality, length of stay and costs for patients undergoing radical cystectomy for bladder cancer. J Urol 187:2011–2017
14. Danna BJ, Wood EL, Kukreja JEB, Shah JB (2016) The future of enhanced recovery for radical cystectomy: current evidence, barriers to adoption, and the next steps. Urology 96:62–68
15. Kehlet H, Wilmore DW (2002) Multimodal strategies to improve surgical outcome. Am J Surg 183:630
16. Kehlet H (1997) Multimodal approach to control postoperative pathophysiology and rehabilitation. Br J Anaesth 78:606–617
17. Cerantola Y, Valerio M, Persson B et al (2013) Guidelines for perioperative care after radical cystectomy for bladder cancer: Enhanced Recovery After Surgery (ERAS(®)) Society recommendations. Clin Nutr 32:879–887
18. Frith C, Wakelam J, Vasdev N, et al (2014) The role of an enhanced recovery protocol in patients undergoing robotic radical cystectomy. Urology 2014
19. Kiecolt-Glaser JK, Page GG, Marucha PT, MacCallum RC, Glaser R (1998) Psychological influences on surgical recovery perspectives from psychoneuroimmunology. Am Psychol 53 (11):1209–1218
20. Egbert LD, Battit GE, Welch CE, Bartlett MK (1964) Reduction of postoperative pain by encouragement and instruction of patients. A study of doctor-patient rapport. N Engl J Med 270:825–827
21. Halaszynski TM, Juda R, Silverman DG (2004) Optimizing postoperative outcomes with efficient preoperative assessment and management. Crit Care Med 32:S76–S86
22. Forster AJ, Clark HD, Menard A et al (2005) Effect of a nurse team coordinator on outcomes for hospitalized medicine patients. Am J Med 118(10):1148–1153
23. Disbrow EA, Bennett HL, Owings JT (1993) Effect of preoperative suggestion on postoperative gastrointestinal motility. West J Med 158(5):488–492
24. Gustafsson UO, Scott MJ, Schwenk W et al (2012) Guidelines for perioperative care in elective colonic surgery: enhanced after surgery (ERAS) Society recommendations. Clin Nutr 31:783–800

25. Smart NJ, White P, Allison AS, Ockrim JB, Kennedy RH, Francis NK (2012) Deviation and failure of enhanced recovery after surgery following laparoscopic colorectal surgery: early prediction model. Colorectal Dis 14(10):727–734
26. Azhar RA, Bochner B, Catto J et al (2016) Enhanced recovery after urological surgery: a contemporary systematic review of outcomes, key elements, and research needs. Eur Urol 70:176–187
27. Nygren J, Thacker J, Carli F et al (2013) Guidelines for perioperative care in elective rectal/pelvic surgery: enhanced recovery after surgery (ERAS) society recommendations. World J Surg 37:285–305
28. Tonnesen H, Kehlet H (1999) Preoperative alcoholism and postoperative morbidity. Br J Surg 86:869–874
29. Tonnesen H, Rosenberg J, Nielsen HJ, Rasmussen V, Hauge C, Pedersen IK et al (1999) Effect of preoperative abstinence on poor postoperative outcome in alcohol misusers: randomised controlled trial. BMJ 318(7194):1311–1316
30. Sorensen LT, Karlsmark T, Gottrup F (2003) Abstinence from smoking reduces incisional wound infection: a randomized controlled trial. Ann Surg 238:1–5
31. Lindstrom D, Sadr Azodi O, Wladis A, Tonnesen H, Linder S, Nasell H et al (2008) Effects of a perioperative smoking cessation intervention on postoperative complications: a randomized trial. Ann Surg 248:739–745
32. Arthur HM, Daniels C, McKelvie R, Hirsh J, Rush B (2000) Effect of a preoperative intervention on preoperative and postoperative outcomes in low-risk patients awaiting elective coronary artery bypass graft surgery. A randomized, controlled trial. Ann Intern Med 133:253–262
33. Carli F, Charlebois P, Stein B et al (2010) Randomized clinical trial of prehabilitation in colorectal surgery. Br J Surg 97(8):1187–1197
34. Dronkers JJ, Lamberts H, Reutelingsperger IM et al (2010) Preoperative therapeutic programme for elderly patients scheduled for elective abdominal oncological surgery: a randomized controlled pilot study. Clin Rehabil 24:614–622
35. Hoogeboom TJ, Dronkers JJ, van den Ende CH, Oosting E, van Meeteren NL (2010) Preoperative therapeutic exercise in frail elderly scheduled for total hip replacement: a randomized pilot trial. Clin Rehabil 24:901–910
36. Hulzebos EH, Helders PJ, Favie NJ et al (2006) Preoperative intensive inspiratory muscle training to prevent postoperative pulmonary complications in high-risk patients undergoing CABG surgery: a randomized clinical trial. JAMA 296(15):1851–1857
37. Weiner P, Zeidan F, Zamir D, Pelled B, Waizman J, Beckerman M et al (1998) Prophylactic inspiratory muscle training in patients undergoing coronary artery bypass graft. World J Surg 22:427–431
38. Weidenhielm L, Mattsson E, Brostrom LA, Wersall-Robertsson E (1993) Effect of preoperative physiotherapy in unicompartmental prosthetic knee replacement. Scand J Rehabil Med 25:33–39
39. Gregg JR, Cookson MS, Phillips S et al (2011) Effect of preoperative nutritional deficiency on mortality after radical cystectomy for bladder cancer. J Urol 185:90–96
40. Garth AK, Newsome CM, Simmance N, Crowe TC (2010) Nutritional status, nutrition practices and post-operative complications in patients with gastrointestinal cancer. J Hum Nutr Diet 23:393–401
41. Bertrand J, Siegler N, Murez T et al (2014) Impact of preoperative immunonutrition on morbidity following cystectomy for bladder cancer: a case-control pilot study. World J Urol 32:233–237
42. Guenaga KF, Matos D, Castro AA, Atallah AN, Wille-Jorgensen P (2005) Mechanical bowel preparation for elective colorectal surgery. Cochrane Database Syst Rev CD001544
43. Tabibi A, Simforoosh N, Basiri A, Ezzatnejad M, Abdi H, Farrokhi F (2007) Bowel preparation versus no preparation before ileal urinary diversion. Urology 70:654–658

44. Xu R, Zhao X, Zhong Z, Zhang L (2010) No advantage is gained by preoperative bowel preparation in radical cystectomy and ileal conduit: a randomized controlled trial of 86 patients. Int Urol Nephrol 42:947–950
45. Raynor MC, Lavien G, Nielsen M, Wallen EM, Pruthi RS (2013) Elimination of preoperative mechanical bowel preparation in patients undergoing cystectomy and urinary diversion. Urol Oncol 31:32–35
46. Aslan G, Baltaci S, Akdogan B et al (2013) A prospective randomized multicenter study of Turkish Society of Urooncology comparing two different mechanical bowel preparation methods for radical cystectomy. Urol Oncol 31:664–670
47. Brady M, Kinn S, Stuart P (2003) Preoperative fasting for adults to prevent perioperative complications. Cochrane Database Syst Rev CD004423
48. Smith I, Kranke P, Murat I et al (2011) Perioperative fasting in adults and children: guidelines from the European society of anaesthesiology. Eur J Anaesthesiol 28:556–569
49. Awad S, Varadhan KK, Ljungqvist O, Lobo DN (2013) A meta-analysis of randomized controlled trials on preoperative oral carbohydrate treatment in elective surgery. Clin Nutr 32:34–44
50. Hausel J, Nygren J, Thorell A, Lagerkranser M, Ljungqvist O (2005) Randomized clinical trial of the effects of oral preoperative carbohydrates on postoperative nausea and vomiting after laparoscopic cholecystectomy. Br J Surg 92:415–421
51. Can MF, Yagci G, Dag B et al (2009) Preoperative administration of oral carbohydrate-rich solutions: comparison of glucometabolic responses and tolerability between patients with and without insulin resistance. Nutrition 25:72–77
52. Maffezzini M, Gerbi G, Campodonico F, Parodi D (2007) Multimodal perioperative plan for radical cystectomy and intestinal urinary diversion. I. Effect on recovery of intestinal function and occurrence of complications. Urology 69:1107–1111
53. Correia MITD, da Silva RG (2004) The impact of early nutrition on metabolic response and postoperative ileus. Curr Opin Clin Nutr Metab Care 7:577–583
54. Kauf TL, Svatek RS, Amiel G et al (2014) Alvimopan, a peripherally acting m-opioid receptor antagonist, is associated with reduced costs after radical cystectomy: economic analysis of a phase 4 randomized, controlled trial. J Urol 191:1721–1727
55. Lee C, Chang S, Kamat A et al (2014) Alvimopan accelerates gastrointestinal recovery after radical cystectomy: a multicenter randomized placebo-controlled trial. Eur Urol 66:265–272
56. Dutton TJ, McGrath JS, Daugherty MO (2014) Use of rectus sheath catheters for pain relief in patients undergoing major pelvic urological surgery. BJU Int 113:246–253
57. Nix J, Smith A, Kurpad R, Nielsen ME, Wallen EM, Pruthi RS (2010) Prospective randomized controlled trial of robotic versus open radical cystectomy for bladder cancer: perioperative and pathologic results. Eur Urol 57:196–201
58. Tobis S, Heinlen JE, Ruel N et al (2014) Effect of alvimopan on return of bowel function after robot-assisted radical cystectomy. J Laparoendosc Adv Surg Tech A 24:693–697
59. Palapattu GS, Haisfield-Wolfe ME, Walker JM et al (2004) Assessment of perioperative psychological distress in patients undergoing radical cystectomy for bladder cancer. J Urol 172:1814–1817
60. Tyson MD, Castle EP, Humphreys MR, Andrews PE (2014) Venous thromboembolism after urologic surgery. J Urol 192:793–797
61. Bergqvist D, Agnelli G, Cohen AT et al (2002) Duration of prophylaxis against venous thromboembolism with enoxaparin after surgery for cancer. N Engl J Med 346:975–980
62. Bratzler DW, Houck PM (2004) Antimicrobial prophylaxis for surgery: an advisory statement from the National Surgical Infection Prevention Project. Clin Infect Dis 38:1706–1715
63. Darouiche RO, Wall MJ Jr, Itani KM et al (2010) Chlorhexidine-Alcohol versus povidone-iodine for surgical-site antisepsis. N Engl J Med 362:18–26
64. Rocos B, Donaldson LJ (2012) Alcohol skin preparation causes surgical fires. Ann R Coll Surg Engl 94:87–89

65. Mir MC, Zargar H, Bolton DM, Murphy DG, Lawrentschuk N (2015) Enhanced recovery after surgery protocols for radical cystectomy surgery: review of current evidence and local protocols. ANZ J Surg 85:514–520
66. Carli F, Kehlet H, Baldinin G et al (2010) Evidence basis for regional anaesthesia in multi-disciplinary fast-track surgical pathways. Reg Anaesth Pain Med 36:63–72
67. Maffezzini M, Campodonico F, Canepa G, Gerbi G, Parodi D (2008) Current perioperative management of radical cystectomy with intestinal urinary reconstruction for muscle-invasive bladder cancer and reduction of the incidence of postoperative ileus. Surg Oncol 17:41–48
68. Pruthi RS, Chun J, Richman M (2003) Reducing time to oral diet and hospital discharge in patients undergoing radical cystectomy using a perioperative care plan. Urology 62:661–665
69. Daneshmand S, Ahmadi H, Schuckman AK et al (2014) Enhanced recovery protocol after radical cystectomy for bladder cancer. J Urol 192:50–55
70. Kurz A, Sessler DI, Lenhardt R (1996) Perioperative normothermia to reduce the incidence of surgical-wound infection and shorten hospitalization. study of wound infection and temperature group. N Engl J Med 334:1209–1215
71. Giglio MT, Marucci M, Testini M, Brienza N (2009) Goal-directed haemodynamic therapy and gastrointestinal complications in major surgery: a meta-analysis of randomized controlled trials. Br J Anaesth 103:637–646
72. Wakeling HG, McFall MR, Jenkins CS et al (2005) Intraoperative oesophageal Doppler guided fluid managements shortens postoperative hospital stay after major bowel surgery. Br J Anaesth 95:634–642
73. Pillai P, McEleavy I, Gaughan M, Snowden C, Nesbitt I, Durkan G et al (2011) A double-blind randomized controlled clinical trial to assess the effect of Doppler optimized intraoperative fluid management on outcome following radical cystectomy. J Urol 186:2201–2206
74. Menon M, Hemal AK, Tewari A et al (2003) Nerve sparing robotic robot-assisted radical cystoprosatectomynad urinary diversion. BJU Int 92:232–236
75. Tang K, Xia D, Li H et al (2014) Robotic vs. open radical cystectomy in bladder cancer: a systematic review and meta-analysis. Eur J Surg Oncol 40:1399–1411
76. Johar RS, Hayn MH, Stegemann AP et al (2013) Complications after robotassisted radical cystectomy: results from the International Robotic Cystectomy Consortium. Eur Urol 64:52–57
77. Parekh DJ, Messer J, Fitzgerald J, Ercole B, Svatek R (2013) Perioperative outcomes and oncologic efficacy from a pilot prospective randomized clinical trial of open versus robotic assisted radical cystectomy. J Urol 189:474–479
78. Bochner BH, Sjoberg DD, Laudone VP (2014) Memorial sloan kettering cancer center bladder cancer surgical trials G. A randomized trial of robot-assisted laparoscopic radical cystectomy. N Engl J Med 371:389–390
79. Novara G, Catto JW, Wilson T et al (2015) Systematic review and cumulative analysis of perioperative outcomes and complications after robot-assisted radical cystectomy. Eur Urol 67:376–401
80. Yuh B, Wilson T, Bochner B et al (2015) Systematic review and cumulative analysis of oncologic and functional outcomes after robot-assisted radical cystectomy. Eur Urol 67:402–422
81. Snow-Lisy DC, Campbell SC, Gill IS et al (2014) Robotic and laparoscopic radical cystectomy for bladder cancer: long-term oncologic outcomes. Eur Urol 65:193–200
82. Nazmy M, Yuh B, Kawachi M et al (2014) Early and late complications of robot-assisted radical cystectomy: a standardized analysis by urinary diversion type. J Urol 191:681–687
83. Erber B, Schrader M, Miller K et al (2011) Morbidity and quality of life in bladder cancer patients following cystectomy and urinary diversion: a single-institution comparison of ileal conduit versus orthotopic neobladder. ISRN Urol 2012:1–8

84. Abe T, Takada N, Shinohara N et al (2014) Comparison of 90-day complications between ileal conduit and neobladder reconstruction after radical cystectomy: a retrospective multi-institutional study in Japan. Int J Urol 21:554–559
85. Lee R, Abol-Enein H, Artibani W et al (2013) Urinary diversion after radical cystectomy for bladder cancer: options, patient selection, and outcomes. BJU Int 113:11–23
86. Ahmed K, Khan SA, Hayn MH et al (2014) Analysis of intracorporeal compared with extracorporeal urinary diversion after robot-assisted radical cystectomy: results from the International Robotic Cystectomy Consortium. Eur Urol 65:340–347
87. Smith N, Castle E, Gonzalgo M et al (2015) The RAZOR (randomized open vs. robotic cystectomy) trial: study design and trial update. BJU Int 115:198–205
88. KarliczeK A, Jesus EC, Matos D, Castro A, Atallah AN, Wiggers T (2006) Drainage or nondrainage in elective colorectal anastomosis: a systematic review and meta-analysis. Colorectal Dis 8:259–265
89. Dutton TJ, Daugherty MO, Mason RG, McGrath JS (2014) Implementation of the Exeter enhanced recovery program for patients undergoing radical cystectomy. BJU Int 113:719–725
90. Smith JB, Meng ZW, Lockyer R et al (2014) Evolution of the Southampton Enhanced Recovery Programme for radical cystectomy and the aggregation of marginal gains. BJU Int 114:375–383
91. Mattei A, Birkhaeuser FD, Baermann C, Warncke SH, Studer UE (2008) To stent or not to stent perioperatively the ureteroileal anastomosis of ileal orthotopic bladder substitutes and ileal conduits? Results of a prospective randomized trial. J Urol 179:582–586
92. Nelson R, Edwards S, Tse B (2007) Prophylactic nasogastric decompression after abdominal surgery. Cochrane Database Syst Rev CD004929
93. Donat SM, Slaton JW, Pisters LL, Swanson DA (1999) Early nasogastric tube removal combined with metoclopramide after radical cystectomy and urinary diversion. J Urol 162:1599–1602
94. Adamakis I, Tyritzis SI, Koutalellis G et al (2011) Early removal of nasogastric tube is beneficial for patients undergoing radical cystectomy with urinary diversion. Int Braz J Urol 37:42–48
95. Choi H, Kang SH, Yoon DK et al (2011) Chewing gum has a stimulatory effect on bowel motility in patients after open or robotic radical cystectomy for bladder cancer: a prospective randomized comparative study. Urology 77:884–890
96. Kouba EJ, Wallen EM, Pruthi RS (2007) Gum chewing stimulates bowel motility in patients undergoing radical cystectomy with urinary diversion. Urology 70:1053–1056
97. Traut U, Brugger L, Kunz R, et al (2008) Systemic prokinetic pharmacologic treatment for postoperative adynamic ileus following abdominal surgery in adults. Cochrane Database Syst Rev CD004930
98. Lightfoot AJ, Eno M, Kreder KJ, O'Donnell MA, Rao SS, Williams RD (2007) Treatment of postoperative ileus after bowel surgery with low-dose intravenous erythromycin. Urology 69:611–615
99. Pruthi RS, Nielsen M, Smith A, Nix J, Schultz H, Wallen EM (2010) Fast track program in patients undergoing radical cystectomy: results in 362 consecutive patients. J Am Coll Surg 210:93–99
100. Smith J, Pruthi RS, McGrath J (2014) Enhanced recovery programs for patients undergoing radical cystectomy. Nat Rev 11:437–444
101. Zingg U, Miskovic D, Pasternak I, Meyer P, Hamel CT, Metzger U (2008) Effect of bisacodyl on postoperative bowel motility in elective colorectal surgery: a prospective, randomized trial. Int J Colorectal Dis 23:1175–1183
102. Schroeder D, Gillanders L, Mahr K, Hill GL (1991) Effects of immediate postoperative enteral nutrition on body composition, muscle function, and wound healing. J Parenter Enter Nutr 15:376–383

103. Behrns KE, Kircher AP, Galanko JA, Brownstein MR, Koruda MJ (2000) Prospective randomized trial of early initiation and hospital discharge on a liquid diet following elective intestinal surgery. J Gastrointest Surg 4:217–221
104. Fearon KCH, Luff R (2003) The nutritional management of surgical patients: enhanced recovery after surgery. Proc Nutr Soc. 62:807–811
105. Osland E, Yunus RM, Khan S, Memon MA (2011) Early versus traditional postoperative feeding in patients undergoing resectional gastrointestinal surgery: a meta-analysis. J Parenter Enter Nutr 35:473–487
106. Holte K (2004) Foss NB, Svensen C, Lund C, Madsen JL, Kehlet H. Epidural anesthesia, hypotension, and changes in intravascular volume. Anesthesiology 100:281–286
107. Soni N (2009) British consensus guidelines on intravenous fluid therapy for adult surgical patients (GIFTASUP): Cassandra's view. Anaesthesia 64:235–238
108. Karl A, Rittler P, Buchner A et al (2009) Prospective assessment of malnutrition in urologic patients. Urology 73:1072–1076
109. Ventham NT, O'Neill S, Johns N, Brady RR, Fearon KC (2014) Evaluation of novel local anesthetic wound infiltration techniques for postoperative pain following colorectal resection surgery: a meta-analysis. Dis Colon Rectum 57:237–250
110. Klein M, Gogenur I, Rosenberg J (2012) Postoperative use of non-steroidal anti-inflammatory drugs in patients with anastomotic leakage requiring reoperation after colorectal resection: cohort study based on prospective data. BMJ 345:61–66
111. Coxib and traditional NSAID Trialists (CNT) Collaboration (2013) Vascular and upper gastrointestinal effects of non-steroidal anti-inflammatory drugs: meta-analyses of individual participant data from randomized trials. Lancet 382:769–779
112. Patel HR, Cerantola Y, Valerio M et al (2014) Enhanced recovery after surgery: are we ready, and can we afford not to implement these pathways for patients undergoing radical cystectomy? Eur Urol 65:263–266
113. Vlug MS, Wind J, Hollmann MW et al (2011) Laparoscopy in combination with fast track management is the best perioperative strategy in patients undergoing colonic surgery: a randomized clinical trial (LAFA-study). Ann Surg 254:868–875
114. Jensen BT, Petersen AK, Jensen JB, Laustsen S, Borre M (2015) Efficacy of a multi-professional rehabilitation programme in radical cystectomy pathways: a prospective randomized controlled trial. Scand J Urol 49:133–141
115. Vasdev N, Pillai P, Snowdon CP, Thorpe AC (2012) Current strategies to enhance recovery following radical cystectomy: single centre initial experience. ISRN Urol 1–6
116. Stowers MD, Lemanu DP, Hill AG (2015) Health economics in enhanced recovery after surgery programs. Can J Anaesth 62:219–230
117. Karl A, Buchner A, Becker A et al (2014) A new concept for early recovery after surgery for patients undergoing radical cystectomy for bladder cancer: results of a prospective randomized study. J Urol 191:335–340
118. Arumainayagam N, McGrath J, Jefferson KP, Gillatt DA (2008) Introduction of an enhanced recovery protocol for radical cystectomy. BJU Int 101:698–701
119. Saar M, Ohlmann C-H, Siemer S et al (2013) Fast-track rehabilitation after robot-assisted laparoscopic cystectomy accelerates postoperative recovery. BJU Int 112:E99–E106
120. Guan X, Liu L, Lei X et al (2014) A comparative study of fast-track verus conventional surgery in patients undergoing laparoscopic radical cystectomy and ileal conduit diversion: Chinese experience. Sci Rep 4:6820
121. Cerruto MA, De Marco V, D'Elia C et al (2014) Introduction of an enhanced recovery protocol to reduce short-term complications following radical cystectomy and intestinal urinary diversion with vescica ileale Padovana neobladder. Urol Int 92:35–40
122. Persson B, Carringer M, Andre′n O, et al (2015) Initial experiences with the enhanced recovery after surgery (ERAS) protocol in open radical cystectomy. Scand J Urol 49:302–307

123. Koupparis A, Villeda-Sandoval C, Weale N et al (2015) Robot-assisted radical cystectomy with intracorporeal urinary diversion: impact on an established enhanced recovery protocol. BJU Int 116:924–931
124. Xu W, Daneshmand S, Bazargani ST et al (2015) Postoperative pain management after radical cystectomy: comparing traditional versus enhanced recovery protocol pathway. J Urol 194:1209–1213
125. Collins JW, Adding C, Hosseini A et al (2016) Introducing an enhanced recovery programme to an established totally intracorporeal robotassisted radical cystectomy service. Scand J Urol 50:39–46
126. Chipollini J, Tang DH, Hussein K, et al (2017) Does implementing an enhanced recovery after surgery protocol increase hospital charges? Comparisons from a radical cystectomy program at a specialty cancer center. https://doi.org/10.1016/j.urology.2017.03.023. [Epub ahead of print]
127. Baack-Kukreja J, Messing E, Shah J (2015) Are we doing "better"? The discrepancy between perception and practice of enhanced recovery after cystectomy principles among urologic oncologists. Urol Oncol Semin Ori 34:120

Current Role of Checkpoint Inhibitors in Urologic Cancers

Kyrollis Attalla, John P. Sfakianos and Matthew D. Galsky

Contents

Abstract

Harnessing the host immune system to combat genitourinary cancers has key theoretical advantages over other anticancer strategies including specificity and memory which should translate to favorable tolerability and response durability

---

K. Attalla · J. P. Sfakianos
Department of Urology, Icahn School of Medicine at Mount Sinai, New York, NY, USA

M. D. Galsky (✉)
Icahn School of Medicine at Mount Sinai, New York, NY, USA
e-mail: matthew.galsky@mssm.edu

M. D. Galsky
Genitourinary Medical Oncology, Tisch Cancer Institute, New York, NY, USA

S. Daneshmand and K. G. Chan (eds.), *Genitourinary Cancers*, Cancer Treatment and Research 175, https://doi.org/10.1007/978-3-319-93339-9_11

in the clinic. Indeed, key examples of the potential for immunotherapeutic treatment of solid tumors are derived from data in genitourinary cancers including Bacillus Calmette–Guerin for urothelial cancer, sipuleucel-T for prostate cancer, and interleukin-2 for renal cancer. Despite these successes, developing effective immunotherapeutic strategies for the treatment of cancer has largely been hampered by an incomplete understanding of tumor immunobiology and mechanisms of immune resistance. In just a few years since entering the clinic, immune checkpoint blockade has dramatically changed the landscaped of treatment for genitourinary cancer and has secured a place as a standard pillar of treatment. Further iterative bench-bedside-bench research is anticipated to extend the benefits of immunotherapeutic-based approaches to additional patients.

Keywords
Urothelial cancer · Prostate cancer · Renal cancer · Immunotherapy
Immune checkpoint blockade · PD-1 · PD-L1

1 Introduction

Exploiting the immune system for cancer treatment likely dates back as early as the 1890s when Dr. William Coley, after observing spontaneous remissions of cancer in patients with severe infections, began to inject a mixture of bacteria and bacterial lysates directly into tumors as a treatment strategy [1, 2]. While the mechanistic basis for some of the treatment successes described by Coley was not know at the time, and remains incompletely defined, Coley's approach likely resulted in the injected pathogen-associated molecular patterns stimulating activation and maturation of tumor-antigen-loaded dendritic cells. Coley's Toxins were used to treat various cancers from the 1890s until the 1960s. As a result of increased regulatory scrutiny of medicinal products, Coley's Toxins were assigned "new drug" status by the United States Food and Drug Administration (US FDA) in the 1960s, restricting the use of this product to clinical trials. Small clinical trials demonstrated mixed results and use of Coley's Toxins subsequently fell by the wayside.

The experience with Coley's Toxins highlighted that in specific scenarios, the immune system could be modulated effectively to induce clinical regressions of cancer. Other immunomodulatory approaches were introduced over the years, similarly based on a hint of mechanistic rationale and a large amount of empiricism, leading to a much greater impact such as intravesical BCG for non-muscle-invasive bladder cancer. However, decades of clinical trials attempting to induce anti-tumor T cell responses were largely disappointing often attributed to poor antigen selection, suboptimal adjuvants, and inappropriate clinical disease states for investigation. It was not until a basic understanding of regulators of T cell function was elucidated that these clinical disappointments were placed in appropriate context. That is, in many patients, the lack of development of an anti-tumor immune response may not be "the problem," but rather the inability of the immune response to "complete the job" due to diverse mechanisms of tumor-related immune resistance.

The immune system has developed a set of checks and balances to control the amplitude and duration of a given immune response. Central to this system are positive and negative co-stimulatory molecules that govern whether a T cell will activate and proliferate or whether the T cell response will be attenuated; these negative signals are mediated by receptors commonly referred to as immune checkpoints. Among the two most well-characterized immune checkpoints are cytotoxic T-lymphocyte-associated antigen 4 (CTLA-4) and program death 1/programmed death ligand 1 (PD-1/PD-L1). Proof of concept in model systems for blocking immune checkpoints as a potential anticancer strategy was initially demonstrated in 1996 when Leach et al. demonstrated that antibodies to CTLA-4 resulted in the rejection of tumors, including pre-established tumors. The clinical development of antibodies directed first against CLTA-4, and later against PD-1/PD-L1, followed demonstrating durable disease control in a subset of patients across a large number of different tumor types harkening an entirely new era in cancer immunotherapy. In this chapter, we review the clinical development of immune checkpoint antibodies for the treatment of genitourinary cancers.

2 Adverse Events with Immune Checkpoint Blockade: General Considerations

While the anticancer activity of immune checkpoint blockade has varied across tumor types, the adverse event profile of this treatment class has been relatively consistent across patient populations. Therefore, given the unique, and potentially life-threatening, adverse events that can occur with immune checkpoint blockade, these considerations are discussed first followed by a discussion of the clinical activity of immune checkpoint blockade in specific genitourinary cancers.

The key adverse events associated with immune checkpoint blockade are commonly referred to as immune-related adverse events. These side effects are manifestations of inflammatory responses that occur in various tissue compartments, the pathophysiology of which are poorly understood. Notably, such events mimic the full range of autoimmune diseases and can involve virtually any organ, though certain events are more common than others. Furthermore, while there is overlap between the immune-related adverse events that occur with CTLA-4 versus PD-1/PD-L1 blockade, there are adverse events that occur more and less commonly with drugs directed against each of these targets. For example, colitis is more much common with CTLA-4 blockade whereas pneumonitis is more common with PD-1 blockade. Combination of CTLA-4 blockade plus PD-1/PD-L1 blockade is associated with a higher frequency of adverse events compared with single-agent

PD-1/PD-L1 blockade. The management of specific immune-related adverse events is based on the organ system involved, the severity, and generally follows algorithms that have been developed based on the extensive clinical experience amassed with these therapies. Management commonly includes holding treatment for less severe side effects and initiation of corticosteroids for more severe side effects, and even anti-tumor necrosis factor (TNF) therapies for steroid-non-responsive events; some adverse events based on the nature and severity require discontinuation of treatment.

To put the potential side effects of PD-1/PD-L1 blockade into perspective, the randomized phase III trials comparing chemotherapy with PD-1/PD-L1 blockade provide some context. In the Keynote-045 study of chemotherapy versus pembrolizumab in patients with metastatic urothelial cancer, 49.4% of patients developed a grade 3–5 adverse event with chemotherapy compared with 15% of patients treated with pembrolizumab [3]. With respect to specific immune-related side effects in patients randomized to pembrolizumab, any grade thyroid abnormalities occurred in 9.4%, pneumonitis in 4.1%, colitis in 2.3%, and adrenal insufficiency in 0.4%. Despite the generally favorable safety profile of single-agent PD-1/PD-L1 blockade, a small subset of patients develop severe immune-related adverse events that can be life-threatening. Early recognition and treatment of immune-related adverse events has become the widely accept dogma in the era of immune checkpoint blockade in an effort to minimize treatment-related morbidity with these agents. As noted, with the combination of PD-1/PD-L1 blockade plus CTLA-4 blockade, the overall safety profile is similar with respect to the types of immune-related events encountered though the incidence of such events is generally much higher than with single-agent therapy.

3 Kidney Cancer

Renal cell carcinoma (RCC) accounts for 3% of adult malignancies and is the eighth leading cause of cancer in the USA [4]. Up to 30% of patients diagnosed with RCC present with synchronous metastases, and recurrence is seen in 30% of patients after complete resection of the primary tumor [5–7]. Patients who present with distant metastases have a dismal 5-year survival rate of less than 10%, and at least half of patients with RCC will eventually require systemic therapy [5, 6, 8]. RCC is generally considered resistant to conventional cytotoxic chemotherapy and radiotherapy but has classically been regarded as an immunogenic tumor as evidenced by occasional spontaneous regressions and mild to moderate success with prior immunotherapeutic approaches [9].

Prior to 2005, the only approved treatment for metastatic RCC (mRCC) was high-dose interleukin-2 (HD IL-2) which exhibited durable responses in approximately 5–10% of patients at the cost of severe acute toxicities as a result of the pro-inflammatory cytokine storm induced by treatment [10]. Low-dose subcutaneous interferon was commonly utilized instead, given its somewhat better safety profile, though durable responses were uncommon. After 2005, the treatment landscape for mRCC shifted from immunotherapeutic approaches to approaches directed at growth factors overexpressed in RCC downstream of altered von Hippel Lindau function, particularly vascular endothelial growth factor (VEGF). Several multitargeted tyrosine kinase inhibitors with activity against the VEGF receptor, antibodies directed against VEGF, and small molecule inhibitors of mammalian target of rapamycin (mTOR) were explored in mRCC leading to FDA approval and integration as standard therapies. Despite the plethora of such therapies introduced to treat mRCC, and the convenience of oral administration offered by many of these drugs, chronic administration is required, adverse effects can substantially impact quality of life, and the vast majority of patients ultimately experience disease progression despite treatment [11].

Ipilimumab, a monoclonal antibody directed at CTLA-4, was investigated in a phase II study of 61 patients with metastatic clear cell RCC treated with two dosing regimens [12]. One patient of the 21 patients treated at a lower dose achieved a partial response compared with 5 out of 40 patients achieving a partial response in the higher-dose cohort. A relationship between anti-tumor activity and the development of immune-related adverse events was observed; patients who experienced grade 3 or 4 toxicities experienced an objective response rate of 30% compared to no patients responding to treatment who did not experience immune-related adverse events.

While the clinical experience with single-agent CTLA-4 blockade in RCC was somewhat disappointing, the proof of concept established led to rapid exploration of PD-1/PD-L1 blockade in the clinic in RCC. Approximately 25% of clear cell RCCs express PD-L1, and upwards of 50% of tumor-infiltrating lymphocytes in RCC express PD-L1, which have been correlated with cancer-specific death, and distant metastatic relapse and poor survival, respectively [13].

Nivolumab is a fully humanized immunoglobulin G4 isotype monoclonal antibody. In the initial phase Ib clinical trial investigating nivolumab as monotherapy, 34 heavily pre-treated patients with metastatic clear cell RCC were enrolled in addition to patients with a variety of other tumor types [14]. Nivolumab was administered intravenously every 2 weeks and doses of 1–10 mg/kg were explored. Remarkably, the objective response rate in patients with metastatic clear cell RCC was 27% at a minimum follow-up of 50.5 months, with 40% of responses ongoing at the time of data lock. The majority of responses were partial responses although one patient did achieve a complete response. These data led to the initiation of a large phase II trial of nivolumab in patients with metastatic clear cell RCC who had progressed despite prior VEGF-targeted therapies [15]. One hundred and sixty-eight patients were randomly assigned to 0.3, 2, or 10 mg/kg of nivolumab administered intravenously once every three weeks. The objective response rate was 20–22% across dose levels, and there was no dose response relationship observed for response rate, progression-free survival, or overall survival. Importantly, responses were generally durable with a median duration of response of 22 months and responses of >24 months in 14 out of 35 responders.

In parallel with the large phase II trial of nivolumab, a "biomarker trial" was initiated to generate insights regarding mechanisms of response and resistance to treatment. In this study, patients underwent a baseline and on-treatment biopsy. A response rate was observed to be 22% in patients with PD-L1-positive tumors (using a $\geq 5\%$ cutoff for PD-L1 as assessed by immunohistochemistry (IHC) in tumor cells) and 8% in patients with PD-L1 "negative" tumors. There were no consistent changes in PD-L1 expression from baseline to on-treatment biopsies; however, post-treatment increases in CD3, CD4, and CD8 cells as assessed by IHC were observed. Transcriptional changes were observed in tumors on nivolumab treatment including an increase in genes associated with innate immunity as well as an increase in genes linked with T cell function.

With both evidence of activity from single-arm studies and some putative predictive biomarkers identified, the CheckMate 025 trial was launched, a phase III trial comparing nivolumab with everolimus in patients with advanced RCC who received one or two prior VEGF-directed therapies [16]. Eight hundred and twenty-one patients were randomized to receive 3 mg/kg of nivolumab administered intravenously every two weeks or everolimus 10 mg orally daily. Treatment with nivolumab was associated with a significantly longer overall survival (median overall survival 25 months versus 19.6 months; hazard ratio (HR) 0.73, $p = 0.002$) and fewer grade 3 or 4 adverse events (19% vs. 37%). Treatment with nivolumab did not lead to an improvement in progression-free survival compared with everolimus, a phenomenon that has been observed across trials with immune checkpoint blockade likely related to a combination of both overall response proportions and response kinetics. Based on these data, nivolumab was approved by the US FDA in November 2015 for the treatment of advanced RCC in patients who received prior anti-angiogenic therapy.

VEGF receptor tyrosine kinase inhibitors (VEGFR TKIs) have served as standard treatments for metastatic RCC in several different lines of therapy since 2004. Preclinical models suggest that targeting the VEGF pathway may antagonize RCC-induced immunosuppression and has provided rationale for strategies combining VEGFR TKIs and immune checkpoint blockade [17]. Several clinical trials combining these therapeutic classes have been conducted revealing generally high-response proportions (Table 1). A randomized phase II study evaluated the PD-L1 antibody atezolizumab with or without the VEGF antibody bevacizumab versus sunitinib in treatment-naïve patients with metastatic RCC [18]. The combination of atezolizumab plus bevacizumab demonstrated an encouraging response rate and survival compared with sunitinib. Ultimately, the role of targeting VEGF signaling plus immune checkpoint blockade in the treatment of metastatic RCC remains to be defined in ongoing randomized phase III trials.

Combining different classes of immunotherapies is also supported by data in model systems and clinical data generated in other malignancies such as metastatic melanoma. The phase I CheckMate 016 trial evaluated nivolumab in combination with the CTLA-4 inhibitor ipilimumab, or the VEGFR TKIs sunitinib or pazopanib [19]. Patients with metastatic RCC were randomized to three dosing strategies with nivolumab plus ipilimumab: nivolumab at 3 mg/kg plus ipilimumab

Table 1 Select clinical trials of combination immune checkpoint blockade and anti-angiogenic agents in metastatic RCC

Citation	Intervention	Setting	Phase	N	Objective response rate
Rini et al. [60]	Tremelimumab + sunitinib	≤1 prior systemic treatment	Phase I	28	43%
Amin et al. [61]	Nivolumab + sunitinib or pazopanib	≤1 prior systemic treatment	Phase I	33	Sunitinib: 52% Pazopanib 45%
Chowdhury et al. [62]	Pembrolizumab + pazopanib	No prior systemic treatment	Phase I	20	40%
Choueiri et al. [63]	Avelumab + axitinib	No prior systemic treatment	Phase Ib	55	54.5%
Atkins et al. [64]	Pembrolizumab + axitinib	No prior systemic treatment	Phase Ib	11	55%

at 1 mg/kg (N3I1 group, $n = 47$), nivolumab at 1 mg/kg plus ipilimumab at 3 mg/kg (N1I3 group, $n = 47$), or nivolumab at 3 mg/kg plus ipilimumab at 3 mg/kg (N3I3 group, $n = 6$) and two nivolumab plus VEGFR TKI groups. All six patients in the N3I3 arm experienced severe toxicities. At approximately two years of follow-up, the overall response rate in both N3I1 and N1I3 arms was 40.4%. Of the 38 responders in both treatment arms, 39.5% ($n = 15$) had an ongoing response at the time of the data lock, with a median duration of response of 20.4 months (95% confidence interval (CI) 8.54—NE) in the N3I1 arm and 19.7 months (95% CI 8.08—NE) in the N1I3 arm. The overall survival rate at 12 months was 81% and 85% for N3I1 arm and N1I3 arm, respectively, and at 24 months was 67% and 70%, respectively.

Given the promising results with CheckMate 016, the CheckMate 214 trial was initiated. CheckMate 214 randomized 1096 patients with treatment-naïve metastatic clear cell RCC to treatment with nivolumab (3 mg/kg) plus ipilimumab (1 mg/kg) × 4 cycles followed by single-agent nivolumab 3 mg/kg every 2 weeks versus sunitinib 50 mg daily for 4 weeks of every 6 week cycle [20]. The randomization was stratified based on the International Metastatic RCC Database Consortium prognostic score and region. The study employed co-primary endpoints of response rate, progression-free survival, and overall survival in intermediate- and poor-risk patients. In intermediate-/poor-risk patients, treatment with ipilimumab plus nivolumab compared to sunitinib was associated with a significantly higher objective response rate (43% vs. 27%, $p < 0.0001$) and longer progression-free survival [HR 0.82 (0.64–1.05), $p = 0.03$] and overall survival [HR 0.63 (0.44–0.89), $p = 0.00003$]. Importantly, grade 3–5 treatment-related adverse events occurred in 46% of patients on ipilimumab plus nivolumab versus 63% of patients on sunitinib. These compelling data have the potential to change the landscape of first-line treatment for patients with metastatic intermediate-/poor-risk RCC.

4 Prostate Cancer

While prostate cancer has not traditionally been considered an immunogenic malignancy like RCC, there have been several characteristics of prostate cancer that have led to extensive studies exploring immunotherapeutic approaches in this disease including the availability of several organ-restricted antigens for immunization (e.g., prostatic acid phosphatase) and a relatively indolent pattern of progression in certain clinical disease states. Indeed, the active cellular immune therapy sipuleucel-T, was shown to improve survival in two randomized trials in men with metastatic castration-resistant prostate cancer (CRPC) representing the only approved "vaccine" to treat patients with an advanced solid tumor [21].

Based on data in model systems suggesting that the abscopal effect is immune-mediated and that CTLA-4 blockade combined with radiation therapy might yield synergistic anticancer activity [22–26] a phase I/II trial examined ipilimumab as monotherapy and in combination with radiotherapy delivered to a site of bone metastasis in patients with CRPC [27]. Post-treatment declines in PSA were observed in 16% of patients treated with ipilimumab +/− radiation, and one patient achieved a complete response. Immune-related adverse events were similar to other trials exploring CTLA-4 blockade and included rash/pruritus, diarrhea, colitis, and hepatitis.

Two phase III trials were subsequently designed to test the efficacy of ipilimumab in patients with metastatic CRPC, one study in patients who had progressed despite docetaxel treatment and the other in chemotherapy-naïve patients. In the post-docetaxel trial [28], men were randomized to radiation therapy to a bone metastasis followed by either ipilimumab or placebo. Compared with placebo, ipilimumab did not yield an improvement in survival, the primary endpoint of the study. However, ipiliumab was associated with a significantly longer progression-free survival (secondary endpoint) and more frequent PSA reductions (exploratory endpoint). A post hoc subgroup analysis demonstrated that ipilimumab offered an overall survival benefit to patients with favorable baseline characteristics, including an alkaline phosphatase <1.5 times the upper limit of normal, hemoglobin >11.0 g/dL, and no visceral metastases. The pre-chemotherapy phase III trial randomized 602 men with CRPC to ipilimumab versus placebo [29]. Again, no significant improvement in overall survival was observed with ipilimumab though anti-tumor activity was observed as evidenced by a modestly longer progression-free survival (5.6 vs. 3.8 months) and a higher PSA response rate (23% vs. 8%). Given the lack of survival benefit with ipilimumab in the context of the adverse event profile, single-agent ipilimumab has not been integrated into standard treatment for CRPC; however, the clear activity in a subset of patients highlights the critical need for predictive biomarkers to identify patients most likely to benefit.

The CLTA-4 antibody tremelimumab has also been explored in patients with prostate cancer. In a phase I trial, tremelimumab was administered to men with castration-naïve non-metastatic biochemically recurrent prostate cancer despite prior local therapy [30]. While no changes in on-treatment versus pre-treatment

PSA doubling time was observed in this small study, 3 patients experienced a marked slowing of PSA rise after completion of treatment highlighting the potential for unusual response kinetics with CTLA-4 blockade as has been seen in other tumor types such as melanoma.

As CTLA-4 blockade yields anticancer activity in only a small subset of patients with CRPC, combination regimens with cancer vaccines have been developed in an attempt to augment these responses [31–34]. Phase I trials have shown that such combinations are feasible, though larger definitive studies have not yet been completed to determine whether combination therapy leads to clinical benefit compared to ipilimumab alone [32, 34].

Given the anticancer activity observed in a subset of patients with prostate cancer treated with CTLA-4 blockade, patients with CRPC were integrated early in the clinical development of the anti-PD-1 antibody nivolumab. Unfortunately, in the phase I trial of nivolumab, no responses were seen in 17 patients with metastatic CRPC limiting enthusiasm for further clinical trials with PD-1/PD-L1 blockade in CRPC for several years in favor of other malignancies [35]. A renewed interest in PD-1/PD-L1 blockade in CRPC emerged based on preliminary data from a phase II trial with the anti-PD-1 antibody pembrolizumab, given in combination with enzalutamide in patients with CRPC progressing despite prior enzalutamide [36]. This study design was based, at least in part, on data suggesting that PD-L1 expression is increased on prostate cancer cells at the time of enzalutamide resistance. Notably, 3 of the initial 10 patients enrolled experienced major post-treatment declines in PSA, 2 of which had regression of measurable disease. Genomic sequencing of archival tumor specimens was possible in a subset of these responding patients indicating that DNA mismatch repair gene alterations/microsatellite instability, a rare finding in prostate cancer, may have been underlying several of these responses. The contribution of continuation of enzalutamide to the activity of this combination regimen is unclear and worthy of further investigation.

Several large phase II and even phase III studies have subsequently been initiated to explore PD-1/PD-L1 blockade in CRPC with results pending. In addition, several combination strategies are being pursued including combinations with androgen deprivation, chemotherapy, and other immunotherapeutic agents. These data are eagerly awaited to determine whether there is a potential role for PD-1/PD-L1-based therapies in the standard management of CRPC.

5 Urothelial Cancer

Translational studies have explored the potential role of immune checkpoints in urothelial cancer dating back to the early appreciation of the role of these molecules in the pathogenesis of cancer. Using IHC testing of frozen tissue from 65 patients who underwent surgical resection of urothelial cancer (bladder and upper tract), Nikinishi et al. correlated expression of PD-L1 with higher grade and stage [37].

Patients with tumors expressing high levels of PD-L1 were also found to have worse overall and recurrence-free survival. Boorjian et al. identified the expression of B7-H3, PD-L1, and PD-1 in 314 radical cystectomy specimens and identified B7-H3 expression in more than 70% of samples and PD-L1 expression in approximately 12% PD-L1 [38]. Clinically, PD-L1 expression was associated with advanced tumor stage and worse all-cause mortality in patients with organ-confined disease. PD-1 expression was identified in 95% of the tumor-infiltrating immune cells and was associated with higher pathologic stage ($p = 0.012$). Subsequent to these two initial studies, further work has been performed to analyze the landscape of immune checkpoint proteins across the continuum of bladder cancer stages. PD-L1 expression has been shown to increase with stage; for example, in one series PD-L1 expression was detected in 7, 16, 23, 30, and 45% of specimens from Ta, T1, T2, T3/4, and CIS tumors, respectively [39]. In a series of 302 consecutive patients treated with radical cystectomy and lymphadenectomy, Xylias et al. analyzed B7-H3, B7-H1 (PD-L1), and PD-1 protein expression by IHC in the primary tumor, 117 matched lymph nodes and 50 adjacent normal urothelium samples. These investigators identified a high degree of correlation between the primary tumor and nodal metastasis with a concordance of 90, 86, and 78% for B7-H3, B7-H1, and PD-1, respectively [40]. In a series of 160 patients, of which 23 (14.4%) were non-invasive tumors, analysis of PD-L1 expression in tumor-infiltrating mononuclear cells using IHC identified no difference in PD-L1 expression between non-invasive and invasive tumors [41].

Ipilimumab was the first-immune checkpoint inhibitor to be explored and was initially approved for the treatment of metastatic melanoma by the US FDA. In urothelial carcinoma, anti-CTL-4 antibiodies were explored in murine model systems of bladder cancer with favorable activity [42]. Despite the intriguing findings in vivo, there have been very few completed clinical trials exploring CLTA-4 blockade in urothelial cancer. A "window of opportunity" study treating patients with invasive bladder cancer was performed [43]. In this study, patients were treated with ipilimumab prior to cystectomy, and pharmacodynamic assessments were performed on the post-treatment tumor specimen. This study revealed that ipilimumab treatment led to a robust infiltration of T cells into the post-treatment tumor specimen compared to the pre-treatment specimen. Given this evidence of pharmacodynamic activity, a phase II study was performed in which patients with chemotherapy-naïve metastatic urothelial cancer were treated with two cycles of gemcitabine plus cisplatin followed by four cycles of gemcitabine, cisplatin, plus ipilimumab [44]. Though the overall outcomes of patients treated on this study were similar to historical patients treated with gemcitabine plus cisplatin alone, on landmark analysis a post-ipilimumab increase in peripheral blood T cells correlated with a much better survival. Though investigation of CTLA-4 blockade in urothelial cancer was quickly supplanted by trials of PD-1/PD-L1 inhibition, additional studies further defining the role of CTLA-4 blockade alone or in combination in this disease are needed.

PD-L1 and PD-1 blockade in urothelial cancer was initially studied in expansion cohorts of phase I studies using atezolizumab and pembrolizumab, respectively [45, 46]. In these studies durable objective responses was identified in a subset of heavily pre-treated patients with metastatic urothelial cancer. Given the evidence of activity and overall safety profile, additional trials of PD-1/PD-L1 blockade in urothelial cancer were rapidly initiated and completed.

As of late 2017, there are five PD-1/PD-L1 inhibitors approved by the US FDA for the treatment of metastatic urothelial cancer (Table 2). The approvals are based largely on phase II trials and a single phase III trial (Table 3). Two phase III trials randomizing patients with metastatic urothelial cancer progressing despite platinum-based chemotherapy to PD-1/PD-L1 blockade versus standard chemotherapy have been completed. Keynote-045 randomized 542 patients to the anti-PD-1 antibody pembrolizumab, or chemotherapy with a co-primary endpoint of progression-free survival and overall survival [3]. Treatment with pembrolizumab was associated with a significant improvement in objective response rate (21.1% vs. 11.4%) and overall survival (10.3 months vs. 7.4 months (HR 0.73; 95% CI 0.59–0.91; $p = 0.002$). Importantly, the benefit of treatment with pembrolizumab was observed not only in the subset of patients with tumors with higher PD-L1 expression but also in the entire study population. IMvigor 211 was a larger phase III study randomizing 931 patients with metastatic urothelial cancer progressing despite prior platinum-based chemotherapy to the anti-PD-L1 antibody atezolizumab, versus standard of care chemotherapy [47]. Based on the results of the IMVigor 210 study, a single-arm phase II study demonstrating higher response rates with atezolizumab based on higher percentage of PD-L1 expression in tumor-infiltrating cells in archival tumor specimens, IMVigor 211 utilized a hierarchical analysis plan that required hypothesis testing be first performed in a subset of patients with increased PD-L1 expression in tumor-infiltrating cells. Only if the primary endpoint was met in this biomarker-defined population could the endpoint be assessed in the overall study population. Treatment with atezolizumab was not associated with an improvement in overall survival in the biomarker-defined population in this study. In an exploratory analysis, median overall survival and 12-month survival rate was better with atezolizumab compared to chemotherapy and the outcomes with atezolizumab were quite consistent with the results from the prior phase II study. Reasons for this trial not meeting the pre-specified primary endpoint include an incomplete understanding of the prognostic versus predictive role of this PD-L1 assay and slightly better performance of chemotherapy than was anticipated.

Two large single-arm phase II trials have also explored PD-1/PD-L1 blockade as first-line treatment for patients with metastatic urothelial cancer deemed ineligible for cisplatin-based chemotherapy [48, 49]. Historically, carboplatin-based regimens have been utilized in such patients but have been associated with inferior outcomes compared to cisplatin-based combinations and have a generally unfavorable toxicity profile [50, 51]. In the IMvigor 210 study, atezolizumab was explored in 119 chemotherapy-naïve cisplatin-ineligible patients and was associated with a response rate of 23% (95% CI 16–31) [52]. Keynote-052 enrolled 270 patients with

Table 2 PD-1/PD-L1 antibodies approved by the United States Food and Drug Administration for treatment of metastatic urothelial cancer as of 2017

Setting	Drug
Metastatic urothelial cancer Chemotherapy-naïve Cisplatin-ineligible	Pembrolizumab (PD-1) Atezolizumab (PD-L1)
Metastatic urothelial cancer Disease progression despite prior platinum-based chemotherapy	Pembrolizumab (PD-1) Nivolumab (PD-1) Atezolizumab (PD-L1) Durvalumab (PD-L1) Avelumab (PD-L1)

Table 3 Major clinical trials of PD-1/PD-L1 blockade in metastatic urothelial cancer

Citation	Drug	Target	Setting	Phase	N	Objective response rate
Balar et al. [52]	Atezolizumab	PD-L1	First-line cisplatin-ineligible	Phase II	119	23% (95% CI 16–31)
O'Donnell et al. [53]	Pembrolizumab	PD-1	First-line cisplatin-ineligible	Phase II	100	29% (95% CI 24–34)
Bellmunt et al. [3]	Pembrolizumab	PD-1	Post-platinum	Phase III	270	21% (95% CI 16–27)
Powles et al. [47]	Atezolizumab	PD-L1	Post-platinum	Phase III	467	13% (95% CI 11–17)
Rosenberg et al. [58]	Atezolizumab	PD-L1	Post-platinum	Phase II	310	15% (95% CI 11–20)
Sharma et al. [59]	Nivolumab	PD-1	Post-platinum	Phase II	270	20% (95% CI 15–25)
Powles et al. [65]	Durvalumab	PD-L1	Post-platinum	Phase I/II	191	18% (95% CI 13–24)
Apolo et al. [66]	Avelumab	PD-L1	Post-platinum	Phase Ib	44	18% (95% CI 8–33)

metastatic urothelial carcinoma who were cisplatin ineligible demonstrating an objective response rate of 29% (95% CI 24–34) [53].

6 Less Common Genitourinary Cancers

The rarity of adrenocortical carcinoma (ACC) has been a barrier to the development of novel therapeutic approaches. A 2015 study examining 28 ACC specimens reported PD-L1 expression on tumor cells in 10.7% and on TILs in 70.4% [54]. The Cancer Genome Atlas (TCGA) data have shown that a subset of ACC harbor a high mutational burden. However, clinical experience with PD-1/PD-L1 blockade in advanced ACC has been mixed. An expansion cohort of a phase Ib study with avelumab, an anti-PD-L1 antibody, enrolled 37 patients with ACC and reported a response rate of 10.5% [55].

Germ cell tumors are generally highly curable with combined modality treatment. However, a subset of patients develop disease progression despite conventional therapy and the prognosis in such patients is poor. Pembrolizumab was investigated in patients with platinum refractory germ cell tumors in a phase II trial presented at the American Society of Clinical Oncology 2017 meeting by Adra et al. Twelve men who had failed or progressed after first-line cisplatin-based chemotherapy and at least one salvage regimen were treated with pembrolizumab until disease progression. Despite being well tolerated, no clinical benefit was observed, with no complete or partial responses seen.

Investigations of PD-L1 expression in penile cancer have been sparse. A retrospective study examining samples collected from 19 patients with squamous cell carcinoma of the penis demonstrated PD-L1 expression in 22% of samples [56]. In a similar study, 23 of 37 (62.2%) of samples tested positive for PD-L1 expression, with PD-L1 expression shown to be associated with advanced disease, nodal metastases, and reduced disease-specific survival [57]. Studies evaluating immune checkpoint blockade in patients with advanced penile cancer are ongoing.

7 Biomarkers Predictive of Response

The vast majority of trials exploring PD-1/PD-L1 blockade in genitourinary cancer have incorporated IHC testing of tumor specimens for expression of PD-L1 in an attempt to develop predictive biomarkers to select patients most likely to derive benefit from treatment. Interpretation of these data across tumor types has been complicated by the use of different assays, different cut-points, quantification of expression in cancer cells versus immune cells versus both, and use of archival tissue typically derived from the primary tumor. Despite these limitations, most initial studies suggested that PD-L1-based IHC testing could be used to enrich the likelihood of patients responding to treatment. However, responses were also observed in patients with "negative" tests, tempering enthusiasm for integration of testing into routine clinical decision-making [46, 52].

The complexity of PD-L1 as a predictive biomarker is epitomized by the manner in which the data has evolved in urothelial cancer. Phase I and II studies exploring various anti-PD-1/PD-L1 generally demonstrated higher response rates in subsets of patients with tumors exhibiting increased PD-L1 expression; however, phase III trials told a different story. In the Keynote-045 randomized study of pembrolizumab versus chemotherapy, a survival benefit with pembrolizumab was observed regardless of PD-L1 expression [3]. In the IMvigor 211 randomized study of atezolizumab versus chemotherapy, there was no benefit with atezolizumab demonstrated in the primary analysis of the high PD-L1 expression subgroup but a survival benefit was observed in the exploratory analysis of the total study population [47]. Currently in genitourinary cancers, PD-L1 testing has limited clinical utility.

Several other potential biomarkers predictive of response to PD-1/PD-L1 blockade have been explored. As tumors harboring a large burden of somatic mutations are hypothesized to generate a greater number of potentially immunogenic antigens, higher tumor mutational burden has been correlated with a higher likelihood of response to treatment [52, 58]. In urothelial cancer, TCGA-defined molecular subtypes have also been explored as potential predictive biomarkers; however, analyses have demonstrated slightly inconsistent findings and have not identified a group with an extremely high or low likelihood of response [58, 59]. Though combinations of biomarkers may ultimately improve the performance of response prediction tools, currently there are no tests with operating characteristics sufficient to routinely inform treatment decisions.

8 Conclusions

Although a renewed enthusiasm for immunotherapy in recent years has resulted in significant strides in the treatment of genitourinary malignancies, ongoing and future clinical trials are eagerly anticipated in order to better integrate immunotherapeutics into the armamentarium against these cancers. Identifying patients most likely to derive benefit from immune checkpoint blockade remains an active area of investigation. Questions regarding optimal dosing, appropriate durations of treatment particularly in patients achieving a response, and the use of sequential versus combination therapies sequence are yet to be answered. Indeed, the rapidly evolving field of cancer immunotherapy has been paralleled with increasing knowledge in tumor immunobiology. Ongoing iterative cycles of bench to bedside and bedside to bench investigations are required to further accelerate progress in the treatment of these diseases.

References

1. Richardson MA, Ramirez T, Russell NC, Moye LA (1999) Coley toxins immunotherapy: a retrospective review. Altern Ther Health Med 5(3):42–47. http://www.ncbi.nlm.nih.gov/pubmed/10234867. Accessed 26 Oct 2017
2. Tsung K, Norton JA (2006) Lessons from Coley's toxin. Surg Oncol 15(1):25–28. https://doi.org/10.1016/j.suronc.2006.05.002
3. Bellmunt J, de Wit R, Vaughn DJ et al (February 2017) Pembrolizumab as second-line therapy for advanced urothelial carcinoma. N Engl J Med https://doi.org/10.1056/nejmoa1613683 (NEJMoa1613683)
4. Siegel R, Naishadham D, Jemal A (2013) Cancer statistics, 2013. CA Cancer J Clin 63(1):11–30. https://doi.org/10.3322/caac.21166
5. Motzer RJ, Bander NH, Nanus DM (1996) Renal-cell carcinoma. N Engl J Med 335(12):865–875. https://doi.org/10.1056/NEJM199609193351207

6. Cohen HT, McGovern FJ (2005) Renal-cell carcinoma. N Engl J Med 353(23):2477–2490. https://doi.org/10.1056/NEJMra043172
7. Motzer RJ, Russo P, Nanus DM, Berg WJ. Renal cell carcinoma. Curr Probl Cancer 21 (4):185–232. http://www.ncbi.nlm.nih.gov/pubmed/9285186. Accessed 5 Sept 2017
8. Dabestani S, Thorstenson A, Lindblad P, Harmenberg U, Ljungberg B, Lundstam S (2016) Renal cell carcinoma recurrences and metastases in primary non-metastatic patients: a population-based study. World J Urol 34(8):1081–1086. https://doi.org/10.1007/s00345-016-1773-y
9. Itsumi M, Tatsugami K (2010) Immunotherapy for renal cell carcinoma. Clin Dev Immunol 2010:1–8. https://doi.org/10.1155/2010/284581
10. Fyfe G, Fisher RI, Rosenberg SA, Sznol M, Parkinson DR, Louie AC (1995) Results of treatment of 255 patients with metastatic renal cell carcinoma who received high-dose recombinant interleukin-2 therapy. J Clin Oncol 13(3):688–696. https://doi.org/10.1200/JCO.1995.13.3.688
11. Vaishampayan U, Vankayala H, Vigneau FD et al (2014) The effect of targeted therapy on overall survival in advanced renal cancer: a study of the national surveillance epidemiology and end results registry database. Clin Genitourin Cancer 12(2):124–129. https://doi.org/10.1016/j.clgc.2013.09.007
12. Yang JC, Hughes M, Kammula U et al (2007) Ipilimumab (anti-CTLA4 antibody) causes regression of metastatic renal cell cancer associated with enteritis and hypophysitis. J Immunother 30(8):825–830. https://doi.org/10.1097/CJI.0b013e318156e47e
13. Thompson RH, Kuntz SM, Leibovich BC et al (2006) Tumor B7-H1 is associated with poor prognosis in renal cell carcinoma patients with long-term follow-up. Cancer Res 66(7):3381–3385. https://doi.org/10.1158/0008-5472.CAN-05-4303
14. Topalian SL, Hodi FS, Brahmer JR et al (2012) Safety, activity, and immune correlates of anti–PD-1 antibody in cancer. N Engl J Med 366(26):2443–2454. https://doi.org/10.1056/NEJMoa1200690
15. Motzer RJ, Rini BI, McDermott DF et al (2015) Nivolumab for metastatic renal cell carcinoma: results of a randomized phase II trial. J Clin Oncol 33(13):1430–1437. https://doi.org/10.1200/JCO.2014.59.0703
16. Motzer RJ, Escudier B, McDermott DF et al (2015) Nivolumab versus everolimus in advanced renal-cell carcinoma. N Engl J Med 373(19):1803–1813. https://doi.org/10.1056/NEJMoa1510665
17. Heine A, Held SAE, Bringmann A, Holderried TAW, Brossart P (2011) Immunomodulatory effects of anti-angiogenic drugs. Leukemia 25(6):899–905. https://doi.org/10.1038/leu.2011.24
18. McDermott DF, Atkins MB, Motzer RJ et al (2017) A phase II study of atezolizumab (atezo) with or without bevacizumab (bev) versus sunitinib (sun) in untreated metastatic renal cell carcinoma (mRCC) patients (pts). J Clin Oncol 35(6_suppl):431–431. https://doi.org/10.1200/jco.2017.35.6_suppl.431
19. Hammers HJ, Plimack ER, Infante JR et al (July 2017) Safety and efficacy of nivolumab in combination with ipilimumab in metastatic renal cell carcinoma: the CheckMate 016 study. J Clin Oncol https://doi.org/10.1200/jco.2016.72.1985 (JCO.2016.72.198)
20. ESMO 2017: Nivolumab plus ipilimumab versus sunitinib in first-line treatment for advanced or metastatic RCC | ESMO. http://www.esmo.org/Conferences/ESMO-2017-Congress/News-Articles/Nivolumab-Plus-Ipilimumab-versus-Sunitinib-in-First-Line-Treatment-for-Advanced-or-Metastatic-RCC. Accessed 8 Oct 2017
21. Kantoff PW, Higano CS, Shore ND et al (2010) Sipuleucel-T immunotherapy for castration-resistant prostate cancer. N Engl J Med 363(5):411–422. https://doi.org/10.1056/NEJMoa1001294
22. Demaria S, Ng B, Devitt ML et al (2004) Ionizing radiation inhibition of distant untreated tumors (abscopal effect) is immune mediated. Int J Radiat Oncol 58(3):862–870. https://doi.org/10.1016/j.ijrobp.2003.09.012

23. Demaria S, Kawashima N, Yang AM et al (2005) Immune-mediated inhibition of metastases after treatment with local radiation and CTLA-4 blockade in a mouse model of breast cancer. Clin Cancer Res 11(2 Pt 1):728–734. http://www.ncbi.nlm.nih.gov/pubmed/15701862. Accessed 2 Apr 2017
24. Dewan MZ, Galloway AE, Kawashima N et al (2009) Fractionated but not single-dose radiotherapy induces an immune-mediated abscopal effect when combined with anti-CTLA-4 antibody. Clin Cancer Res 15(17):5379–5388. https://doi.org/10.1158/1078-0432.CCR-09-0265
25. Finkelstein SE, Salenius S, Mantz CA et al (2015) Combining immunotherapy and radiation for prostate cancer. Clin Genitourin Cancer 13(1):1–9. https://doi.org/10.1016/j.clgc.2014.09.001
26. Sharabi AB, Lim M, DeWeese TL, Drake CG (2015) Radiation and checkpoint blockade immunotherapy: radiosensitisation and potential mechanisms of synergy. Lancet Oncol 16 (13):e498–e509. https://doi.org/10.1016/S1470-2045(15)00007-8
27. Slovin SF, Higano CS, Hamid O et al (2013) Ipilimumab alone or in combination with radiotherapy in metastatic castration-resistant prostate cancer: results from an open-label, multicenter phase I/II study. Ann Oncol 24(7):1813–1821. https://doi.org/10.1093/annonc/mdt107
28. Kwon ED, Drake CG, Scher HI et al (2014) Ipilimumab versus placebo after radiotherapy in patients with metastatic castration-resistant prostate cancer that had progressed after docetaxel chemotherapy (CA184-043): a multicentre, randomised, double-blind, phase 3 trial. Lancet Oncol 15(7):700–712. https://doi.org/10.1016/S1470-2045(14)70189-5
29. Beer TM, Kwon ED, Drake CG et al (2017) Randomized, double-blind, phase III trial of ipilimumab versus placebo in asymptomatic or minimally symptomatic patients with metastatic chemotherapy-naive castration-resistant prostate cancer. J Clin Oncol 35(1):40–47. https://doi.org/10.1200/JCO.2016.69.1584
30. McNeel DG, Smith HA, Eickhoff JC et al (2012) Phase I trial of tremelimumab in combination with short-term androgen deprivation in patients with PSA-recurrent prostate cancer. Cancer Immunol Immunother 61(7):1137–1147. https://doi.org/10.1007/s00262-011-1193-1
31. Fong L, Kwek SS, O'Brien S et al (2009) Potentiating endogenous antitumor immunity to prostate cancer through combination immunotherapy with CTLA4 blockade and GM-CSF. Cancer Res 69(2):609–615. https://doi.org/10.1158/0008-5472.CAN-08-3529
32. van den Eertwegh AJ, Versluis J, van den Berg HP et al (2012) Combined immunotherapy with granulocyte-macrophage colony-stimulating factor-transduced allogeneic prostate cancer cells and ipilimumab in patients with metastatic castration-resistant prostate cancer: a phase 1 dose-escalation trial. Lancet Oncol 13(5):509–517. https://doi.org/10.1016/S1470-2045(12)70007-4
33. Jochems C, Tucker JA, Tsang K-Y et al (2014) A combination trial of vaccine plus ipilimumab in metastatic castration-resistant prostate cancer patients: immune correlates. Cancer Immunol Immunother 63(4):407–418. https://doi.org/10.1007/s00262-014-1524-0
34. Madan RA, Mohebtash M, Arlen PM et al (2012) Ipilimumab and a poxviral vaccine targeting prostate-specific antigen in metastatic castration-resistant prostate cancer: a phase 1 dose-escalation trial. Lancet Oncol 13(5):501–508. https://doi.org/10.1016/S1470-2045(12)70006-2
35. Brahmer JR, Drake CG, Wollner I et al (2010) Phase I study of single-agent anti-programmed death-1 (MDX-1106) in refractory solid tumors: safety, clinical activity, pharmacodynamics, and immunologic correlates. J Clin Oncol 28(19):3167–3175. https://doi.org/10.1200/JCO.2009.26.7609
36. Graff JN, Alumkal JJ, Drake CG et al (2016) Early evidence of anti-PD-1 activity in enzalutamide-resistant prostate cancer. Oncotarget 7(33):52810–52817. https://doi.org/10.18632/oncotarget.10547

37. Nakanishi J, Wada Y, Matsumoto K, Azuma M, Kikuchi K, Ueda S (2007) Overexpression of B7-H1 (PD-L1) significantly associates with tumor grade and postoperative prognosis in human urothelial cancers. Cancer Immunol Immunother 56(8):1173–1182. https://doi.org/10.1007/s00262-006-0266-z
38. Boorjian SA, Sheinin Y, Crispen PL et al (2008) T-cell coregulatory molecule expression in urothelial cell carcinoma: clinicopathologic correlations and association with survival. Clin Cancer Res 14(15):4800–4808. https://doi.org/10.1158/1078-0432.CCR-08-0731
39. Inman BA, Sebo TJ, Frigola X et al (2007) PD-L1 (B7-H1) expression by urothelial carcinoma of the bladder and BCG-induced granulomata: associations with localized stage progression. Cancer 109(8):1499–1505. https://doi.org/10.1002/cncr.22588
40. Xylinas E, Robinson BD, Kluth LA et al (2014) Association of T-cell co-regulatory protein expression with clinical outcomes following radical cystectomy for urothelial carcinoma of the bladder. Eur J Surg Oncol 40(1):121–127. https://doi.org/10.1016/j.ejso.2013.08.023
41. Bellmunt J, Mullane SA, Werner L et al (2015) Association of PD-L1 expression on tumor-infiltrating mononuclear cells and overall survival in patients with urothelial carcinoma. Ann Oncol Off J Eur Soc Med Oncol 26(4):812–817. https://doi.org/10.1093/annonc/mdv009
42. Mangsbo SM, Sandin LC, Anger K, Korman AJ, Loskog A, Totterman TH (2010) Enhanced tumor eradication by combining CTLA-4 or PD-1 blockade with CpG therapy. J Immunother 33(3):225–235. https://doi.org/10.1097/CJI.0b013e3181c01fcb00002371-201004000-00001 [pii]
43. Carthon BC, Wolchok JD, Yuan J et al (2010) Preoperative CTLA-4 blockade: tolerability and immune monitoring in the setting of a presurgical clinical trial. Clin Cancer Res 16 (10):2861–2871. https://doi.org/10.1158/1078-0432.ccr-10-0569 (1078-0432.CCR-10-0569 [pii])
44. Galsky MD, Hahn NM, Albany C et al (2016) Phase II trial of gemcitabine + cisplatin + ipilimumab in patients with metastatic urothelial cancer. ASCO Meet Abstr 34(2_suppl):357
45. Powles T, Eder JP, Fine GD et al (2014) MPDL3280A (anti-PD-L1) treatment leads to clinical activity in metastatic bladder cancer. Nature 515(7528):558–562. https://doi.org/10.1038/nature13904
46. Plimack ER, Bellmunt J, Gupta S et al (2017) Safety and activity of pembrolizumab in patients with locally advanced or metastatic urothelial cancer (KEYNOTE-012): a non-randomised, open-label, phase 1b study. Lancet Oncol 18(2):212–220. https://doi.org/10.1016/S1470-2045(17)30007-4
47. Powles T, Loriot Y, Duran I et al (2017) IMvigor 211: a phase III randomized study examining atezolizumab versus chemotherapy for platinum-treated advanced urothelial cancer. In: EACR-AACR-SIC
48. Galsky MD, Hahn NM, Rosenberg J et al (2011) A consensus definition of patients with metastatic urothelial carcinoma who are unfit for cisplatin-based chemotherapy. Lancet Oncol 12(3):211–214. https://doi.org/10.1016/S1470-2045(10)70275-8
49. Galsky MD, Hahn NM, Rosenberg J et al (2011) Treatment of patients with metastatic urothelial cancer "unfit" for cisplatin-based chemotherapy. J Clin Oncol 29(17):2432–2438. https://doi.org/10.1200/JCO.2011.34.8433
50. Galsky MD, Chen GJ, Oh WK et al (2011) Comparative effectiveness of cisplatin-based and carboplatin-based chemotherapy for treatment of advanced urothelial carcinoma. Ann Oncol 23(2):406–410. https://doi.org/10.1093/annonc/mdr156 (mdr156 [pii])
51. De Santis M, Bellmunt J, Mead G et al (2012) Randomized phase II/III trial assessing gemcitabine/carboplatin and methotrexate/carboplatin/vinblastine in patients with advanced urothelial cancer who are unfit for cisplatin-based chemotherapy: EORTC study 30986. J Clin Oncol 30(2):191–199. https://doi.org/10.1200/jco.2011.37.3571 (JCO.2011.37.3571 [pii])
52. Balar AV, Galsky MD, Rosenberg JE et al (2017) Atezolizumab as first-line treatment in cisplatin-ineligible patients with locally advanced and metastatic urothelial carcinoma: a single-arm, multicentre, phase 2 trial. Lancet 389(10064):67–76. https://doi.org/10.1016/S0140-6736(16)32455-2

53. O'Donnell PH, Grivas P, Balar AV et al (2017) Biomarker findings and mature clinical results from KEYNOTE-052: First-line pembrolizumab (pembro) in cisplatin-ineligible advanced urothelial cancer (UC). J Clin Oncol 35(15_suppl):4502. https://doi.org/10.1200/jco.2017.35.15_suppl.4502
54. Fay AP, Signoretti S, Callea M et al (2015) Programmed death ligand-1 expression in adrenocortical carcinoma: an exploratory biomarker study. J Immunother Cancer 3(1):3. https://doi.org/10.1186/s40425-015-0047-3
55. Le Tourneau C, Hoimes CJ, Zarwan C, Wong DJL, Bauer S, Wermke M, Claus R, Chin KM, von Heydebreck A, Cuillerot J-M, JLG. Avelumab (MSB0010718C; anti-PD-L1) in patients with advanced adrenocortical carcinoma from the JAVELIN solid tumor phase Ib trial: safety and clinical activity. https://doi.org/10.1200/jco.2016.34.15_suppl.4516
56. Wang J, Rodriguez J, Rao P, Pettaway CA, Pagliaro LC (2015) Programmed death ligand-1 (PD-L1) expression in penile squamous cell carcinoma. J Clin Oncol 33(7_suppl):393–393. https://doi.org/10.1200/jco.2015.33.7_suppl.393
57. Udager AM, Liu T-Y, Skala SL et al (2016) Frequent PD-L1 expression in primary and metastatic penile squamous cell carcinoma: potential opportunities for immunotherapeutic approaches. Ann Oncol 27(9):1706–1712. https://doi.org/10.1093/annonc/mdw216
58. Rosenberg JE, Hoffman-Censits J, Powles T et al (March 2016) Atezolizumab in patients with locally advanced and metastatic urothelial carcinoma who have progressed following treatment with platinum-based chemotherapy: a single-arm, multicentre, phase 2 trial. Lancet (London, England). https://doi.org/10.1016/s0140-6736(16)00561-4
59. Sharma P, Retz M, Siefker-Radtke A et al (2017) Nivolumab in metastatic urothelial carcinoma after platinum therapy (CheckMate 275): a multicentre, single-arm, phase 2 trial. Lancet Oncol. https://doi.org/10.1016/S1470-2045(17)30065-7
60. Rini BI, Stein M, Shannon P et al (2011) Phase 1 dose-escalation trial of tremelimumab plus sunitinib in patients with metastatic renal cell carcinoma. Cancer 117(4):758–767. https://doi.org/10.1002/cncr.25639
61. Meeting Library | Nivolumab (anti-PD-1; BMS-936558, ONO-4538) in combination with sunitinib or pazopanib in patients (pts) with metastatic renal cell carcinoma (mRCC). http://meetinglibrary.asco.org/record/94621/abstract. Accessed 6 Oct 6 2017
62. Meeting Library | A phase I/II study to assess the safety and efficacy of pazopanib (PAZ) and pembrolizumab (PEM) in patients (pts) with advanced renal cell carcinoma (aRCC). http://meetinglibrary.asco.org/record/152938/abstract. Accessed 6 Oct 2017
63. Meeting Library | First-line avelumab + axitinib therapy in patients (pts) with advanced renal cell carcinoma (aRCC): Results from a phase Ib trial. http://meetinglibrary.asco.org/record/144685/abstract. Accessed 6 Oct 2017
64. Atkins MB, Gupta S, Choueiri TK et al (2015) Phase Ib dose-finding study of axitinib plus pembrolizumab in treatment-naïve patients with advanced renal cell carcinoma. J Immunother Cancer 3(Suppl 2):P353. https://doi.org/10.1186/2051-1426-3-S2-P353
65. Powles T, O'Donnell PH, Massard C et al (2017) Efficacy and safety of durvalumab in locally advanced or metastatic urothelial carcinoma. JAMA Oncol 45(2):e172411. https://doi.org/10.1001/jamaoncol.2017.2411
66. Apolo AB, Infante JR, Balmanoukian A et al (April 2017) Avelumab, an anti-programmed death-ligand 1 antibody, in patients with refractory metastatic urothelial carcinoma: results from a multicenter, phase Ib study. J Clin Oncol https://doi.org/10.1200/jco.2016.71.6795 (JCO2016716795)

The Cancer Genome Atlas Project in Bladder Cancer

Alejo Rodriguez-Vida, Seth P. Lerner and Joaquim Bellmunt

Contents

A. Rodriguez-Vida · J. Bellmunt
Medical Oncology Department, Institut Hospital del Mar d'Investigacions Mèdiques (IMIM), Hospital del Mar, Barcelona, Spain

S. P. Lerner
Scott Department of Urology, Dan L Duncan Cancer Center, Baylor College of Medicine, Houston, USA

J. Bellmunt (✉)
Harvard Medical School, Bladder Cancer Center, Dana-Farber Cancer Institute/Brigham and Women's Cancer Center, Boston, USA
e-mail: Joaquim_bellmunt@dfci.harvard.edu

S. Daneshmand and K. G. Chan (eds.), *Genitourinary Cancers*, Cancer Treatment and Research 175, https://doi.org/10.1007/978-3-319-93339-9_12

Abstract

Bladder cancer (BC) remains an aggressive disease with a poor prognosis, especially for patients with metastatic disease who have a limited median overall survival of 14 months. Urothelial carcinomas harbor frequent molecular dysregulations including recurrent mutations and copy number alteration, some of which could be potential therapeutic targets. However, no molecularly targeted agents have been approved to date for the treatment of advanced BC. Gaining new insights into the molecular landscape of BC will be critical to tailor future targeted agents for the treatment of advanced disease. The Cancer Genome Atlas (TCGA) project is cataloguing the genetic and epigenetic alterations responsible for cancer through the application of high-throughput genome analysis techniques. After the landmark paper profiling 131 patients was published in 2014, additional patients have been added with an updated TCGA analysis now including 412 patients. This chapter will review the previously described genomic alterations reported in the first manuscript and the new major highlights found in the expanded analyses recently published. The aim will be to review how this comprehensive integrated genomic analysis can inform the design of precision medicine targeted therapy for the treatment of advanced disease.

Keywords

The cancer genome atlas project · Urothelial carcinoma · Cancer genomics Whole-genome and RNA sequencing · Molecular subtypes · Mutational load Molecular biomarkers · Molecular therapeutic targets

1 Introduction

Bladder cancer (BC) is the ninth most common tumor worldwide, with an incidence of more than 330,000 new cases each year and an annual mortality rate of 130,000 [1]. Urothelial carcinoma (UC) accounts for nearly 90% of bladder cancers. It is associated with tobacco smoking in 65–70% of cases and is three times more prevalent in men than in women. At the initial diagnosis of BC, 30% of cases present as muscle-invasive bladder cancer (MIBC), with approximately one-third of them having distant metastases at presentation. Among patients who undergo radical cystectomy, around 25% will have pathologic lymph node metastasis at the time of surgery [2]. Despite the improvements seen during the last decade in terms of both surgical quality and systemic therapy, BC remains an aggressive disease with a poor prognosis, especially for patients with locally advanced or metastatic disease who have a reduced median overall survival (OS) of around 14 months [3, 4]. Therefore, there is an important unmet need for effective anticancer treatment in order to improve outcome and survival for patients with advanced BC.

The first focused molecular analyses of patients with BC revealed that urothelial carcinomas harbor frequent molecular alterations including recurrent mutations and multiple regions of somatic copy number alteration (CNA), some of which could be potential therapeutic targets [5–8]. Moreover, it has been shown that MIBC and non-MIBC (NMIBC) each have a distinctive molecular landscape, where low-grade NMIBC is characterized by a high incidence of FGFR3 mutations and high-grade MIBC has a higher frequency of many types of mutations [9, 10]. However, no molecularly targeted agents have so far been approved for the treatment of advanced BC. Recently, pembrolizumab, an immune checkpoint inhibitor targeting the programmed cell death-1 (PD-1) receptor, showed for the first time in history an improvement in OS compared to investigator-choice standard chemotherapy (paclitaxel, docetaxel, vinflunine) as second or third line for patients with advanced UC progressing to platinum-based chemotherapy [11]. However, the population recruited for PD-1 inhibitors studies in BC have not been selected according to any specific molecular findings and programmed cell death ligand-1 (PD-L1) expression has not found to be a predictive biomarker of treatment benefit. Gaining new insights into the disease biology and the molecular landscape of BC will therefore be critical to molecularly tailor future targeted agents for the treatment of advanced disease.

The Cancer Genome Atlas (TCGA) project is a collaboration that begun in 2005, between the National Cancer Institute and the National Human Genome Research Institute with the purpose of cataloguing the genetic and epigenetic alterations responsible for cancer through the application of high-throughput genome analysis techniques, including large-scale genome sequencing and bioinformatics [12]. The final goal of TCGA is to deepen our understanding of the molecular basis of cancer in order to improve our ability to diagnose, treat, and prevent this lethal disease. Thus far, the TCGA has generated comprehensive, multidimensional maps of the key genomic alterations in 33 types of cancer, including urothelial carcinomas. The TCGA dataset, comprising more than two petabytes of genomic data of tumor tissue and matched normal tissues from more than 11,000 patients, has been made publically available and can be accessed through the TCGA Data Portal [13].

The first comprehensive molecular landscape study of BC by the TCGA was published in 2014 and integrated data from 131 patients with chemotherapy-naïve high-grade muscle-invasive urothelial bladder carcinomas (T2–T4a, N0, M0) undergoing surgical resection with either transurethral resection or radical cystectomy [14]. This first study included data on DNA copy number, somatic mutations, gene fusions, messenger RNA expression, protein expression, DNA methylation, transcript splice variants, viral integration and pathway alterations as well as a thorough description of four expression-based molecular subtypes of BC. In 2017, a second comprehensive TCGA study was published, analyzing an expanded cohort of 412 patients with either localized or metastatic chemotherapy-naïve muscle-invasive bladder carcinoma [15]. This second analysis is derived from a threefold increase in the number of tumors, thus improving the power to detect less frequent molecular abnormalities. Moreover, this updated study provides several new analyses that were not part of the first paper including mutation burden and neoantigen load, an integrated analysis of non-coding RNA and new analytic detection of pathogens in BC. Finally, it reports for the first time a robust correlation of mutation signature clusters and expression-based subtypes in a univariate and multivariate association with survival. This chapter will review the major highlights described in these two important TCGA studies on the molecular characterization of BC and how the findings can inform the design of precision medicine targeted therapy for the treatment of advanced disease.

2 Somatic DNA Alterations

The TCGA studies confirmed that MIBC is characterized by a high overall mutation rate, similar to that of lung cancer or melanoma. This is an important result since several studies have shown that mutation load is a biomarker of response to immune checkpoint inhibitors [16, 17]. In the first TCGA analysis, there were on average 302 exonic mutations, 204 segmental alterations in genomic copy number, and 22 genomic rearrangements per sample. Whole-exome sequencing (WES) targeted 186,260 exons in 18,091 genes and identified 39,312 somatic mutations (including 38,012 point mutations and 1138 insertions or deletions) [14]. These results were internally validated by a targeted re-sequencing of all significantly mutated genes and by a comparison with whole-genome sequencing (WGS) of 18 samples, with a validation rate of 99% [14]. WES of the 412 tumors included in the second TCGA analysis increased the number of targeted exons to 193,094 and the number of genes to 18,862. It identified 131,660 somatic mutations, including 128,772 single nucleotide variants, and 2888 insertions or deletions [15]. Many of the focal mutations involved genes previously known in bladder cancer such as TP53 (49%), PIK3CA (20%), RB1 (13%), FGFR3 (12%), ERCC2 (12%), and TSC1 (8%). In addition, several other genes that have not previously been reported as significantly mutated in BC were identified, such as MLL2 (27%), CDKN1A (14%), or STAG2 (11%) [14]. Similarly, the second TCGA study identified 58 genes mutated at a frequency statistically significantly higher than background, 34 of which had not been previously identified as significantly mutated in the first study, including KMT2C (18%), ATM (14%), and FAT1 (12%) [15].

The second TCGA study tried to detect processes contributing to the high mutation rate, using a Bayesian approach. It identified five differential mutation signatures (APOBEC-a and APOBEC-b, ERCC2, C > T at CpG, POLE), which correlated with different subsets of BC with different mutation burdens and mechanisms. Clustering of four of these five mutation signatures (APOBEC-a and APOBEC-b, ERCC2 and C > T at CpG) identified four mutational signature clusters, MSig1 to MSig4. Interestingly, the activity of an endogenous mutagen, the DNA cytidine deaminase APOBEC accounted for 67% of the overall mutations. The majority of APOBEC-mediated mutations were clonal, suggesting that APOBEC activity is an early event in the carcinogenic development of BC. Moreover, the mutation signature cluster of high-APOBEC mutagenesis and high mutation burden (MSig1) was strongly associated with an improved OS ($p = 1.4 \times 10^{-4}$) with 75% of subjects alive 5 years after diagnosis of MIBC [15]. The authors hypothesize that the unusually good survival of this subset is due to the high mutation burden, boosting the host immune antitumor response. On the other hand, MSig2 cancers had the lowest mutation rate and the poorest 5-year survival (22%). The identification of APOBEC as the main driver of mutagenesis in BC is extremely relevant since a better understanding of its expression and activity could have a major benefit for selecting patients for clinical trials of immunotherapy.

The high mutation rate seen in BC as in lung cancer has been associated with smoking habit in several studies [18]. Moreover, several clinical trials in both BC and other advanced cancers have shown a relationship between smoking status and the relative benefit of immunotherapy and it has been postulated that this benefit is due to the high mutational load induced by smoking [11, 19]. Consequently, the TCGA has analyzed the correlation between smoking status and the presence of molecular alterations. In the first TCGA study, 72% of patients were current or past smokers. However, there was no statistically significant association between smoking status and the mutational load, frequency of mutations in any significantly mutated gene, occurrence of CNAs, or expression subtype [14]. This misbalance may reflect the fact that not all mutations might have the same potential to act as neoepitopes and consequently neoantigen load could be a more robust predictive biomarker for immunotherapy than mutational load. Hence, the second TCGA study included a neoantigen prediction analysis by enumerating peptides bearing somatic mutations and assessing their binding against the patient's inferred HLA type. The effect of the neoantigen load was then analyzed in a univariate and multivariate analysis. Interestingly, neoantigen load did strongly correlate with mutation burden and was associated with improved survival ($p = 5.2 \times 10^{-4}$). On multivariate analysis, neoantigen load remained an independent predictor of survival after adjusting for age, tumor stage, histology, and node status ($p = 8 \times 10^{-4}$) [15].

3 MRNA Expression and Molecular Subtypes

Analysis of RNA-sequencing data from the 129 tumors included in the first TCGA study identified the well-known distinction between luminal and basal subtypes of BC [20–22], and divided them into four clusters, clusters I–II being luminal and clusters III–IV being basal [14]. Luminal cluster I (or papillary-like cluster) was enriched in tumors with papillary morphology ($p = 0.0002$), FGFR3 mutations ($p = 0.0007$), FGFR3 copy number gain ($p = 0.04$), and elevated FGFR3 expression ($p < 0.0001$). Consequently, the authors hypothesized that tumors with cluster I expression and/or FGFR3 alterations could benefit from FGFR inhibitors. Moreover, luminal clusters I and II showed high protein expression of HER2, comparable to those found in TCGA HER2-positive breast cancers [23], and an elevated estrogen receptor beta signaling, flagging them as potential responders to hormone therapy and HER2 inhibitors. Luminal clusters I and II also showed characteristics similar to those of luminal A breast cancer, with high mRNA and protein expression of luminal breast differentiation markers, including GATA3 and FOXA1. On the other hand, the signature of basal cluster III (or basal/squamous-like cluster) showed molecular features similar to that of basal-like breast cancers and squamous cell cancers of the head and neck and lung [23, 24], such as high expression of KRT14, KRT5, KRT6A, and EGFR. These distinctive expression-based clusters were then externally validated using an external data set of 308 MIBC tumor samples from a prior study which confirmed the same four distinctive cluster subgroups [14, 22].

A similar RNA-sequencing analysis was undertaken on the second TCGA study in the expanded cohort of 412 patients, recapitulating the same two major luminal and basal transcriptional subtypes identified in the first study [15]. Moreover, this expanded analysis provided further discrimination within these subgroups which led to a re-cataloguing of the different subtypes into five entities: luminal-papillary ($n = 142$), luminal-infiltrated ($n = 78$), luminal ($n = 26$), basal-squamous ($n = 142$), and to the identification of a novel neuronal subtype ($n = 20$). As described before, the luminal-papillary cluster was enriched with papillary tumors (58% vs. 20% in the other subtypes; $p < 10^{-13}$) and with lower-stage T1 or T2 tumors (55% vs. 23%, $p < 10^{-8}$). Similarly, it was characterized by frequent FGFR3 alterations (44%), either mutations, amplification, overexpression, or fusions, which indicates that many tumors of the luminal-papillary cluster tumors might have developed from a precursor non-MIBC. This subtype was also characterized by a major loss of DNA methylation and included cases that were almost all node-negative, from younger patients (median age 61 vs. 69; $p < 4 \times 10^{-3}$), and had better survival ($p < 0.05$) [15].

The luminal-infiltrated subtype, on the other hand, was distinguished from other luminal subtypes by a strong expression of smooth muscle and myofibroblast gene signatures and a p53-like expression which has previously been associated with chemoresistance [21]. The luminal-infiltrated subtype correlated with the prior luminal cluster II, which has been reported to benefit from anti-PDL1 inhibitor atezolizumab [16, 17]. The basal-squamous subtype was characterized by high expression of basal and stem-like markers (KRT5, KRT6A, KRT14) and squamous differentiation markers (TGM1, DSC3, PI3) and included 82% of tumors containing squamous cell features ($p < 10^{-11}$). This subtype was enriched in TP53 mutations ($p = 5 \times 10^{-3}$) and had a high carcinoma-in situ (CIS) expression signature score, indicating that they may have originated from bladder basal cells through CIS lesions. The basal-squamous subtype also showed the strongest immune expression signature, including T cell markers and inflammation genes, indicating the presence of lymphocytic infiltrates. Interestingly, the basal-squamous subtype correlated with the prior clusters III and IV, which were the clusters showing greatest benefit from anti-PDL1 inhibitor atezolizumab after cluster II [16, 17].

The neuronal subtype, finally, included three of four histologic small cell neuroendocrine tumors found in the whole cohort, but showed no apparent histologic distinction from other types of MIBC in the majority of cases (85%). This subtype was characterized by a high expression of many neuronal differentiation genes, as well as neuroendocrine markers. Half of the samples had mutations in both TP53 and RB1, which is a genetic hallmark of small cell neuroendocrine cancer, regardless of the primary origin. This subtype was the most infrequent cluster (5%) and had the highest CIS expression signature score, also indicating it may have originated from CIS lesions. Importantly, the neuronal subtype had the poorest survival compared to the other four subgroups ($p = 1.4 \times 10^{-3}$) in keeping with the known aggressive behavior of neuroendocrine BCs [15].

The identification of these mRNA expression subtypes as five distinctive molecular entities is a critical discovery that will promote gaining new insights into the specific biology of each subtype, a critical requisite to using molecular correlates to tailor future tumor-personalized targeted therapies.

4 Pathway Analysis and Therapeutic Targeting

The information obtained from the somatic mutation analysis and copy number data was integrated in order to identify the more frequently altered pathways and potential targets amenable for therapeutic intervention. Importantly, most of the canonical signaling pathways that were consistently altered in both TCGA studies provide significant opportunities for a molecular-targeted therapeutic blockade [14, 15]. Integrated analysis revealed three frequently dysregulated pathways: p53/cell cycle regulation (89%), RTK/RAS/PI3 K signaling (71%), and chromatin remodeling pathways with alterations in the histone-modifying genes in 52% of cases, and in the nucleosome remodeling complex in 26% [15]. p53/cell cycle alterations included TP53 mutations in 48% of cases, MDM2 amplification (copy number >4) in 6%, and MDM2 overexpression (>twofold above the median) in 19%, with strong mutual exclusivity between these events ($p < 10^{-16}$) [15]. Mutations in chromatin-modifying and regulatory genes were common, with 10 such genes having a mutation frequency greater than 5%, and with 66% of samples showing a mutation in one or more genes. Of note, 10 of the 39 significantly mutated genes with mutation frequency >5% were either chromatin-modifying or chromatin-regulatory genes, such as KDM6A (a histone de-methylase), histone methyltransferases (KMT2A, KMT2C, KMT2D), or histone acetylases (CREBBP, EP300, KANSL1) [15]. Mutations in these ten genes were predominantly inactivating, which suggests that they are functionally relevant. Taken together, this data indicate that dysregulation of gene expression mediated by alterations in chromatin-regulatory genes is a driver of BC development [15]. Moreover, the presence of abnormalities in chromatin-modifying enzymes identifies a subset of BC patients who could benefit from drugs targeting chromatin modifications, such as agents that bind acetyl-lysine binding motifs (bromodomains) [25, 26].

PI3K signaling alterations included activating point mutations in PIK3CA (22%), which could potentially benefit from PI3K inhibitors; mutations or deletions of TSC1 (8%), which could potentially benefit from mTOR inhibitors [15] and overexpression of AKT3 (10%), potentially responsive to AKT inhibitors [14]. As mentioned earlier, FGFR3 pathway was also frequently altered, including mutations (14%) and fusions (2%), all potentially responsive to FGFR inhibitors [15]. FGFR3 mutations were more frequent in lower-stage tumors (21% in T1–T2 vs. 10% in T3–T4; $p = 0.003$) and correlated with better survival ($p = 0.04$) [15]. Other frequent altered pathways with therapeutic implications included amplification of EGFR (9%, potentially responsive to EGFR inhibitors), mutations of HER3 (6%, potentially sensitive to HER inhibitors), and mutation or amplification of HER2 (9%, potentially sensitive to HER2 inhibitors) [14]. Of note, the frequency of HER2 alterations was comparable to that of the TCGA HER2-positive breast cancers, albeit with less amplifications and more mutations [23]. DNA repair pathways also showed frequent genomic alterations (16%) including mutations in ATM (14%) and ERCC2 (9%), and deletions in RAD51B (2%) [15], and could indicate responsiveness to platinum agents or PARP inhibitors.

5 Other Significant Findings

- *Viral DNA integration*: RNA-sequencing and WGS data were used to identify evidence of viral DNA genomic integration due to infection by several virus, such as cytomegalovirus (CMV), BK polyomavirus, human papilloma virus (HPV), or human herpes virus (HHV) [14, 15]. The first analysis identified viral DNAs in 7 of 122 tumors (6%), and viral transcripts in 5 of 122 (4%) [14]. Taking both studies together, there was evidence of infection by CMV ($n = 3$), HPV ($n = 11$), HHV4 ($n = 6$), HHV5 ($n = 6$), and polyomavirus ($n = 1$), indicating that viral infection might have a role in the development of a small subset of BC [14, 15].
- *Non-coding RNAs (lncRNAs and miRNAs) subdivide mRNA expression subtypes*: The second TCGA study provided for the first time an integrated analysis of non-coding RNA, including long non-coding RNA (lncRNA) and microRNA (miRNA). Clustering by lncRNA and miRNA expression was concordant with the mRNA subtypes while providing further discrimination within them, with differential epithelial-mesenchymal transition (EMT), CIS scores, histologic features, and survival [15]. For example, lncRNA cluster 3 was a subset of the luminal-papillary subtype with a better survival. It was characterized by a low frequency of TP53 mutations and high frequency of FGRF3 mutations/fusions and was associated with papillary histology, node-negative disease, or low T-stage/node-positive cases. Similarly, the four miRNA clusters were concordant with subtypes for mRNA ($p = 2.4 \times 10^{-52}$), lncRNA ($p = 1.5 \times 10^{-45}$), hypomethylation ($p = 4.5 \times 10^{-30}$) and were associated with histological subtype (papillary vs. non-papillary), combined T-stage/node+, node positive/negative, and CIS gene sets [15]. miRNA subtype 3 was enriched in lncRNA 3, and had better survival, consistent with low EMT scores. On the other hand, miRNA subtype 4 and 2 contained most of the basal/squamous

mRNA subtype, and had relatively poor survival, consistent with relatively high EMT scores.

- *Proteomic data subtypes*: The second TCGA study also included for the first time an unsupervised clustering using reverse phase protein array (RPPA) proteomic data analysis. This analysis identified five robust clusters with differential protein expression profiles, pathway activities, and overall survival ($p = 0.019$), several of them displaying alterations suitable for therapeutic intervention [15]. Proteomic cluster C1 (epithelial/papillary) was associated with low EMT scores, papillary differentiation, and improved survival. Cluster C2 (epithelial/intermediate) had a more intermediate outcome profile. Both clusters C1 and C2 are enriched in HER2 expression levels, indicating they might benefit from HER2 inhibitors [15]. Cluster C3 (proliferative/low signaling) had a high cell cycle pathway score, low PI3K and mTOR pathway signaling, but high EGFR expression levels, making it a potential candidate for EGFR-directed therapies. Clusters C4 and C5 had higher EMT pathway scores, of which cluster C4 (EMT/hormone signaling) had the worst outcome and was associated with non-papillary samples and pathologic advanced stage 3 and 4.

6 Survival Univariate and Multivariate Analysis

The second TCGA analysis assessed the correlation of 101 clinical and molecular variables with overall survival in a univariate and multivariate log-rank test. Of the 101 covariates analyzed by univariate log-rank tests, 13 were selected for multivariate Cox regression analysis. LASSO regression analysis was chosen to fit a multivariate model. The best-survival subtype was set as the reference variable for each of mRNA, lncRNA, miRNA, and MSig.

The variables with largest coefficients were AJCC stages III and IV, the mRNA neuronal and luminal subtypes, the low mutation rate MSig 2, and miRNA subtype 4, which is a subset of basal-squamous cases, and KLF4 regulon activity, all of which were associated with poorer survival. The mRNA luminal-infiltrated subtype, age, GATA3 regulon activity, and MSig4 were retained with smaller coefficients. The ranking order from poorer to better survival were: mRNA neuronal subtype, AJCC stage IV, MSig2, miRNA subtype 4, AJCC stage III, mRNA luminal subtype, KLF4 regulon, mRNA luminal-infiltrated, age, GATA3 regulon, and MSig 4.15. Tumor stages III and IV correlated with worse survival and were associated with a 45% and 112% higher risk of death, respectively, than stage I and II tumors combined. Mutational signature cluster MSig1 showed a 47% lower risk of death than MSig4, while cluster MSig2 had a 38% higher risk of death. The mRNA neuronal subtype had the worse survival outcome and had a 63% higher risk of death than the basal/squamous subtype. This latter showed no significant risk differences with the three luminal subtypes. Finally, miRNA cluster 4, a poorer-survival subset of the basal/squamous mRNA subtype as mentioned earlier, had a 36% higher risk of death than miRNA subtype 1 [5].

7 Subtype-Stratified Potential Treatments

By integrating mRNA subtype classification, altered pathways data, EMT and CIS signatures, and immune infiltrate analyses, the second study of the TCGA proposed potential specific therapeutic recommendations for each subtype of MIBC, depending on their specific molecular landscape, that can be tested in prospective clinical trials:

- *Luminal-papillary subtype*: It is characterized by FGFR3 mutation, fusions and/or amplification, papillary histology and a very low CIS score. This subtype can be assessed as having relatively low risk for progression, and when diagnosed as localized disease, it might not need to be treated with neoadjuvant chemotherapy (NAC). On the other hand, FGFR3 tyrosine kinase inhibitors should be tested in patients with metastatic disease.
- *Luminal-infiltrated subtype*: It has high expression of both EMT and myofibroblast markers. It is enriched on immune markers such as PD-L1 and CTLA4, which is in keeping with the fact this subtype has been reported to benefit from anti-PDL1 inhibitor atezolizumab [16, 17], as mentioned earlier. Thus, patients presenting with this molecular subtype could not only benefit from PD-L1 inhibitors on the metastatic setting but also in both the neoadjuvant and postoperative adjuvant settings. Neoadjuvant cisplatin-based chemotherapy could also be used but is expected to produce infrequent tumor responses, as this subtype has been associated with chemoresistance.
- *Luminal subtype*: It is characterized by a very high expression of luminal markers (uroplakins). Because this subtype had not been previously described as a separate entity, the potential therapies are not well defined. Consequently, it could benefit from NAC for localized disease and/or therapies targeting each specific molecular alteration.
- *Basal-squamous subtype*: It is characterized by female enrichment, squamous differentiation, and basal keratin expression. This subtype has the strongest immune expression signature (indicating the presence of lymphocytic infiltrates) and is enriched on immune markers such as PD-L1 and CTLA4. This is illustrated by the fact that this subtype also showed benefit in the atezolizumab trials [16, 17]. This subtype could benefit from NAC for localized disease and from immune checkpoint inhibitors for the metastatic setting.
- *Neuronal subtype*: It is characterized by expression of both neuroendocrine and neuronal markers and a high cell cycle signature indicating a high proliferative status. Similarly to small cell neuroendocrine tumors originating from other organs, etoposide-platinum combination chemotherapy should be the preferred option, in both the neoadjuvant and metastatic setting.

Finally, the authors suggest that this molecularly driven therapeutic sub-classification should be prospectively validated in future clinical trials, as well as tested retrospectively in ongoing or completed clinical trials that assessed similar treatment strategies.

8 Conclusions

In the past 30 years, the treatment of advanced bladder cancer has barely moved beyond platinum-based combination chemotherapy and surgery. The recent approval of the immune checkpoint inhibitor pembrolizumab as second or third line in the metastatic setting, after showing an improved overall survival, has been the major breakthrough revolution in bladder cancer therapy of the last decades [11]. However, this immune therapy, in the same way as classical platinum chemotherapy, is administered to all patients in an unselected manner and no robust predictive biomarkers of response have been identified. Consequently, a significant proportion of patients will never benefit from these therapies but we are unable to predict that in advance given the lack of clinical or molecular biomarkers. That is why the main objective of the TCGA studies is to provide a comprehensive molecular characterization of the genetic landscape of MIBC in order to improve our ability to personalize the therapy of this lethal disease. The two TCGA studies on urothelial cancer have shown that the molecular landscape of this disease is rich in several genetic and epigenetic alterations and that up to two-thirds of patients have potentially actionable mutations. The first TCGA analysis integrated genomic data from 131 MIBC samples and showed several relevant findings: a high somatic mutation rate, similar to that of lung cancer and melanoma; statistically significant recurrent mutations in 32 genes; four mRNA expression subtypes showing a distinctive molecular landscape; and potential therapeutic targets in 69% of the samples [14]. The second TCGA study expanded the cohort to 412 samples and demonstrated several other relevant findings: The high mutational load in BC is mainly driven by the APOBEC-mediated mutagenesis; tumors with high-APOBEC and high mutation load had an extraordinary improved survival; mRNA clustering identified a novel neuronal subtype with small cell neuroendocrine features and poor survival. Finally, the integration of mRNA subtype classification, altered pathways data, EMT and CIS signatures, and immune infiltrate analyses provided one the most important findings of this second TCGA study: the identification of five expression-based distinctive molecular subtypes with different developmental mechanisms and distinct therapeutic potential [15]. Although this molecular sub-classification still needs to be prospectively validated in future clinical trials, it opens a massive window of opportunities into personalized treatment of bladder cancer.

References

1. Sobin LH, Gospodariwicz M, Wittekind C (eds) (2009) TNM classification of malignant tumors. UICC International Union Against Cancer, 7th edn. Wiley-Blackwell, pp 262–265
2. Witjes JA, Compérat E, Cowan NC et al (2014) EAU guidelines on muscle-invasive and metastatic bladder cancer: summary of the 2013 guidelines. Eur Urol 65(4):778–792
3. Loehrer PJ, Einhorn LH, Elson PJ et al (1992) A randomized comparison of cisplatin alone or in combination with methotrexate, vinblastine, and doxorubicin in patients with metastatic urothelial carcinoma: a cooperative group study. J Clin Oncol 10(7):1066–1073
4. von der Maase H, Sengelov L, Roberts JT et al (2005) Long-term survival results of a randomized trial comparing gemcitabine plus cisplatin, with methotrexate, vinblastine, doxorubicin, plus cisplatin in patients with bladder cancer. J Clin Oncol 23(21):4602–4608
5. Goebell PJ, Knowles MA (2010) Bladder cancer or bladder cancers? Genetically distinct malignant conditions of the urothelium. Urol Oncol 28(4):409–428
6. Forbes SA, Bindal N, Bamford S et al (2011) COSMIC: mining complete cancer genomes in the catalogue of somatic mutations in cancer. Nucleic Acids Res 39(Database issue):D945–950
7. Lindgren D, Sjödahl G, Lauss M et al (2012) Integrated genomic and gene expression profiling identifies two major genomic circuits in urothelial carcinoma. PLoS ONE 7(6): e38863
8. Hurst CD, Platt FM, Taylor CF, Knowles MA (2012) Novel tumor subgroups of urothelial carcinoma of the bladder defined by integrated genomic analysis. Clin Cancer Res 18 (21):5865–5877
9. van Rhijn BW, Lurkin I, Radvanyi F, Kirkels WJ, van der Kwast TH, Zwarthoff EC (2001) The fibroblast growth factor receptor 3 (FGFR3) mutation is a strong indicator of superficial bladder cancer with low recurrence rate. Cancer Res 61(4):1265–1268
10. Knowles MA, Hurst CD (2015) Molecular biology of bladder cancer: new insights into pathogenesis and clinical diversity. Nat Rev Cancer 15(1):25–41
11. Bellmunt J, de Wit R, Vaughn DJ et al (2017) Pembrolizumab as second-line therapy for advanced urothelial carcinoma. N Engl J Med
12. https://cancergenome.nih.gov/. Last accessed June 2017
13. https://tcga-data.nci.nih.gov/docs/publications/tcga/. Last accessed June 2017
14. Network CGAR (2014) Comprehensive molecular characterization of urothelial bladder carcinoma. Nature 507(7492):315–322
15. Robertson G, Kim J, Al-Ahmadie H et al (2017) Comprehensive molecular characterization of muscle-invasive urothelial carcinoma. Cell
16. Rosenberg JE, Hoffman-Censits J, Powles T et al (2016) Atezolizumab in patients with locally advanced and metastatic urothelial carcinoma who have progressed following treatment with platinum-based chemotherapy: a single-arm, multicentre, phase 2 trial. Lancet 387 (10031):1909–1920
17. Balar AV, Galsky MD, Rosenberg JE et al (2016) Atezolizumab as first-line treatment in cisplatin-ineligible patients with locally advanced and metastatic urothelial carcinoma: a single-arm, multicentre, phase 2 trial. Lancet
18. Lawrence MS, Stojanov P, Polak P et al (2013) Mutational heterogeneity in cancer and the search for new cancer-associated genes. Nature 499(7457):214–218
19. Yang Y, Pang Z, Ding N et al (2016) The efficacy and potential predictive factors of PD-1/PD-L1 blockades in epithelial carcinoma patients: a systematic review and meta analysis. Oncotarget 7(45):74350–74361
20. Choi W, Czerniak B, Ochoa A et al (2014) Intrinsic basal and luminal subtypes of muscle-invasive bladder cancer. Nat Rev Urol 11(7):400–410
21. Choi W, Porten S, Kim S et al (2014) Identification of distinct basal and luminal subtypes of muscle-invasive bladder cancer with different sensitivities to frontline chemotherapy. Cancer Cell 25(2):152–165

22. Sjödahl G, Lauss M, Lövgren K et al (2012) A molecular taxonomy for urothelial carcinoma. Clin Cancer Res 18(12):3377–3386
23. Network CGA (2012) Comprehensive molecular portraits of human breast tumours. Nature 490(7418):61–70
24. Network CGAR (2012) Comprehensive genomic characterization of squamous cell lung cancers. Nature 489(7417):519–525
25. Filippakopoulos P, Qi J, Picaud S et al (2010) Selective inhibition of BET bromodomains. Nature 468(7327):1067–1073
26. Wu X, Liu D, Tao D et al (2016) BRD4 regulates EZH2 transcription through upregulation of C-MYC and represents a novel therapeutic target in bladder cancer. Mol Cancer Ther 15 (5):1029–1042

Modern Management of Testicular Cancer

Jian Chen and Siamak Daneshmand

Contents

J. Chen · S. Daneshmand (✉)
University of Southern California Norris Comprehensive Cancer Center,
Los Angeles, CA, USA
e-mail: daneshma@med.usc.edu

S. Daneshmand and K. G. Chan (eds.), *Genitourinary Cancers*, Cancer
Treatment and Research 175, https://doi.org/10.1007/978-3-319-93339-9_13

Abstract

Testicular cancer is a rare urological malignancy with high cure rate. The development of highly effective systemic treatment regimens along with advances in surgical treatment of advanced disease has led to continued improvement in outcomes. Patients with testicular cancer who are treated following the treatment guideline mostly achieved high quality of life and long-term survival. However, patients who were identified as having non-guideline directed care were at significantly higher risk of relapse. In this book chapter, we introduce in depth the modern management of testicular cancer, including diagnosis, staging and risk stratification, treatment strategies of seminoma and non-seminoma germ cell tumors, follow-up protocols, and salvage treatment for disease relapse. We also review new studies and updates on medical and surgical management of advanced testicular cancer.

Keywords

Germ cell tumor · Non-seminoma · Seminoma · Active surveillance
Chemotherapy · Retroperitoneal lymph node dissection · Radiotherapy
Relapse · Salvage treatment

1 Introduction

Testicular cancer is a rare urological malignancy in the USA, with 8850 new diagnoses and 410 deaths estimated in 2017 [1]. Testicular cancer is also one of the most curable solid malignancies with cure rates of 99–100% for Stage I disease and 70–80% for Stage II and III disease. The development of highly effective chemotherapy regimens along with advances in surgical treatment of advanced disease has led to continued improvement in outcomes. Today, most patients presenting with disease confined to the testicle will not require any further therapy and are appropriate candidates for surveillance [2]. Patients presenting with disseminated disease can be cured with a combination of risk-adapted chemotherapy and surgery for significant residual masses. Testicular cancer is a highly curable disease even in its most advanced stages. Also, the patients at presentation are at typical young age. This means patients can enjoy high-quality, long-term survival, and thus, treatment decisions are of paramount importance in this disease. The modern concept of testicular cancer management is achieving high and durable cure rates while minimizing the burden of treatment given the potential long-term toxicities associated with systemic therapies.

Following the treatment guideline, most patients achieved high quality of life and long-term survival. However, patients who were identified as having non-guideline directed care were at significantly higher risk of relapse [3]. This chapter focuses on the diagnosis and modern management of testicular germ cell tumors (GCTs).

2 Pathology Classification

The 2004 World Health Organization classification of testicular tumors is based on morphology [4] and includes two main groups: testicular germ cell tumors (GCTs) and sex cord–stromal tumors (SCSTs), accounting for approximately 95 and 4% of all testicular tumors, respectively.

2.1 Germ Cell Tumors (GCTs)

Seminoma

Pure seminoma constitutes 45–50% of all post-pubertal GCTs. They can also arise mixed with other morphological types [5]. Some seminoma may contain syncytiotrophoblastic cells without other elements, and these may be associated with mild elevation of serum β-human chorionic gonadotropin (β-hCG).

Non-seminoma

- *Embryonal carcinoma (ECCs)*
  Pure ECCs account for only 3% of all GCTs, but are seen in 80–90% of all non-seminoma germ cell tumors (NSGCTs). Pure ECCs occur in the third to fourth decade [6] and are rare in pre-pubertal boys [7].
- *Yolk sac tumor (YSTs)*
  Pure YSTs are the most common GCTs of infants and young boys. In post-pubertal boys, they are usually seen as a component of NSGCTs in about 50% of cases [8]. However, the YSTs in infants are ontogenically and clinically different from post-pubertal YSTs and have a better prognosis. Ninety-five to 100% of patients with YSTs components have elevated serum α-fetoprotein (AFP) levels.

- *Choriocarcinoma*
  Choriocarcinoma is uncommon in its pure form (<1% of GCTs) and may be a component of mixed GCTs in up to 15% of cases. In its pure form, it is associated with high β-hCG levels and usually presents with visceral metastasis.
- *Teratoma*
  Testicular teratomas in their pure form occur in children aged <4 years and are ontogenically and clinically different from their post-pubertal counterparts. Post-pubertal teratomas are seen as a component of mixed GCTs. Irrespective of their degree of differentiation (mature or immature), all post-pubertal teratomas are considered malignant. In mixed GCTs, teratomatous components are often the only recognizable part of the tumor after spontaneous regression or chemotherapy.

2.2 Sex Cord–Stromal Tumors (SCST)

Leydig cell tumor

Leydig cell tumors are the most common testicular SCST and account for up to 3% of all testicular neoplasms [9]. Most occur in adults and may be accompanied by hyperestrinism and gynecomastia. In boys, they are usually associated with precocious puberty. Ten percent of Leydig cell tumors will metastasize.

Sertoli cell tumor

Sertoli cell tumors comprise <1% of all testicular tumors and have no age predilection. Gynecomastia is evident in one-third of patients, and 10% of these tumors can metastasize.

3 Diagnosis

3.1 Symptoms

Germ cell tumors (GCTs) usually present as asymptomatic testicular enlargements or defined intratesticular lesions. Although most patients present with a painless testicular mass, pain can be present in about 25% of patients.

3.2 Basic Evaluation

Any patient who presents with signs or symptoms of testicular cancer should undergo a testicular ultrasound and serum tumor markers: β-hCG, AFP, and lactate dehydrogenase (LDH).

Testicular ultrasound

Combined with a physical examination, the sensitivity of ultrasound to detect testicular tumors approximates 100%. It is critical to image both testicles to document the status of the contralateral testicle as a small percentage of patients can present with bilateral testicular tumors. In addition, 2–3% of patients will develop a contralateral tumor during follow-up and comparison to the scans at presentation can prove critical [10]. Patient who have equivocal lesions particularly those <1 cm with normal tumor markers should undergo a repeat evaluation with ultrasound within 6 weeks [11].

The majority of testicular tumors <1 cm will prove to be benign. Benign testicular masses that can mimic malignant tumor on imaging include hematomas, focal infarction or infection, or epidermoid cysts, which have a very characteristic appearance on ultrasound [12].

More advanced ultrasound imaging such as contrast-enhanced ultrasonography (CEUS) and real-time sonoelastography (RTSE) can improve diagnostic accuracy. CEUS uses microbubbles injected intravenously to assess vascularity of lesions, and RTSE assesses tissue elasticity [13–15]. However, neither of these modalities is widely available and has not become a standard part of imaging for the primary testicular tumors.

Tumor markers

Tumor markers are secreted by the testicular cancer and should be measured before, during, and after treatment. These markers are capable of detecting tumors that cannot be demonstrated by currently available imaging techniques. Also, the tumor cell population may change, resulting in a different expression pattern of markers. For example, the primary tumor may secrete only AFP, while metastases may produce only β-hCG, or vice versa.

AFP and/or β-hCG are elevated in 65–80% of patients with advanced NSGCTs. β-hCG is elevated in around 25% of seminoma, but AFP is never elevated in pure seminoma [16]. LDH is used as a serum tumor marker for seminoma, although LDH is less specific than AFP or β-hCG. However, elevated serum LDH can be used as an independent prognostic variable in advanced disease [17].

The American Society of Clinical Oncology (ASCO) has suggested the followings on the use of serum tumor markers in adult men with GCTs [16]:

- Markers cannot be used to screen for GCTs, to decide whether orchiectomy is indicated, or to select treatment for patients with cancer of unknown primary origin.

Table 1 Tumor marker half life

AFP	3.5–6 days
β-hCG	16–24 h
LDH	24 h

- To stage patients with non-seminoma germ cell tumors (NSGCTs), it is recommended to measure AFP, β-hCG, and LDH before and after orchiectomy and before chemotherapy for those with extragonadal NSGCTs.
- AFP and β-hCG should be measured shortly before retroperitoneal lymph node dissection and at the start of each chemotherapy cycle for NSGCTs, and periodically to monitor for relapse.
- Post-orchiectomy β-hCG and LDH measurements are recommended for patients with seminoma and pre-orchiectomy elevations.
- Tumor markers should not be used to guide or monitor treatment for seminoma or to detect relapse in those treated for Stage I disease. However, measuring β-hCG and AFP to monitor relapse in patients treated for advanced seminoma is recommended (Table 1).

3.3 Imaging

Computed tomography (CT)
The imaging of choice in assessment of metastatic GCTs is computed tomography (CT). CT is readily available at most hospitals, does not require specialized protocols, has excellent reproducibility, and affords comparison evaluation even when done at different centers [18]. The concern about radiation exposure is subjugated by the subsequent need for systemic treatment of disseminated disease. Many centers are now routinely offering low-dose CT techniques to minimize the risk of radiation exposure, particularly since young patients with metastatic disease will require multiple scans during treatment and follow-up surveillance. Low-dose protocols can still produce high-quality scans which can be used to measure tumor size and treatment response [19].

Initial evaluation of patient with GCTs should include a CT scan of the chest, abdomen, and pelvis with intravenous contrast which is the basis for clinical staging and risk stratification.

- *CT abdomen and pelvis*
  The determination of nodal enlargement is critical in the staging of metastatic GCTs. In the Response Evaluation Criteria in Solid Tumors (RECIST) version 1.1, a lymph node greater than 15 mm would be considered abnormal [20]. Certainly, smaller lymph nodes may harbor metastatic disease and the size of normal lymph nodes varies in the retroperitoneum of healthy young patients. In one study using 10 mm diameter as the threshold, there was a 37% sensitivity for malignancy although the specificity was 100% [21]. Another study looked at 8 mm as the cutoff for a normal lymph node in the retroperitoneum, with the sensitivity and specificity being about 70% [22]. There is no true consensus on

the threshold for abnormal lymph nodes in the retroperitoneum. The most accepted measurement is the short diameter on axial section, although studies have varying measuring criteria. The clinician needs to consider additional criteria such as nodal shape, distribution, presence of fat within the node (seen in normal lymph nodes), as well as location. The isolated presence of enlarged lymph nodes within the landing zone for the affected testicle laterality should raise suspicion for metastatic disease. The decision to treat patients with chemotherapy however should not rely solely on enlarged lymph nodes since 20–30% of patients with clinical Stage II disease based on radiographic findings will be found to have normal lymph nodes on pathology [23, 24].

- *CT chest*

  A full evaluation of metastatic disease should include a CT scan of the chest given the high prevalence of pulmonary nodules [25]. Most identifiable pulmonary nodules are due to metastatic disease except for rare calcified foci [26]. Over half of the patients with retroperitoneal lymph node metastases have concomitant pulmonary metastases, while about 10% have isolated disease in the lungs [27]. However, the incidence of pulmonary involvement in patients with pure seminoma is far less common (<5%) [28].

Bone scan

The incidence of bone metastases is rare, and bone scan should be limited to patients with symptoms or suspicion of bone involvement on CT scan [29].

Positron emission tomography (PET)

PET scans should not be used routinely in initial evaluation of patients with metastatic GCTs since it does not add to the staging information or clinical decision making.

PET scans have been increasingly used in the evaluation and follow-up of patients with metastatic cancer. The most common tracer used is 2–18 fluoro-2-deoxy-D-glucose (FDG) performed in conjunction with CT images. In metastatic GCTs, the major three limitations of PET scan are (1) extensive FDG uptake with inflammation; (2) poor detection of small lesions; (3) cannot distinguish mature teratoma from necrosis in the evaluation of treated disease [30]. Although GCTs generally have high FDG uptake, several prospective trials have proven the limitations of PET scans to detect teratomas or metastatic lesions <1 cm [31–33]. Theoretically, PET scan should help distinguish necrosis from active residual disease, and the inflammatory reaction associated with treatment response leads to significant false positive results [31]. Even with sufficient time to allow inflammation to subside, PET scans will not distinguish fibrosis from teratoma in NSGCTs and hence do not change the management in this setting.

PET scans have also been extensively used to predict pathologic response to chemotherapy. The German multicenter PET study group reported on 121 patients with NSGCTs who underwent post-chemotherapy residual tumor resection. The prediction of pathological viable residual disease based on PET scan was only 56% and not superior to CT or serum tumor markers [34]. In prospective clinical trials including 85 lesions from 45 patients, the positive and negative predictive values for PET scan to detect viable disease were 91 and 62%, respectively. Importantly, in patients with multiple residual masses, increased FDG uptake in all lesions was a strong predictor of pathologic viable disease [35]. However, expert consensus is that there is very little role for FDG-PET imaging in the management of NSGCTs given the above-mentioned limitations and lack of guidance on whether to proceed with resection tumor resection [36].

In the pure seminoma setting, where there is no concern about finding teratoma and surgery is often more difficult and morbid, PET scans may have a role in detection of residual viable disease. In the SEMPET trial, 127 patients with residual masses following chemotherapy had an FDG-PET scan for metastatic seminoma. The sensitivity, specificity, negative predictive value (NPV), and positive predictive value (PPV) for viable disease were 82, 90, 95, and 69%, respectively, when the PET scan was performed 6 weeks following chemotherapy [37, 38]. In a recent meta-analysis, 375 PET scans or PET/CTs were evaluated in nine studies showing sensitivity of 78%, specificity of 86% with a PPV of 58% and NPV of 94%.

Thus, for seminoma, given the high probability of finding fibrosis/necrosis in the post-chemotherapy setting for residual masses <3 cm, the current recommendation is to obtain an FDG-PET scan for masses >3 cm at least 6–8 weeks following completion of chemotherapy. Lesions which are not avid on FDG-PET can be followed carefully. If the mass is <3 cm, the use of an FDG-PET scan is optional, since the general recommendation is careful surveillance. It is important to note that false positives are common and management should be individualized. In equivocal cases, a biopsy can be performed to rule out viable disease.

Table 2 Serum tumor marker staging (S)

	LDH (U/liter)	β-hCG (mIU/ml)	AFP (ng/ml)
SX	Marker studies not available or not done		
S0	Normal	Normal	Normal
S1[a]	<1.5 × normal	<5000	<1000
S2[b]	1.5–10 × normal	5000–50,000	1000–10,000
S3[b]	>10 × normal	>50,000	>10,000

For staging, serum levels of tumor markers are measured **after** radical orchiectomy
[a]All the markers must be in the stated range to be considered S1
[b]Only one marker needs to be in the stated range to be considered S2 or S3
AFP α-fetoprotein; *β-hCG* β-human chorionic gonadotropin; *LDH* lactate dehydrogenase

Table 3 Stage grouping

Stage	T	N	M	S
Stage 0	Tis (in situ)	N0	M0	S0
Stage I	T1–T4	N0	M0	SX
Stage IA	T1	N0	M0	S0
Stage IB	T2–T4	N0	M0	S0
Stage IS	Any T	N0	M0	S1–S3
Stage II	Any T	N1–N3	M0	SX
Stage IIA	Any T	N1	M0	S0–S1
Stage IIB	Any T	N2	M0	S0–S1
Stage IIC	Any T	N3	M0	S0–S1
Stage III	Any T	Any N	M1	SX
Stage IIIA	Any T	Any N	M1a	S0–S1
Stage IIIB	Any T	N1–N3	M0	S2
	Any T	Any N	M1a	S2
Stage IIIC	Any T	N1–N3	M0	S3
	Any T	Any N	M1a	S3
	Any T	Any N	M1b	Any S

Table 4 IGCCCG criteria defining good, intermediate, and poor risk germ cell tumors

	AFP	β-hCG	LDH	Tumor site
Good risk	<1000 ng/mL	<5000 mU/mL	<1.5 × ULN	Gonadal or retroperitoneal primary
Intermediate risk	1000–10,000 ng/mL	5000–50,000 mU/mL	1.5–10.0 × ULN	Gonadal or retroperitoneal primary
Poor risk	≥ 10,000 ng/mL	≥ 50,000 mU/mL	≥ 10.0 × ULN	Mediastinal primary site; Non-pulmonary visceral metastases

Intermediate and poor risk patients should receive 4 cycles of PEB, whereas good risk can be treated with 3 cycles of PEB. *Note* Seminoma patients can only be classified as poor risk due to presence of mediastinal primary, not by markers alone

AFP α-fetoprotein; *β-hCG* β-human chorionic gonadotropin; *LDH* lactate dehydrogenase

Indication for brain imaging

Brain metastases are rare in GCTs, and brain imaging should only be considered in patients with neurologic symptoms or those with International Germ Cell Cancer Collaborative Group (IGCCCG) poor risk disease [17]. Patients with pure choriocarcinoma also carry an increased risk of brain metastases [39]. Magnetic resonance imaging (MRI) is the modality of choice for evaluation of the central nervous system which has a higher sensitivity than CT scan in detection of metastatic disease [40].

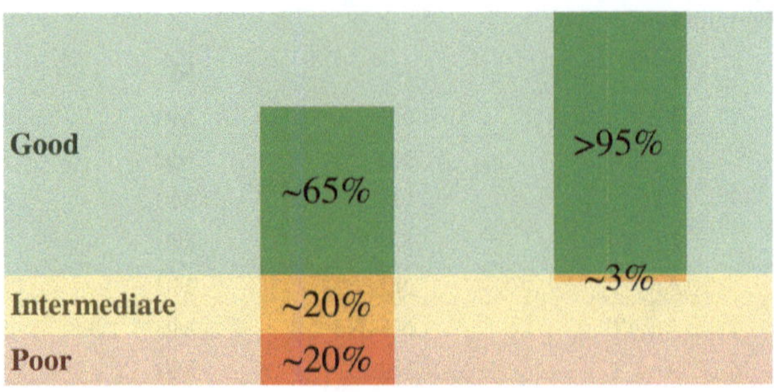

Fig. 1 IGCCCG risk group distribution of metastatic non-seminomas and metastatic seminoma

4 Staging and Risk Stratification

Testicular cancers are staged using the TNM classification as with most other cancers. Additional stratification includes histologic type (seminoma/non-seminoma), tumor marker level, primary site (testicular/extragonadal), and the presence or absence of non-pulmonary visceral metastasis. The TNM stage along with the tumor marker elevation (measured post-orchiectomy) called the S stage is combined to form the stage group (Tables 2 and 3).

To develop reliable prognostic groups, a new staging classification is prevalently used. The International Germ Cell Cancer Collaborative Group (IGCCCG) pooled data from 5862 patients with metastatic GCTs from 10 countries which formed the IGCCCG risk classification (Table 4) [17]. The IGCCCG classifies patients into good, intermediate, or poor prognosis groups based on level of marker elevation and site of disease which in turn has been incorporated into the TNM system. Approximately 65% of patients with metastatic non-seminomas in modern series fall into the good prognosis group with survival rates of about 97% [41, 42] (Fig. 1). Most patients (>95%) of patients with metastatic seminoma fall into the good prognosis group with survival rates of >95% [43]. Intermediate risk patients include about 20% of the metastatic non-seminomas and only 3% of seminomas with overall survival rates of about 90% [44, 45]. Only non-seminomas have poor prognosis grouping comprising of about 20% of patients with metastatic disease with survival rates of 65–70% [46].

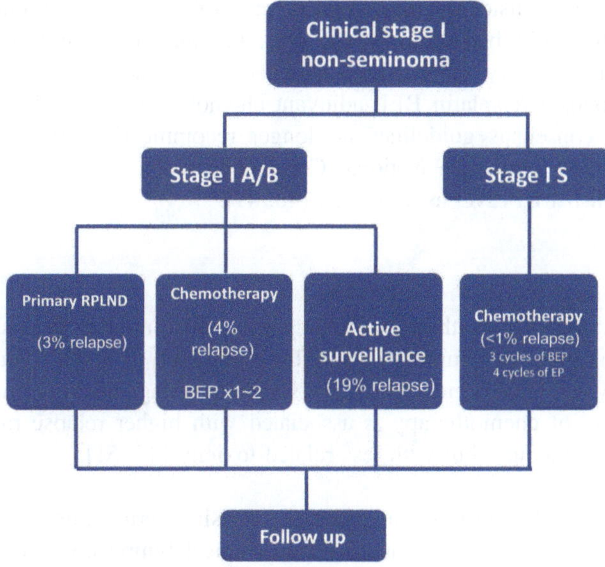

Fig. 2 Management of clinical Stage I NSGCTs

5 Management for non-seminoma germ cell tumors (NSGCTs)

5.1 Clinical Stage I

Three post-orchiectomy management strategies are recommended, active surveillance (AS), primary retroperitoneal lymph node dissection (RPLND), and adjuvant chemotherapy with one or two cycles of bleomycin, etoposide, and cisplatin (BEP) (Fig. 2). Either of these three management strategies has a cure rates approaching 100%.

<u>Retroperitoneal lymph node dissection (RPLND)</u>
RPLND has been utilized for treating germ cell tumors (GCTs) since the 1900s, and there is ample data on its long-term efficacy and safety. As opposed to chemotherapy, surgery is not associated with cardiopulmonary disease, secondary malignancy, or metabolic syndrome. The procedure alone reduces the probability of requiring subsequent chemotherapy by half and eliminates the need for abdominal CT scans during follow-up. However, primary RPLND does not eliminate the risk of recurrence outside the retroperitoneum (5–8% of all recurrences in Stage I and 30% of patients with pathological Stage II disease).

RPLND carried outside the high-volume centers is associated with higher infield recurrence rate and higher morbidity [47]. In addition, if positive lymph nodes are detected on primary RPLND, patients still need two cycles of bleomycin/etoposide/cisplatin BEP adjuvant chemotherapy. Therefore, in Europe and Canada, consensus guidelines no longer recommend primary RPLND for Stage I NSGCTs, while the National Comprehensive Cancer Network (NCCN) guidelines still list RPLND as an option [48, 49].

Adjuvant chemotherapy

Adjuvant chemotherapy with one or two cycles of BEP reduces the risk of Stage I non-seminoma germ cell tumors (NSGCTs) recurrence to 3–4%. Thus, adjuvant chemotherapy has since been considered a standard management option [47, 50, 51, 52]. One cycle of chemotherapy is associated with higher relapse rate than two cycles of chemotherapy, but with less related toxicity [47, 51].

Clinical Stage IS refers to the presence of rising serum tumor markers after orchiectomy without visible enlarged retroperitoneal lymph nodes or distant disease. In this setting, chemotherapy (three cycles of BEP or four cycles of etoposide/cisplatin (EP)) is preferred over RPLND since the site of disease cannot be confirmed. RPLND for Stage I NSGCTs has relapse rates up to 50%, compared to <1% relapse when managed with chemotherapy [53].

Active surveillance (AS)

The main rationale for AS is that, even when disease replase, systemic chemotherapy is highly effective and thus, the majority of patients with Stage I NSGCTs after orchiectomy can be spared the primary RPLND or the adjuvant chemotherapy.

Large prospective studies of AS showed overall Stage I NSGCTs cure rates exceeding 98% and were compared favorably with RPLND and adjuvant chemotherapy. Relapse and survival rates were similar among trials [54–61]. Fifty to 85% of patients are unnecessarily exposed to RPLND due to the failure of current preoperative staging evaluations to predict pathological Stage I disease reliably. Similar proportion of patients are exposed to unnecessary chemotherapy and associated toxicity. AS spares 70–75% of all unselected patients the burden of any active treatment and thus minimizes treatment-related morbidity.

5.2 Clinical Stage IIA (Tumor Marker Negative)

The majority of Stage IIA NSGCTs patients are treated with chemotherapy as per the International Germ Cell Cancer Collaborative Group (IGCCCG) recommendations [62]. However, 12–35% of these patients are found to have pathologically

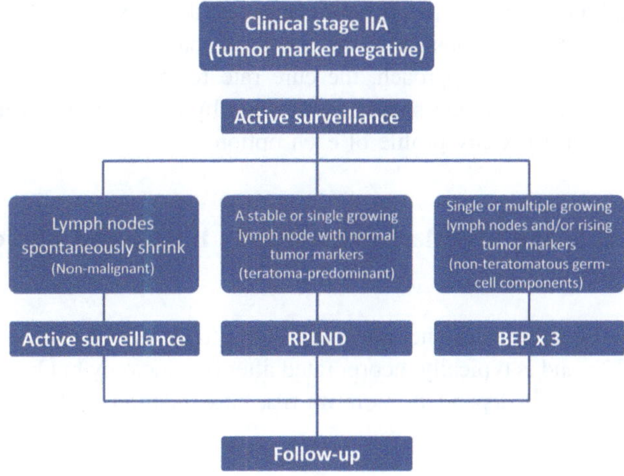

Fig. 3 Management of clinical Stage IIA non-seminoma germ cell tumors (tumor marker negative)

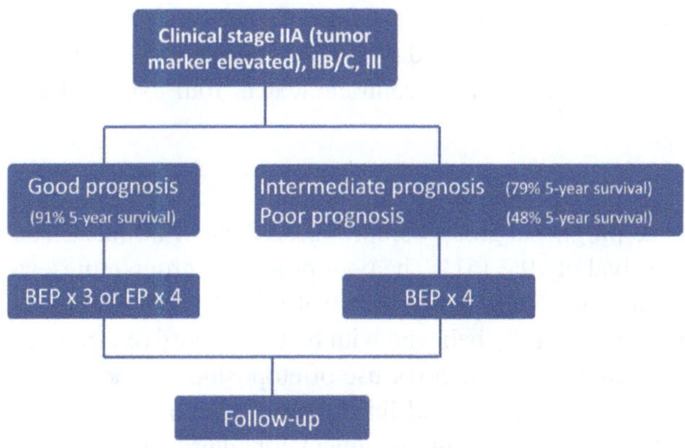

Fig. 4 Management of clinical Stage IIA (marker elevated), Stage IIB/C, and Stage III non-seminoma

negative lymph nodes (pathological Stage I) at RPLND [62–65]. Moreover, 30% of patients can have retroperitoneal teratoma that is resistant to chemotherapy [62]. Hence, to avoid overtreatment, patients with borderline-enlarged 1–2 cm retroperitoneal lymph nodes and negative tumor markers may be treated with initial AS or primary RPLND to clarify stage, reserving chemotherapy for progressing lymph nodes or increasing marker levels (Fig. 3).

If initial AS is chosen, abdominal imaging should be performed within 6–12 weeks. If lymph nodes spontaneously shrink, it is likely to be non-malignant and the patient can continue AS. A stable or single growing lymph node with normal tumor markers is possibly teratoma-predominant disease, and RPLND should be performed, with the goal of curative monotherapy. In case of single or multiple growing lymph nodes and/or rising tumor markers, three cycles of BEP should be offered because of higher possibility of non-teratomatous germ cell components. Regardless of the chosen approach, the cure rate for Stage IIA NSGCTs is 98–100%, and therefore treatment should be decided by taking into consideration the acute and long-term toxicity profile of each option.

5.3 Clinical Stage IIA (Marker Elevated), II B/C, and Clinical Stage III

Cisplatin-based combination chemotherapy is the treatment of choice for Stage II and III NSGCTs and is typically incorporated after orchiectomy but before RPLND. The chance of cure is dependent more on risk classification by IGCCCG than by stage (Fig. 4).

Good prognosis group

The good prognosis group comprises 60% of all metastatic testicular germ cell tumors (TGCTs) patients and has an excellent 5-year survival rate of 91% [61]. The standard first-line treatment for good prognosis patients is three cycles of BEP or, in selected cases where bleomycin is contraindicated, four cycles of EP.

Intermediate and poor prognosis group

The intermediate prognosis group compromised 26% of all metastatic patients and had a 5-year survival of 79% [61]. The poor prognosis group represented 14% of all metastatic patients and had a 5-year survival of only 48% in the IGCCCC study [61]. However, it is generally believed with better supportive care (e.g., antiemetics, or colony-stimulating factor support), use of etoposide in place of vinblastine, and improvements with salvage second-line therapy, the outcomes are better in the modern era. The standard first-line treatment for intermediate and poor prognosis patients is four cycles of BEP, or if bleomycin is contraindicated, four cycles of etoposide, ifosfamide, and cisplatin (VeIP).

Benefit and side effects of eliminating bleomycin

Concern about pulmonary toxicity has resulted in evaluation of four cycles of EP as an alternative to BEP. Pulmonary toxicity presents with a multitude of syndromes, including bronchiolitis obliterans with organizing pneumonia (BOOP) [66], eosinophilic hypersensitivity [67], and interstitial pneumonitis with progression to pulmonary fibrosis [68]. Mortality from bleomycin interstitial pneumonitis is estimated at 3% [69]. Patients at higher risk of developing bleomycin toxicity include those with lower glomerular filtration rate (GFR) and older age [69, 70]. This concern led to study of EP for four cycles as an alternative to BEP three cycles in good risk patients (GETUG T93BP) [42]. Of the 270 subjects randomized, the four-year event-free survival rate was 91% for three cycles of BEP and 86% for four cycles of EP (HR 0.58, 95% CI 0.29–1.19, $p = 0.135$). Although not statistically significant, the trend clearly favors inclusion of bleomycin. Pulmonary toxicity occurred in 9% of subjects on the cycles of BEP arm and 6% of subjects on four cycles of EP arm with no fatal toxicity in either group.

Toxicities which occur at higher rates when a forth cycle of cisplatin is administered include peripheral neuropathy, ototoxicity, and infertility [71, 72]. Both cisplatin and etoposide cumulative doses are also associated with increasing risk of secondary malignancy, primarily myelodysplastic syndrome and leukemia [73, 74]. For these reasons, it is often preferable to give three cycles of BEP, but these trade-offs can be discussed with patients to facilitate informed shared decision making.

The salvage regimen of pacliTaxel, Ifosfamide, and cisPlatin (TIP) is being investigated as frontline regimen for intermediate and poor risk patients, to provide an alternative to PEB. The multi-institutional phase II surpassed its benchmark, with 68% of patients achieving complete response, and now TIP is being compared directly to four cycles of PEB for intermediate and poor risk testis cancer patients in a randomized trial (NCT01873326) [75].

Alternative regimens for platinum ineligible patients

Because carboplatin has been associated with inferior rates of cure when substituted for cisplatin in both BEP and EP for testis cancer, every effort is made to utilize cisplatin [76, 77]. The fractionated nature of the BEP or EP regimens makes it feasible to dose cisplatin even in renal impaired patients.

Table 5 Follow-up schedule for testicular germ cell tumors (TGCTs)

	Follow-up year			
	1	2	3–5	6–10
Physical examination	Every 3 months	Every 3 months	Every 6 months	Every 12 months
Tumor markers	Every 3 months	Every 3 months	Every 6 months	Every 12 months
Chest X-ray	Every 3 months	Every 3 months	Every 6 months	Every 12 months
CT abdomen and pelvis	Every 6 months	Every 6 months	As indicated	As indicated
CT chest	As indicated	As indicated	As indicated	As indicated

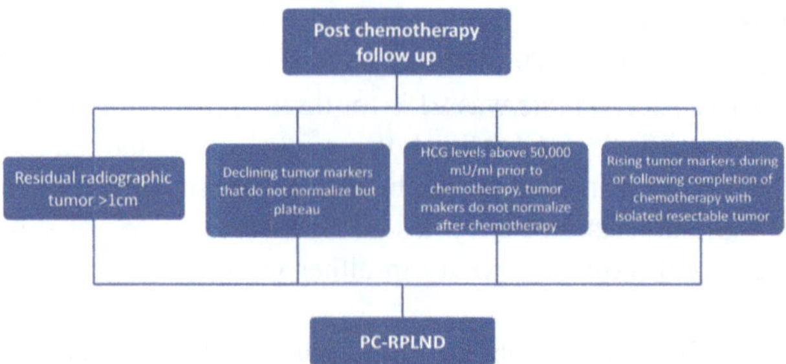

Fig. 5 Indications of post-chemotherapy RPLND

5.4 Follow-up

Four to eight weeks after the completion of first-line chemotherapy, determination of tumor markers and re-staging CT should be performed. Seventy to 90% of metastatic GCTs will achieve complete remission with normalization of tumor markers and complete radiographic response [78–80], require no further treatment and surveillance is a preferred option [80]. For those who have persistently high or increasing levels of tumor markers and/or residual masses, post-chemotherapy RPLND (PC-RPLND) is warranted.

The objectives of follow-up are detection of disease recurrence, treatment-related morbidity, and prevention and detection of long-term complications such as secondary malignancies and cardiovascular disease. Follow-up visits should include regular physical examination, tumor marker measurement, and repeat imaging. The frequency and option of imaging depend on the estimated relapse risk, and the time that has elapsed since treatment completion. However, follow-up schedules have never been validated prospectively and therefore several schedules exist and may be valid. Table 5 gives an example of one follow-up schedule.

5.5 Post-chemotherapy RPLND (PC-RPLND)

Indications

PC-RPLND is one of the most technically challenging operations in urology and requires significant expertise in retroperitoneal surgery as well as vascular techniques. A thorough understanding of the abdominal and retroperitoneal anatomy is critical in assuring optimal outcomes (Fig. 5).

- In patients with NSGCTs, any residual radiographic tumor >1 cm is indication for a PC-RPLND. Several models have been developed to predict the retroperitoneal histology and streamline indications for resection of the residual mass. These models have included predictors of necrosis, which include the

Table 6 Outcome of patients undergoing surveillance following complete or partial response <1 cm residual retroperitoneal mass) with induction chemotherapy

	Patients	Median follow-up (years)	RFS (%)	CSS (%)	DOD	Unnecessary RPLND
Indiana	141	15.5	90	97	4 (3%)	135 (96%)
Oregon/UBC	161	4.3	94	100	0 (0%)	153 (95%)
PMH	129	7	92	99	1 (0.8%)	119 (92%)

PMH Princess Margaret Hospital; *UBC* University of British Columbia; *RFS* recurrence-free survival; *CSS* cancer-specific survival; *DOD* dead of disease

absence of teratoma in the orchiectomy specimen, normal β-hCG levels, small masses prior to surgery, and significant response to chemotherapy in terms of volume. An update of this model in more than 1000 patients did not reliably predict necrosis to change recommendations for resection [81].

- Patients who have declining tumor markers that do not normalize but plateau should also be considered for PC-RPLND. Cystic teratomas may contain elevated tumor markers that can continuously leak into the bloodstream which explain the elevated but stable tumor markers in this setting [82].
- Patients who present with significantly elevated β-hCG levels above 50,000 mU/ml prior to initiation of chemotherapy may not completely normalize their markers following adequate chemotherapy and should be considered for PC-RPLND if there is a residual mass present [83].
- Patients with obvious rising tumor markers during or following completion of chemotherapy may have cisplatin-resistant disease or progression of disease and should be considered for salvage therapy (salvage ifosfamide-based therapy or high-dose chemotherapy with autologous stem cell transplantation). Surgical resection should only be considered in select cases of isolated resectable disease [36].

Situations that PC-RPLND can be withheld

It is imperative that expert radiologist as well as the surgeon reviews the cross-sectional imaging prior to as well as following response to chemotherapy to determine the extent of residual disease. Patients who achieve complete serologic and radiographic complete response to first-line chemotherapy are at very low risk for relapse. As many as 30% of patients with residual lymph nodes <1 cm may harbor teratoma or even viable GCTs, prompting a few centers to recommend PC-RPLND for all patients following risk-adapted chemotherapy regardless of radiographic response [84]. Recent series from several centers however suggest that patient with residual disease <1 cm may be safely observed with a cancer-specific survival of 97–100%. From a total of 431 patients in these series, there were only 22 retroperitoneal recurrences all of whom were salvaged by delayed PC-RPLND if the mass contained residual teratoma [85] (Table 6).

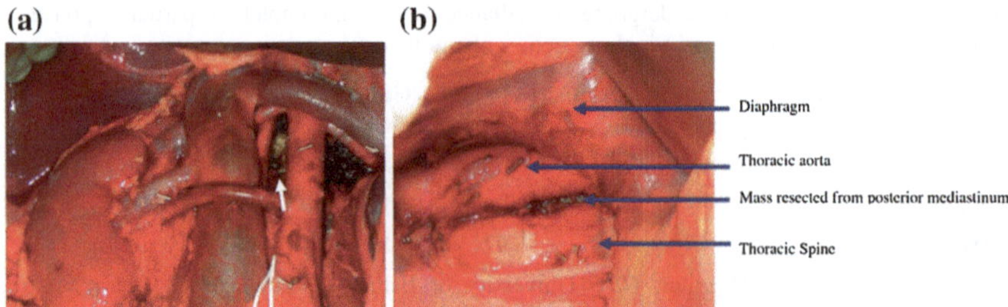

Fig. 6 Thoracoabdominal incision allowing dissection of mass in the retrocrural area (white arrow, filled with hemostatic agents) (**a**), contiguous with the posterior mediastinum (**b**)

Fig. 7 Two-team approach to simultaneous neck and abdominal resection

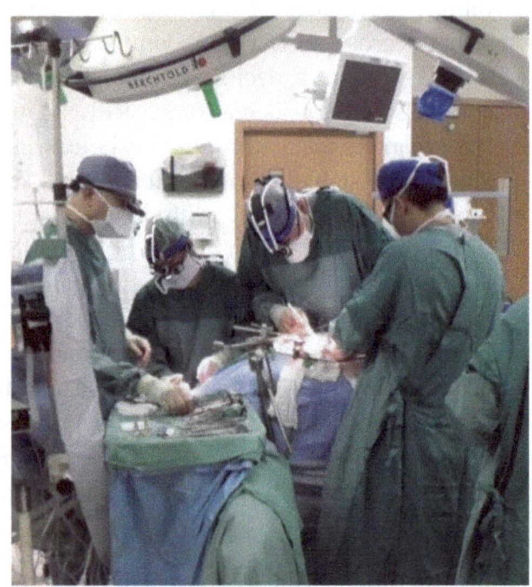

Surgical approach and templates

Controversy still exists regarding the exact template of dissection in PC-RPLND. Depending on the template used, extra-template disease has been detected in 7–32% of cases in a series from Memorial Sloan Kettering [86]. However, several retrospective series have shown that bilateral dissection may not be required in all cases of PC-RPLND [87–90]. In 98 patients undergoing a modified template, Heindenreich found eight recurrences during a mean follow-up of 39 months, only one of which had an infield relapse [88]. In another study from Indiana University, the authors reported a relapse rate of 4% in a series of 100 patients who underwent modified template PC-RPLND with all recurrences outside the boundaries of a full

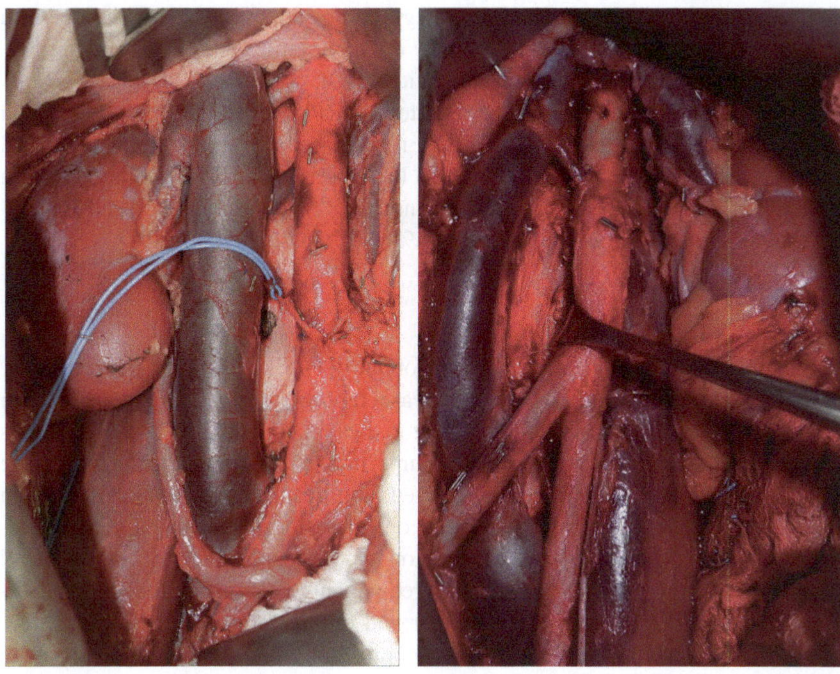

(a) Bilateral template on the right **(b)** Bilateral template on the left

Fig. 8 Midline extraperitoneal (EP) PC-RPLND

bilateral template [89]. Modified template PC-RPLND may be appropriate for patients with unilateral localized tumors <5 cm or no palpable residual disease, left-sided primaries, and right-sided testis cancer with absence of mature teratoma or viable cancer in the residual masses [87–89].

The surgical approach should also be adapted to the size and location of the mass. Most PC-RPLND can be approached through a midline incision. Those requiring suprahilar dissection, large masses requiring a nephrectomy, or significant retrocrural disease may be best approached through a thoracoabdominal incision or a midline incision extended to the costochondral margin. Thoracoabdominal incisions allow for concomitant resection of ipsilateral lung lesion or lower posterior mediastinal lesions, (Fig. 6). If a neck dissection is indicated, it can be performed simultaneously along with a PC-RPLND (Fig. 7); however, complex mediastinal masses are probably best approached in a staged manner to reduce complication rates. In patients with known teratoma or viable GCTs metastasis, all visible extraretroperitoneal disease should be resected. In patients with necrosis in the retroperitoneum, extraretroperitoneal disease should be excised if feasible, although surveillance represents an alternative strategy for select patients. An individualized surgical approach should be made based on metastatic pattern, prior disorders, patient factors, and institutional considerations [90].

University of Southern California reported on RPLND using a midline incision that is completely extraperitoneal (EP) to minimize the complications associated with entering the peritoneal cavity (Fig. 8). In this series of EP-RPLND comprising 69 patients (41 PC-RPLNDs), there were no cases of ileus and the mean hospital stay was three days. Nineteen patients (28%) had masses >10 cm [91].

Minimally invasive RPLND

Minimally invasive (laparoscopic or robotic) PC-RPLND is a technically demanding procedure, and so far only case reports or small series have been reported by a few experienced surgeons at dedicated centers. Most of these series have generally been limited to small-volume masses. Although techniques have evolved, earlier laparoscopic series reported significant conversion rates to open surgery. Calestroupat et al. [92] reported on 26 patients who underwent laparoscopic PC-RPLND which included excision of the residual mass plus unilateral template dissection only. In this series, three patients were converted to open surgery and there were eight lymphovascular and one intestinal complication. More recently Steiner et al. reported on laparoscopic PC-RPLND on 100 patients with low-volume Stage II disease. Although complication and open conversion rates were low, 71% had unilateral template dissections and the mean transverse diameter of the residual mass was only 1.4 cm, with 57 patients having residual masses <1 cm in size, which we would consider for surveillance [93]. More recently,

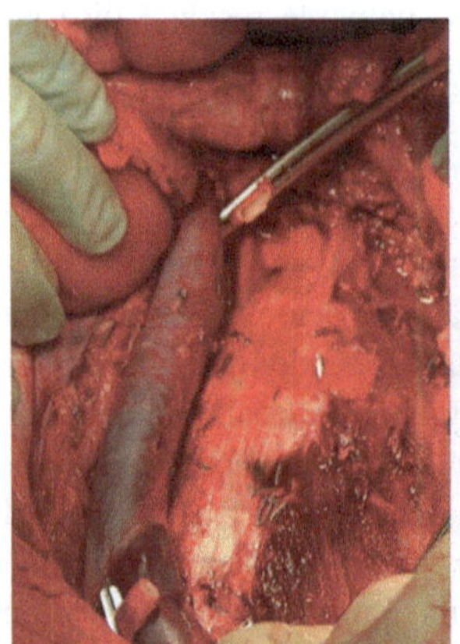

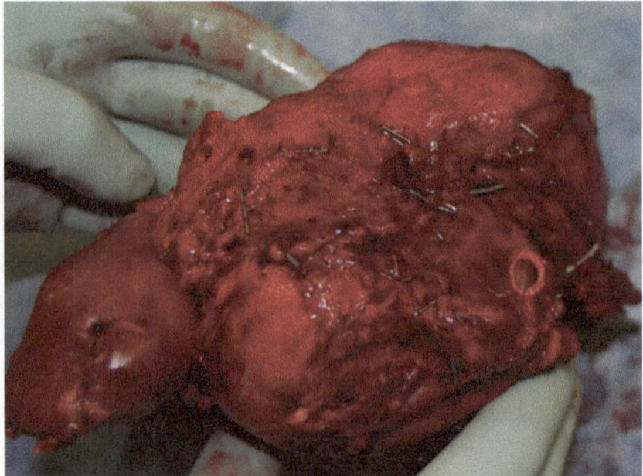

Fig. 9 Adjuvant surgery **a** bilateral template on the right and **b** bilateral template on the left

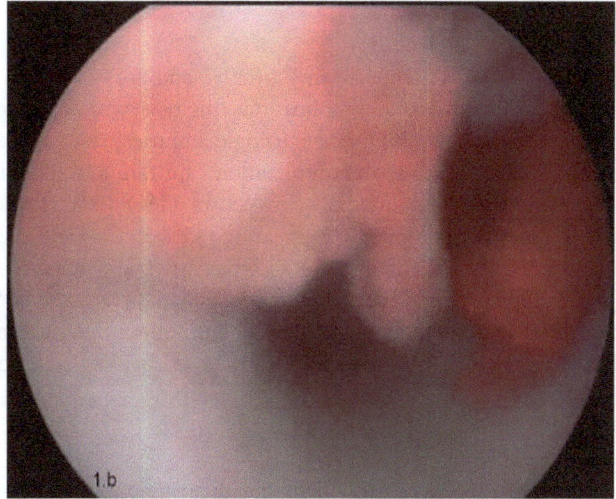

Fig. 10 Intraoperative vena cavoscopy revealing intraluminal mass

several surgeons have described their experience with robotic-assisted laparoscopic RPLND with fewer conversions and complications [94, 95]. Stepanian et al. reported 20 procedures in 19 patients. There were no open conversions or transfusions. There was one ureteral transection that was repaired at the time of surgery. Two patients had ejaculatory dysfunction after surgery [94]. Pearce et al. reported a multicenter series of primary R-RPLND for low-stage NSGCTs. Of the 47 patients studied, there were two intraoperative complications (4%), four early postoperative complications (9%), no late complications, and the rate of antegrade ejaculation was 100% [95]. The patients in these two studies had predominantly Stage I (80%) or II (17%) disease, and only two cases were post-chemotherapy. In that regard, although minimally invasive PC-RPLND may be technically feasible in select cases, the results may not be generalizable or reproducible at other lower-volume centers.

Adjuvant surgery

Twenty percent patients undergoing PC-RPLND need adjuvant surgery. The most commonly performed additional procedure is a left nephrectomy followed by vascular resection including en bloc vena cava and/or aortic resection (Fig. 9) [96]. These procedures are necessary when the residual masses cannot be safely separated from adjoining structures. The need for adjuvant procedures escalates with increasing complexity of the residual tumor and worse IGCCCG risk classification. Complete surgical resection of all residual disease is critical to assure optimal outcomes. Teratomas can invade the vena cava, presenting as a filling defect within the lumen of the great vessel (Fig. 10). Resection of the residual mass along with tumor thrombectomy or vena cavectomy is often curative.

Complications of PC-RPLND

Complications of PC-RPLND range from 7 to 30% and are obviously higher than for primary RPLND. Short-term complications include wound infection, ileus, chylous ascites, renovascular injury, neurologic injuries, with mortality rates of <1% in expert centers. Long-term complications are rare and include incisional hernia, bowel obstruction, and ureteral obstruction (1%) [97]. Tumor size and location are the primary predictors of complication rates. Retrograde ejaculation is a common consequence of bilateral PC-RPLND; however, experts performing nerve-sparing techniques can achieve antegrade ejaculation rates of >80% [97]. Modifications to the RPLND technique, such as with an extraperitoneal approach, have been shown to reduce short-term morbidity in particular, significantly lower rates of ileus [91].

Growing teratoma syndrome

A small subset of patients have growth of the metastatic tumor despite normalization of tumor markers. It is important to recognize this clinical scenario known as growing teratoma syndrome (GTS) since they may be erroneously categorized as non-response to primary chemotherapy. The masses all have cystic features with necrosis elements on radiographic evaluation signifying response of the malignant elements to treatment with chemo-resistant teratoma in the cystic portions. Growth rates are variable with median growth rate of 0.5 cm/month in our series, with only 40% of the patients harboring teratoma in the primary orchiectomy specimen [98]. Appropriate management is completion of planned chemotherapy (unless the mass is symptomatic), followed by complete surgical resection. The prognosis is excellent when pathology contains only mature teratoma.

Resection of residual retroperitoneal mass following salvage chemotherapy. Mass was circumferentially surrounding and densely adherent to aorta and left renal

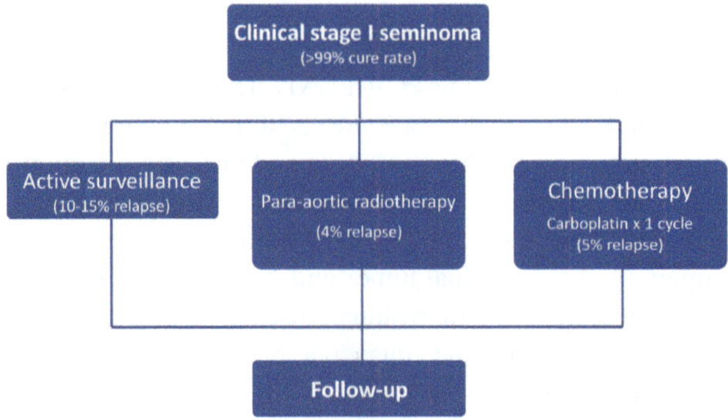

Fig. 11 Management of clinical Stage I seminoma

hilum necessitating nephrectomy and en bloc aortic resection. An aorto-bi-iliac graft was placed as interposition.

6 Management for Seminoma

6.1 Clinical Stage I

Eight-five percent of all seminomas are clinically Stage I at the time of diagnosis [99]. Compared to non-seminomas, seminomas are less likely to metastasize and are sensitive to both radiation and chemotherapy. The recurrence rate after radical orchiectomy was 15–20%, with the most predominant site of relapse being the retroperitoneal lymph nodes (up to 95% of cases), followed by mediastinal, supraclavicular nodes, and lung [43, 100, 101, 102, 103]. With prolonged disease-free survival in early-stage seminoma, long-term quality of life, and treatment-related side effects have become increasingly significant in selecting management options. Three management options after radical orchiectomy are adjuvant radiotherapy, adjuvant chemotherapy, and AS (Fig. 11); If carried out properly, all three management options lead to nearly uniform cure rates of >99%.

Adjuvant radiotherapy

Adjuvant para-aortic radiation reduces the relapse rate to 2–4%, with almost all of those being cured with subsequent chemotherapy [101, 104, 105]. However, 85% of patients are unnecessarily over-treated since they are cured with orchiectomy alone. To date, radiation doses have been gradually reduced to 20–25 Gy in 1.5–2 Gy fractions through consecutive clinical trials [105]. Similarly, radiotherapy volume has been reduced to the para-aortic field alone without ipsilateral pelvic lymph node radiation [106]. Infield relapses are rare, and if suspected, a biopsy should be taken to exclude non-germ-cell malignancies.

Long-term side effects of radiotherapy exist, particularly for young patients with a high likelihood of long-term survival. Long-term survivors of Stage I seminoma after adjuvant radiotherapy are at excess risk of death due to cardiac disease and secondary malignancies [107–109]. Although the association of cardiac toxicity and radiotherapy has been questioned, patients need to be informed of this increased risk [110]. Travis et al. combined 14 population-based registries, including 10, 534 patients with seminoma (all stages) treated with radiotherapy. For a 35-year-old patient with seminoma, the cumulative 40-year risk of a second malignancy was 36% versus 23% among general population [107]. Due to these long-term side effects, adjuvant radiotherapy is no longer considered a standard option by most groups and guidelines, but remains an option for highly selected patients, for example, those who are not candidates for salvage chemotherapy.

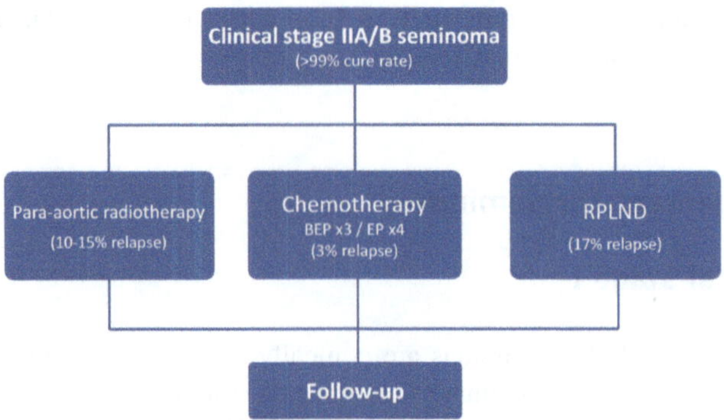

Fig. 12 Management of clinical Stage IIA/B seminoma (CSIIA/B-SEM)

Adjuvant carboplatin

Based on a large randomized trial, carboplatin is not inferior to radiotherapy, with similar relapse rates of 5.3 versus 4% [111, 112]. However, compared to AS, the relative risk reduction is only about one to two-thirds, from 15% with AS to 5–9% with adjuvant carboplatin [111, 113]. Similar to radiotherapy, about 85% of patients receive unnecessary treatment, while exposing to the risk of long-term toxicity and side effects.

Active surveillance (AS)

Several major series have demonstrated the safety and efficacy of AS, making this approach the preferred treatment option [58, 100, 102, 113, 114, 115]. Over 95% of relapses occur within the first 2–3 years after orchiectomy. At relapse, nearly all of these treatment-naïve patients can be treated successfully with either cisplatin-based chemotherapy or radiotherapy. AS enables 85% of patients to avoid treatment-related toxicity, and the remaining 10–15% of patients with relapse can effectively be salvaged with either radiotherapy or chemotherapy.

6.2 Clinical Stage IIA/B

Fifteen to twenty percent seminoma patients have Stage II disease at diagnosis, with involvement of infra-diaphragmatic lymph nodes on imaging. The most important prognostic factor in Stage II seminoma is the extent of retroperitoneal disease (lymph node size) [116]. Majority of patients (70%) with Stage II disease have low bulk disease (lymph nodes <5 cm, Stage IIA/B). Stage II, together with Stage I seminoma who relapse on surveillance or after adjuvant carboplatin, can be managed with radiotherapy, chemotherapy, or RPLND, achieving close to 100% cure rate (Fig. 12).

Main issues taken into consideration when choosing management option are treatment efficacy, the proportion relapse and additional therapy, and the acute/late morbidity of each treatment strategy.

Radiotherapy

The results with radiotherapy in the management of low-volume nodal disease are excellent with relapse rates of 10–15% in most series. In a retrospective series from Princess Margaret Cancer Centre in Toronto, Canada, 106 patients with low-volume retroperitoneal disease were treated between 1995 and 2010. Of the 106 patients, 59 patients had relapsed on surveillance and 47 had Stage II disease at presentation [117]. Eighty-seven were treated with radiotherapy and 19 were treated with primary chemotherapy. In the radiotherapy cohort, relapse rate was 8.6% for patients with lymph nodes <2 cm, and 10% for those with lymph nodes 2–5 cm. All patients were salvaged, and there were no deaths from seminoma or associated with treatment.

Chemotherapy

The results with cisplatin-based chemotherapy regimens: bleomycin/etoposide/cisplatin (BEP) or etoposide/cisplatin (EP) for low-volume nodal disease are excellent in most series, with few relapses and most patients being cured. Tanstadt et al. [43] reported on 73 patients treated between 2000 and 2006 with no relapses or deaths associated with treatment. Kollmannsberger et al. [102] reported on 65 patients with Stage II disease treated between 1999 and 2008 with chemotherapy (39% had Stage IIC disease). The relapse rate was 3%; however, 5% of patients died of treatment-related toxicity. In the Princess Margaret series mentioned above, of the 19 patients treated with chemotherapy, only one relapsed and was salvaged with second-line chemotherapy [117]. The Spanish Germ Cell Cancer Group reported on 72 patients treated between 1994 and 2003 with chemotherapy. Six patients relapsed, and one patient died of the disease [118].

Retroperitoneal lymph node dissection (RPLND)

RPLND is a standard treatment for non-seminoma germ cell tumors (NSGCTs). Unlike radiotherapy and systemic chemotherapy, which are associated with cardiovascular disease, insulin resistance, and secondary malignancy, RPLND has minimal long-term morbidity. Given the efficacy of RPLND in management of NSGCTs, interest has developed in this surgery as a frontline treatment for seminoma with isolated lymph node metastasis to the retroperitoneum.

Four retrospective studies have shown promising results when surgery is performed for seminomas with low-volume retroperitoneal metastases. The first study was reported by Warszawski et al. in 1997 from Germany [119]. This study retrospectively reviewed the results of 63 patients with Stage I ($n = 45$) and II seminoma ($n = 18$) after RPLND from 1975 to 1985 and compared the results with patient who received radiation. For patients with Stage I or IIA seminoma, with a median follow-up of 79 months, there was a 5.7% recurrence rate. The surgery provided excellent regional control with all the recurrences being identified as out of the retroperitoneal field. The efficacy of RPLND with larger nodal disease (>2 cm) decreased, with 6/11 (55%) patients recurring in the retroperitoneum. Mezvrishvili et al. [120] evaluated the outcomes of four patients with Stage IIA disease managed with RPLND. With a mean follow-up of 56 months, they did not have any local or distant recurrence. Hu et al. [121] reported on the outcomes of four patients with clinical Stage II pure testicular seminoma after RPLND. No patients underwent adjuvant therapy. With a median follow-up of 25 months, there were no recurrences or deaths. Lusch et al. [122] have recently presented a series on open or robotic RPLND in patients with Stage IIA/B seminoma. They identified 11 patients who underwent RPLND. Three of these patients (22%) received one cycle of carboplatin prior to RPLND. With a mean follow-up of 18 months, they had a 36% recurrence rate. One of the patients with recurrence had more advanced

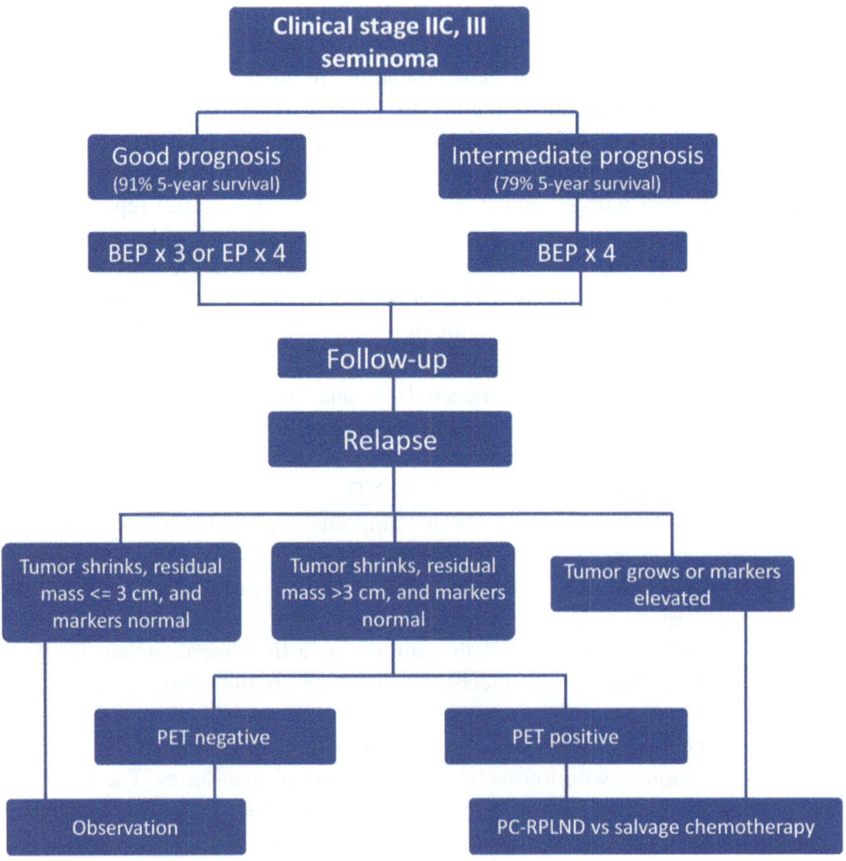

Fig. 13 Management of clinical Stage IIC, III seminoma

disease with clinical Stage IIC disease, an initial lymph node metastasis >6 cm, and a clinically positive inguinal lymph node. All patients who recurred were salvaged with radiotherapy and chemotherapy, and three out of four have no evidence of disease. Taken together, these studies include a total of 92 patients with Stage I-IIC seminoma and 14 who experienced recurrence. The overall recurrence rate for all patients was 14% with patients having higher stage disease being at greater risk of recurrence.

To better determine if RPLND can be recommended as a primary treatment option, two prospective clinical trials (SEMS and PRIMETEST) are underway. The SEMS trial is multi-institutional effort in the USA that includes patients with lymph nodes 1–3 cm in size. The PRIMETEST trial from Germany includes patients with lymph nodes <5 cm in size. The results of these studies will help determine if patients with metastatic seminoma will have a treatment option with minimal long-term morbidity.

6.3 Clinical Stage IIC and III

It managed the same as clinical Stage IIA (marker elevated), IIB/C and Stage III NSGCTs.

The indication for PC-RPLND in advanced seminoma is different and often individualized (Fig. 13). Pure seminomas generally respond well to systemic chemotherapy, and the concern for residual teratoma does not exist. Following chemotherapy, there is generally an intense desmoplastic reaction in a sheet like distribution around the great vessels, and discrete residual masses are uncommon. Viable cancer is almost never found in masses <3 cm, and therefore, PET scans have no utility and these patients should undergo continued surveillance. In patients with residual masses >3 cm viable cancer can be found in approximately 20% of patients and PC-RPLND can be curative [123]. PET scans can be useful in this setting and can guide further management. Surgical resection of these densely fibrotic masses is extremely challenging and often requires adjunctive surgery and/or vascular resection.

7 Salvage Treatment for Disease Relapse

7.1 Salvage Chemotherapy for Relapse

When relapse occurs, salvage treatment may be offered using a standard dose chemotherapy (SDC) regimen or high-dose chemotherapy (HDC) with autologous stem cell rescue (ASCR). Prospective randomized data are lacking to directly compare the two approaches. The single prospective randomized study that compared HDC (etoposide, ifosfamide and cisplatin/vinblastine, ifosfamide, and cisplatin × three cycles with one HDC-ASCR) to SDC (etoposide, ifosfamide and cisplatin (VeIP)/vinblastine, ifosfamide and cisplatin (VIP) × four cycles) for first relapse did not show an event-free or overall survival advantage [124]. However, this study has been criticized because a large number of patients did not receive the intended HDC and because single HDC-ASCR was used, which has been associated with inferior outcomes compared to tandem transplant approaches [125].

Furthermore, retrospective data suggest that HDC with tandem ASCR may be preferred. In a retrospective analysis of the International Prognostic Factors study group database 821 patients with relapsed testicular cancer who received HDC were compared to 773 patients who received SDC at first relapse [126]. The two-year event-free survival was significantly better with HDC vs SDC (55 vs. 44.1%, $p < 0.001$) in all five risk groups, and there was an overall survival advantage (60.6 vs. 46.3%, $p < 0.001$) except for patients in the lowest risk groups. These results must be viewed with the caveat of the potential bias inherent in retrospective analyses.

More individualized treatment decision making is of course desirable. Factors that predict for a favorable cure rate with SDC are pure seminoma, prior complete response to cisplatin therapy, low-volume metastases, and testicular primary [127–130]. It is also important to consider that HDC-ASCR may be more effective for first relapse, even in populations expected to respond to SDC salvage, and may also be safer when administered earlier. For example, in a series of patients with relapsed seminoma treated with HDC 92% treated at initial relapse achieved a cure response versus 67% treated in the third or fourth line setting [12]. There have been reports of greater toxicity from ASCR in patients with germ cell tumor with greater prior cisplatin exposure [131]. Definitive recommendations cannot be made until additional randomized studies are completed. The ongoing CTSU (Cancer Trials Support Unit) trial A031102 comparing paclitaxel, ifosfamide, and cisplatin (TIP; standard dose arm) to carboplatin–etoposide (TI-CE; high-dose/stem cell transplant arm) will provide much needed level one evidence to guide decision making for salvage therapy (NCT02375204).

7.2 Late Relapse

Late relapse is defined as any recurrence at least two years following complete response to primary treatment. Rates of late relapse range from 1 to 3% with seminomas having less risk. The retroperitoneum was the primary site of recurrence in over 50% of 521 patients in one reported series [132]. There can be significant lag time between treatment of primary disease and relapse of 10 years or more, and primary RPLND does not seem to be protective. Late relapses are generally detected by symptoms since patients are often no longer under close surveillance and up to half can present with elevated tumor markers. Most experts recommend upfront surgical resection since many patients have somatic differentiated teratoma and will be resistant to chemotherapy [133].

7.3 RPLND After Salvage Chemotherapy

Patients who have undergone salvage chemotherapy have limited options. Those who have resectable retroperitoneal disease should be considered for surgical resection or so-called desperation PC-RPLND. Up to half of these patients will have mature teratoma in the resected specimen despite elevated tumor markers and long-term survival rates can be 30–70% depending on prognostic factors [81]. Up to one-third of patients with viable cancer in the resected tumor may have long-term disease specific survival [134]. Surgery in this setting can be extremely challenging and all efforts should be made to completely resect all residual tumor since incomplete resection portends a very poor prognosis [135].

References

1. Siegel R, Miller K, Jemal A (2017) Cancer statistics. CA Cancer J Clin 67:7–30
2. Nichols C, Roth B, Albers P et al (2013) Active surveillance is the preferred approach to clinical stage I testicular cancer. J Clinic Onc 31:3490
3. Wymer K, Pearce S, Harris K et al (2017) Adherence to national comprehensive cancer network® guidelines for testicular cancer. J Urol 197:684
4. Eble J, Sauter G, Epstein J (2004) World Health Organization classification of tumors, pathology and genetics of tumors of the urinary system and male genital organs. WHO histological classification of testis Tumors. IARC Press, Lyon, France, p 218
5. Ulbright TBD (2010) Testicular and paratesticular tumors. In: SE M (ed) Diagnostic surgical pathology. Philadelphia: Lippincott Williams and Wilkins, pp 1944–2004
6. Krag Jacobsen G, Barlebo H, Olsen J, Schultz HP, Starklint H, Søgaard H et al (1984) Testicular germ cell tumours in Denmark 1976–1980. Pathology of 1058 consecutive cases. Acta Radiol Oncol 23(4):239–247. PubMed PMID: 6093440. eng
7. Hawkins EP, Finegold MJ, Hawkins HK (1986) Nonseminomatous malignant germ cell tumors in children. A review of 89 cases from the pediatric oncology group, 1971–1984. Cancer 58:2579–2584
8. Talerman A (1980) Endodermal sinus (yolk sac) tumor elements in testicular germ-cell tumors in adults: comparison of prospective and retrospective studies. Cancer 46(5):1213–1217. PubMed PMID: 6163519. eng
9. Kim I, Young RH, Scully RE (1985) Leydig cell tumors of the testis. A clinicopathological analysis of 40 cases and review of the literature. Am J Surg Pathol 9(3):177–192. PubMed PMID: 3993830. eng
10. Stief C, Fizazi K, Evans C (2015) Medical treatment of urologic malignancies. International Consultation on Urologic Diseases
11. Albers P, Albrecht W, Algaba F et al (2011) EAU guidelines on testicular cancer: 2011 update. Eur Urol 60:304
12. Aganovic L, Cassidy F (2012) Imaging of the scrotum. Radiol Clin North Am 50:1145
13. De Zordo T, Stronegger D, Pallwein-Prettner L et al (2013) Nature reviews. Urology 10:135
14. Aigner F, De Zordo T, Pallwein-Prettner L et al (2012) Real-time sonoelastography for the evaluation of testicular lesions. Radiology 263(2):584
15. Huang DY, Sidhu PS (2012) Focal testicular lesions: colour Doppler ultrasound, contrast-enhanced ultrasound and tissue elastography as adjuvants to the diagnosis. Brit J Radiol 85:S41

16. Gilligan TD, Hayes DF, Seidenfeld J, Temin S (2010) ASCO clinical practice guideline on uses of serum tumor markers in adult males with germ cell tumors. J Oncol Pract 6(4):199–202
17. International Germ Cell Cancer Collaborative Group: International Germ Cell Consensus Classification (1997) A prognostic factor-based staging system for metastatic germ cell cancer. J Clin Oncol 15, 594
18. Schnall M, Rosen M (2006) Primer on imaging technologies for cancer. J Clin Oncol 24:3225
19. O'Malley ME, Chung P, Haider M et al (2010) Comparison of low dose with standard dose abdominal/pelvic multidetector CT in patients with stage 1 testicular cancer under surveillance. Eur Radiol 20:1624
20. Chalian H, Tore HG, Horowitz JM et al (2011) Radiographics: a review publication of the radiological society of North America. Inc. 31:2093
21. Hilton S, Herr HW, Teitcher JB et al (1997) CT detection of retroperitoneal lymph node metastases in patients with clinical stage I testicular nonseminomatous germ cell cancer: assessment of size and distribution criteria. Am J Roentgenol 169:521
22. Hudolin T, Kastelan Z, Knezevic N et al (2012) Correlation between retroperitoneal lymph node size and presence of metastases in nonseminomatous germ cell tumors. Int J Surg Path 20:15
23. Donohue JP, Thornhill JA, Foster RS et al (1995) The role of retroperitoneal lymphadenectomy in clinical stage B testis cancer: the Indiana University experience (1965 to 1989). J Urol 153:85
24. Stephenson AJ, Bosl GJ, Motzer RJ et al (2005) Retroperitoneal lymph node dissection for nonseminomatous germ cell testicular cancer: impact of patient selection factors on outcome. J Clin Onc 23:2781
25. Beyer J, Albers P, Altena R et al (2013) Maintaining success, reducing treatment burden, focusing on survivorship: highlights from the third European consensus conference on diagnosis and treatment of germ-cell cancer. Ann Onc 24:878
26. See WA, Hoxie L (1993) Chest staging in testis cancer patients: imaging modality selection based upon risk assessment as determined by abdominal computerized tomography scan results. J Urol 150:874
27. Cagini L, Nicholson AG, Horwich A et al (1998) Thoracic metastasectomy for germ cell tumours: long term survival and prognostic factors. Ann Onc 9:1185
28. White PM, Adamson DJ, Howard et al (1999) Imaging of the thorax in the management of germ cell testicular tumours. Clin Radiol 54:207
29. Motzer RJ, Agarwal N, Beard C et al (2012) Testicular cancer. J Nat Compr Cancer Netw JNCCN 10:502
30. De Santis M, Pont J (2004) The role of positron emission tomography in germ cell cancer. World J Urol 22:41
31. Spermon JR, De Geus-Oei LF, Kiemeney LA et al (2002) The role of (18) fluoro-2-deoxyglucose positron emission tomography in initial staging and re-staging after chemotherapy for testicular germ cell tumours. BJU Int 89:549
32. Tsatalpas P, Beuthien-Baumann B, Kropp J et al (2002) Diagnostic value of 18F-FDG positron emission tomography for detection and treatment control of malignant germ cell tumors. Urol Int 68:157
33. de Wit M, Brenner W, Hartmann M et al (2008) [18F]-FDG-PET in clinical stage I/II non-seminomatous germ cell tumours: results of the German multicentre trial. Ann Onc 19:1619
34. Oechsle K, Hartmann M, Brenner W et al (2008) [18F] Fluorodeoxyglucose positron emission tomography in nonseminomatous germ cell tumors after chemotherapy: the German multicenter positron emission tomography study group. J Clin Onc 20(26):5930
35. Kollmannsberger C, Oechsle K, Dohmen BM et al (2002) Prospective comparison of [18F] fluorodeoxyglucose positron emission tomography with conventional assessment by

computed tomography scans and serum tumor markers for the evaluation of residual masses in patients with non-seminomatous germ cell carcinoma. Cancer 94:2353

36. Daneshmand S, Albers P, Fosså SD et al (2012) Contemporary management of postchemotherapy testis cancer. Eur Urol 62:867
37. Bachner M, Loriot Y, Gross-Goupil M et al (2012) 2-18fluoro-deoxy-D- glucose positron emission tomography (FDG-PET) for postchemotherapy seminoma residual lesions: a retrospective validation of the SEMPET trial. Ann Oncol 23:59
38. De Santis M, Becherer A, Bokemeyer C et al (2004) 2-18fluoro-deoxy-D-glucose positron emission tomography is a reliable predictor for viable tumor in postchemotherapy seminoma: an update of the prospective multicentric SEMPET trial. J Clin Oncol 22:1034
39. Kollmannsberger C, Nichols C, Bamberg M et al (2000) First-line high-dose chemotherapy ± radiation therapy in patients with metastatic germ-cell cancer and brain metastases. Ann Oncol 11:553
40. Davis PC, Hudgins PA, Peterman SB et al (1991) Diagnosis of cerebral metastases: double-dose delayed CT vs contrast-enhanced MR imaging. Am J Neurorad 12:293
41. Olofsson SE, Tandstad T, Jerkeman M et al (2011) Population-based study of treatment guided by tumor marker decline in patients with metastatic nonseminomatous germ cell tumor: a report from the Swedish-Norwegian testicular cancer group. J Clin Oncol 29:2032
42. Culine S, Kerbrat P, Kramar A et al (2007) Refining the optimal chemotherapy regimen for good-risk metastatic nonseminomatous germ-cell tumors: a randomized trial of the Genito-Urinary Group of the French Federation of Cancer Centers (GETUG T93BP). Ann Oncol 18:917
43. Tandstad T, Smaaland R, Solberg A et al (2011) Management of seminomatous testicular cancer: a binational prospective population-based study from the Swedish Norwegian testicular cancer study group. J Clin Oncol 29:719
44. de Wit R, Skoneczna I, Daugaard G et al (2012) Randomized phase III study comparing paclitaxel-bleomycin, etoposide, and cisplatin (BEP) to standard BEP in intermediate-prognosis germ-cell cancer: intergroup study EORTC 30983. J Clin Oncol 30:792
45. Fizazi K, Delva R, Caty A et al (2014) A risk-adapted study of cisplatin and etoposide, with or without ifosfamide, in patients with metastatic seminoma: results of the GETUG S99 multicenter prospective study. Eur Urol 65:381
46. Fizazi K, Pagliaro L, Flechon A et al (2014) A phase III trial of personalized chemotherapy based on serum tumor marker decline in poor-prognosis germ-cell tumors: Results of GETUG 13. Lancet Oncol 15:1442
47. Albers P, Siener R, Krege S et al (2008) Randomized phase III trial comparing retroperitoneal lymph node dissection with one course of bleomycin and etoposide plus cisplatin chemotherapy in the adjuvant treatment of clinical stage I Nonseminomatous testicular germ cell tumors: AUO trial AH 01/94 by the German Testicular Cancer Study Group. J Clin Oncol 26:2966–2972
48. Krege S, Beyer J, Souchon R et al (2008) European consensus conference on diagnosis and treatment of germ cell cancer: a report of the second meeting of the European Germ Cell Cancer Consensus group (EGCCCG): part I. Eur Urol 53:478–496
49. National-Comprehensive-Cancer-Network (2012) CCN-Clinical-Practice-Guidelines-in Oncology—Testicular Cancer. http://www.nccn.org/professionals/physician_gls/pdf/testicular.pdf Version 1, 2012
50. Cullen MH, Stenning SP, Parkinson MC et al (1996) Short-course adjuvant chemotherapy in high-risk stage I nonseminomatous germ cell tumors of the testis: a medical research council report. J Clin Oncol 14:1106–1113
51. Tandstad T, Dahl O, Cohn-Cedermark G et al (2009) Risk-adapted treatment in clinical stage I nonseminomatous germ cell testicular cancer: the SWENOTECA management program. J Clin Oncol 27:2122–2128

52. Pont J, Albrecht W, Postner G et al (1996) Adjuvant chemotherapy for high-risk clinical stage I nonseminomatous testicular germ cell cancer: long-term results of a prospective trial. J Clin Oncol 14:441–448
53. Jewett MAS, Lange PH, Raghavan D (1997) Controversies in the treatment of early stage nonseminomatous testicular cancer. In: Raghavan D, Leibel S, Scher H (eds) Principles and practice of genitourinary oncology. Lippincott Raven
54. Kollmannsberger C, Moore C, Chi KN et al (2010) Non-risk-adapted surveillance for patients with stage I nonseminomatous testicular germ-cell tumors: diminishing treatment-related morbidity while maintaining efficacy. Ann Oncol 21:1296–1301
55. Sturgeon JF, Moore MJ, Kakiashvili DM et al (2011) Non-risk-adapted surveillance in clinical stage I nonseminomatous germ cell tumors: the Princess Margaret Hospital's experience. Eur Urol 59:556–562
56. Colls BM, Harvey VJ, Skelton L et al (1999) Late results of surveillance of clinical stage I nonseminoma germ cell testicular tumours: 17 years' experience in a national study in New Zealand. BJU Int 83:76–82
57. Roeleveld TA, Horenblas S, Meinhardt W et al (2001) Surveillance can be the standard of care for stage I nonseminomatous testicular tumors and even high risk patients. J Urol 166:2166–2170
58. Daugaard G, Petersen PM, Rorth M (2003) Surveillance in stage I testicular cancer. Apmis 111:76–83
59. Atsu N, Eskicorapci S, Uner A et al (2003) A novel surveillance protocol for stage I nonseminomatous germ cell testicular tumours. BJU Int 92:32–35
60. Sweeney CJ, Hermans BP, Heilman DK et al (2000) Results and outcome of retroperitoneal lymph node dissection for clinical stage I embryonal carcinoma–predominant testis cancer. J Clin Oncol 18:358–362
61. Hermans BP, Sweeney CJ, Foster RS et al (2000) Risk of systemic metastases in clinical stage I nonseminoma germ cell testis tumor managed by retroperitoneal lymph node dissection. J Urol 163:1721–1724
62. Stephenson AJ, Bosl GJ, Motzer RJ, Bajorin DF, Stasi JP, Sheinfeld J (2007) Nonrandomized comparison of primary chemotherapy and retroperitoneal lymph node dissection for clinical stage IIA and IIB nonseminomatous germ cell testicular cancer. J Clin Oncol 25(35):5597–5602
63. Weissbach L, Bussar-Maatz R, Flechtner H, Pichlmeier U, Hartmann M, Keller L (2000) RPLND or primary chemotherapy in clinical stage IIA/B nonseminomatous germ cell tumors? Results of a prospective multicenter trial including quality of life assessment. Eur Urol 37(5):582–594
64. Donohue JP, Thornhill JA, Foster RS, Rowland RG, Bihrle R (1995) Clinical stage B non-seminomatous germ cell testis cancer: the Indiana University experience (1965–1989) using routine primary retroperitoneal lymph node dissection. Eur J Cancer 31A(10):1599–1604
65. Pizzocaro G (1987) Retroperitoneal lymph node dissection in clinical stage IIA and IIB nonseminomatous germ cell tumours of the testis. Int J Androl 10(1):269–275
66. Santrach PJ, Askin FB, Wells RJ, Azizkhan RG, Merten DF (1989) Nodular form of bleomycin related pulmonary injury in patients with osteogenic sarcoma. Cancer 64:806
67. Holoye PY, Luna MA, MacKay B, Bedrossian CW (1978) Bleomycin hypersensitivity pneumonitis. Ann Intern Med 88(1):47–49
68. Jules-Elysee K, White DA (1990) Bleomycin-induced pulmonary toxicity. Clin Chest Med 11:1
69. Simpson AB, Paul J, Graham J et al (1998) Fatal bleomycin pulmonary toxicity in the west of Scotland 1991–95: a review of patients with germ cell tumours. Br J Cancer 78:1061
70. O'Sullivan JM, Huddart RA, Norman AR et al (2003) Predicting the risk of bleomycin lung toxicity in patients with germ-cell tumours. Ann Oncol 14:91

71. von Schlippe M, Fowler CJ, Harland SJ (2001) Cisplatin neurotoxicity in the treatment of metastatic germ cell tumour: time course and prognosis. Br J Cancer 85:823
72. Pont J, Albrecht W (1997) Fertility after chemotherapy for testicular germ cell cancer. Fertil Steril 68:1
73. Travis LB, Andersson M, Gospodarowicz M et al (2000) Treatment-associated leukemia following testicular cancer. J Natl Cancer Inst 92:1165
74. Nichols CR, Breeden ES, Loehrer PJ et al (1993) Secondary leukemia associated with a conventional dose of etoposide: review of serial germ cell tumor protocols. J Natl Cancer Inst 85:36
75. Feldman DR, Hu J, Dorff TB, Lim K, Patil S, Woo KM, Carousso M et al (2016) Paclitaxel, ifosfamide and cisplatin efficacy for first-line treatment of patients with intermediate- or poor-risk germ cell tumors. J Clin Oncol 34:2478–2483
76. Horwich A, Sleijfer DT, Fossa SD et al (1997) Randomized trial of bleomycin, etoposide, and cisplatin compared with bleomycin, etoposide, and carboplatin in good-prognosis metastatic nonseminomatous germ cell cancer: a Multiinstitutional Medical Research Council/European Organization for Research and Treatment of Cancer Trial. J Clin Oncol 15:1844
77. Bajorin DF, Sarosdy MF, Pfister DG et al (1993) Randomized trial of etoposide and cisplatin versus etoposide and carboplatin in patients with good-risk germ cell tumors: a multiinstitutional study. J Clin Oncol 11:598
78. Williams SD, Birch R, Einhorn LH, Irwin L, Greco FA, Loehrer PJ (1987) Treatment of disseminated germ-cell tumors with cisplatin, bleomycin, and either vinblastine or etoposide. N Engl J Med 316(23):1435–1440
79. de Wit R, Stoter G, Sleijfer DT et al (1998) Four cycles of BEP vs four cycles of VIP in patients with intermediate-prognosis metastatic testicular non-seminoma: a randomized study of the EORTC Genitourinary Tract Cancer Cooperative Group. European Organization for Research and Treatment of Cancer. Br J Cancer 78(6):828–832
80. Ravi P, Gray KP, O'Donnell EK, Sweeney CJ (2014) A meta-analysis of patient outcomes with subcentimeter disease after chemotherapy for metastatic non-seminomatous germ cell tumor. Ann Oncol 25(2):331–338
81. Vergouwe Y, Steyerberg EW, Foster RS et al (2007) Predicting retroperitoneal histology in postchemotherapy testicular germ cell cancer: a model update and multicentre validation with more than 1000 patients. Eur Urol 51:424
82. Beck SD, Foster RS, Bihrle R et al (2007) Post chemotherapy RPLND in patients with elevated markers: current concepts and clinical outcome. Urol Clin North Am 34:219
83. Zon RT, Nichols C, Einhorn LH (1998) Management strategies and outcomes of germ cell tumor patients with very high human chorionic gonadotropin levels. J Clin Oncol 16:1294
84. Tarin T, Carver B, Sheinfeld J (2011) The role of lymphadenectomy for testicular cancer: indications, controversies, and complications. Urol Clin North Am 38:439
85. Daneshmand S, Stephenson AJ, Sheinfeld J, Jewett MA (2011) The management of subcentimeter residual mass in NSGCT: pcRPLND vs. observation. Urol Oncol 29:842
86. Carver BS, Shayegan B, Eggener S et al (2007) Incidence of metastatic nonseminomatous germ cell tumor outside the boundaries of a modified postchemotherapy retroperitoneal lymph node dissection. J Clin Oncol 25:4365
87. Rabbani F, Goldenberg SL, Gleave ME et al (1998) Retroperitoneal lymphadenectomy for post-chemotherapy residual masses: is a modified dissection and resection of residual masses sufficient? Br J Urol 81:295
88. Heidenreich A, Pfister D, Witthuhn R et al (2009) Postchemotherapy retroperitoneal lymph node dissection in advanced testicular cancer: radical or modified template resection. Eur Urol 55:217
89. Beck SD, Foster RS, Bihrle R et al (2007) Is full bilateral retroperitoneal lymph node dissection always necessary for postchemotherapy residual tumor? Cancer 110:1235

90. Hu B, Daneshmand S (2015) Role of extraretroperitoneal surgery in patients with metastatic germ cell tumors. Urol Clin North Am 42:369
91. Syan-Bhanvadia S, Bazargani ST, Clifford TG et al (2017) Midline extraperitoneal approach to retroperitoneal lymph node dissection in testicular cancer: minimizing surgical morbidity. Eur Urol (Epub ahead of print)
92. Calestroupat JP, Sanchez-Salas R, Cathelineau X et al (2009) Postche- motherapy laparoscopic retroperitoneal lymph node dissection in nonseminomatous germ-cell tumor. J Endourol 23:645
93. Steiner H, Leonhartsberger N, Stoehr B et al (2013) Postchemotherapy laparoscopic retroperitoneal lymph node dissection for low-volume, stage II, nonseminomatous germ cell tumor: first 100 patients. Eur Urol 63:1013
94. Stepanian S, Patel M, Porter J (2016) Robot-assisted laparoscopic retroperitoneal lymph node dissection for testicular cancer: evolution of the technique. Eur Urol 70:661
95. Pearce SM, Golan S, Gorin MA et al (2017) Safety and early oncologic effectiveness of primary robotic retroperitoneal lymph node dissection for nonseminomatous germ cell testicular cancer. Eur Urol 71(3):476
96. Djaladat H, Nichols C, Daneshmand S (2012) Adjuvant surgery in testicular cancer patients undergoing postchemotherapy retroperitoneal lymph node dissection. Ann Surg Oncol 19:2388
97. Nguyen CT, Stephenson AJ (2011) Role of postchemotherapy retroperitoneal lymph node dissection in advanced germ cell tumors. Hematol Oncol Clin North Am 25:593
98. Lee DJ, Djaladat H, Tadros NN et al (2014) Growing teratoma syndrome: clinical and radiographic characteristics. Int J Urol 21:905
99. Powles TB, Bhardwa J, Shamash J et al (2005) The changing presentation of germ cell tumours of the testis between 1983 and 2002. BJU Int 95:1197–1200
100. Warde P, Gospodarowicz MK, Panzarella T et al (1995) Stage I testicular seminoma: results of adjuvant irradiation and surveillance. J Clin Oncol 13:2255–2262
101. Chung P, Mayhew LA, Warde P et al (2010) Management of stage I seminomatous testicular cancer: a systematic review. Clin Oncol (R Coll Radiol) 22:6–16
102. Kollmannsberger C, Tyldesley S, Moore C et al (2011) Evolution in management of testicular seminoma: population-based outcomes with selective utilization of active therapies. Ann Oncol 22:808–814
103. Santoni R, Barbera F, Bertoni F et al (2003) Stage I seminoma of the testis: a bi-institutional retrospective analysis of patients treated with radiation therapy only. BJU Int 92:47–52
104. Jones WG, Fossa SD, Mead GM et al (2005) Randomized trial of 30 versus 20 Gy in the adjuvant treatment of stage I testicular seminoma: a report on Medical Research Council Trial TE18, European Organisation for the Research and Treatment of Cancer Trial 30942 (ISRCTN18525328). J Clin Oncol 23:1200–1208
105. Fossa SD, Horwich A, Russell JM et al (1999) Optimal planning target volume for stage I testicular seminoma: A Medical Research Council randomized trial. Medical Research Council Testicular Tumor Working Group. J Clin Oncol 17:1146
106. Travis LB, Curtis RE, Storm H et al (1997) Risk of second malignant neoplasms among long-term survivors of testicular cancer. J Natl Cancer Inst 89:1429–1439
107. Zagars GK, Ballo MT, Lee AK et al (2004) Mortality after cure of testicular seminoma. J Clin Oncol 22:640–647
108. Horwich A, Fossa SD, Stenning SP et al (2010) Risk of second cancers among a cohort of 2,703 long-term survivors of testicular seminoma treated with radiotherapy. J Clin Oncol 28: 15 s: (suppl; abstr 4538)
109. van den Belt-Dusebout AW, de Wit R, Gietema JA et al (2007) Treatment-specific risks of second malignancies and cardiovascular disease in 5-year survivors of testicular cancer. J Clin Oncol 25:4370–4378
110. Oliver RT, Mason MD, Mead GM et al (2005) Radiotherapy versus single-dose carboplatin in adjuvant treatment of stage I seminoma: a randomised trial. Lancet 366:293–300

111. Oliver RT, Mead GM, Rustin GJ et al (2011) Randomized trial of carboplatin versus radiotherapy for stage I seminoma: mature results on relapse and contralateral testis cancer rates in MRC TE19/EORTC 30982 study (ISRCTN27163214). J Clin Oncol 29:957–962
112. Tandstad T, Cavallin-Stahl E, Dahl O, et al (2014) Management of clinical stage I seminomatous testicular cancer: a report from SWENOTECA. J Clin Oncol 32:5 s (suppl; abstr 4508)
113. Warde P, Specht L, Horwich A et al (2002) Prognostic factors for relapse in stage I seminoma managed by surveillance: a pooled analysis. J Clin Oncol 20:4448–4452
114. van der Maase H, Specht L, Jacobson GK et al (1993) Surveillance following orchiectomy for stage I seminoma of the testis. Eur J Cancer 29:1931–1934
115. Germa-Lluch JR, Garcia del Muro X, Maroto P et al (2002) Clinical pattern and therapeutic results achieved in 1490 patients with germ-cell tumours of the testis: the experience of the Spanish Germ-Cell Cancer Group (GG). Eur Urol 42:553–562
116. Chung PW, Gospodarowicz MK, Panzarella T et al (2004) Stage II testicular seminoma: patterns of recurrence and outcome of treatment. Eur Urol 45:754–759; discussion 759–760
117. Chung PW, Sridharan S, Jewett M et al (2013) Contemporary management of stage I and stage II seminoma. Int J Radiat Oncol Biol Phys 87:2s (Suppl; abstr 206)
118. Garcia-del-Muro X, Maroto P, Guma J, et al (2008) Chemotherapy as an alternative to radiotherapy in the treatment of stage IIA and IIB testicular seminoma: a Spanish Germ
119. Warszawski N, Schmucking M (1997) Relapses in early-stage testicular seminoma: radiation therapy versus retroperitoneal lymphadenectomy. Scand J Urol Nephrol 31:355–359
120. Mezvrishvili Z, Managadze L (2006) Retroperitoneal lymph node dissection for high-risk stage I and stage IIA seminoma. Int Urol Nephrol 38:615–619
121. Hu B, Shah S, Shojaei S, Daneshmand S (2015) Retroperitoneal lymph node dissection as first-line treatment of node-positive seminoma. Clin Genitourin Cancer
122. Lusch G (2017) Winter, Albers. PD53-11 Primary retroperitoneal lymph node dissection (RPLND) in stage II A/B seminoma patients without adjuvant therapy: a phase II trial (PRIMETEST). J Urol 197:e1044–e1045
123. Heidenreich A, Thuer D, Polyakov S (2008) Postchemotherapy retroperitoneal lymph node dissection in advanced germ cell tumours of the testis. Eur Urol 53:260
124. Pico J-L, Rosti G, Kramar A et al (2005) A randomized trial of high-dose chemotherapy in the salvage treatment of patients failing first-line platinum chemotherapy for advanced germ cell tumors. Ann Oncol 16:1152
125. Lorch A, Kleinhans A, Kramar A et al (2012) Sequential versus single high-dose chemotherapy in patients with relapsed or refractory germ cell tumors: long-term results of a prospective randomized trial. J Clin Oncol 30:800
126. Lorch A, Bacoul-Mollevi C, Kramar A et al (2011) Conventional-dose versus high-dose chemotherapy as first salvage treatment in male patients with metastatic germ cell tumors: evidence from a large international database. J Clin Oncol 29:2178
127. Miller KD, Loehrer PJ, Gonin R et al (1997) Salvage chemotherapy with vinblastine, ifosfamide, and cisplatin in recurrent seminoma. J Clin Oncol 15:1427
128. Motzer RJ, Geller NL, Tan CC et al (1991) Salvage chemotherapy for patients with germ cell tumors. The memorial sloan-kettering cancer center experience (1979–89). Cancer 67:1305
129. Pizzocaro G, Salvioni R, Piva L et al (1992) Modified cisplatin, etoposide (or vinblastine) and ifosfamide salvage therapy for male germ cell tumors. Long-term results. Ann Oncol 3:211
130. Loehrer P, Johnson D, Elson P et al (1995) Importance of bleomycin in favorable-prognosis disseminated germ cell tumors: an Eastern Cooperative Oncology Group trial. J Clin Oncol 13:470
131. Motzer RJ, Mazumdar M, Bosl GJ et al (1996) High-dose carboplatin, etoposide, and cyclophosphamide for patients with refractory germ cell tumors: treatment results and prognostic factors for survival and toxicity. J Clin Oncol 14:1098

132. Oldenburg J, Martin JM, Fossa SD (2006) Late relapses of germ cell malignancies: incidence, management, and prognosis. J Clin Oncol 24:5503
133. Lutke Holzik MF, Hoekstra HJ, Mulder NH et al (2003) Non-germ cell malignancy in residual or recurrent mass after chemotherapy for nonseminomatous testicular germ cell tumor. Ann Surg Oncol 10:131
134. Beck SD, Foster RS, Bihrle R et al (2005) Pathologic findings and therapeutic outcome of desperation post-chemotherapy retroperitoneal lymph node dissection in advanced germ cell cancer. Urol Oncol 23:423
135. Daneshmand S (2015) Role of surgical resection for refractory germ cell tumors. Urol Oncol 33:370